"Trauma Bonded is a book that car you how to recognize and reconcile you have failed you. Sarah's story helps you know that you deserve the love that you are shown, even at your worst and that you can persevere and thrive, no matter what challenges life throws at you.

—Alex Vidales, Podcast producer and host of StageCraft on WERA-LP

The power of Westbrook's vulnerability is breathtaking. It is a rare thing to go so deeply inside someone's personal experience of abuse and trauma. It is at once harrowing and profoundly cathartic."

—Aaron Toronto, Producer and Director of "The Brilliant Darkness!"

TRAUMA BONDED

A **TRUE STORY** OF NAVIGATING
ATTACHMENTS **FORGED** IN **COMPLEX PTSD**

TRAUMA BONDED

SARAH WESTBROOK, LPC

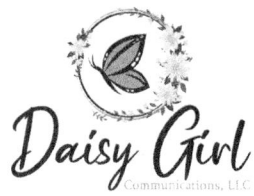

Contact information for Daisy Girl Communications, LLC– daisygirlcommunications@gmail.com
P.O. Box 322 Osage Beach, MO 65065

ISBN: 979-8-9879219-0-6 (paperback)
ISBN: 979-8-9879219-1-3 (ebook)
ISBN: 979-8-9879219-2-0 (hardcover)
ISBN: 979-8-9879219-3-7 (audiobook)

Library of Congress Control Number: 2023911379

Printed in the United States of America

Ordering Information:
Special discounts are available on quantity purchases by corporations, associations, and others. For details, contact www.daisygirlcommunications.com

Most names in this memoir have been changed to honor the privacy of the individuals portrayed in my story.

Content Warning:

This book is for mature audiences.

Child Abuse

Sexual Content

Marital Affairs

Suicidal Ideation

Language

*Dedicated to friends who are closer than family.
Thank you for wading through the shit life has
thrown me and for keeping me laughing at irony.
You know who you are.*

ACKNOWLEDGEMENTS

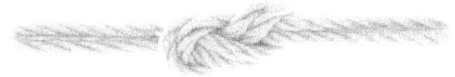

First to Mason, my sexy husband. I am so humbled that you continue to embrace me despite the darkness I have brought (and will likely bring again) into our marriage. Thank you for using beard oil daily so we can kiss without exfoliating all the tender spots. To Zuri Brown, for walking into my head and having the courage to stay awhile and fight my demons by my side. To Jean Strolberg, for taking over line-edits when reading through my own story, once again, felt daunting. (I'm saving my bandwidth for recording the audiobook.) To my children for forcing me to grow up and be better. To my Army family who showed up for us over and over again. To Lisa Peck @ www.stepitupqueen.com. You tore my book apart and helped me rebuild it. Thanks for sticking with me through my triggers and helping me discover even deeper healing. To Tammy Mehr, Joan Stradling and my peeps at Jefferson City Novelist Group (JCNG) for your support, beta reading, and feedback. You ROCK! And finally to the entire team at Book Launchers @ www.booklaunchers.com, for turning my dream into a reality and letting me stay in the driver's seat of this project.

TABLE OF CONTENTS

PROLOGUE

MAY 1997

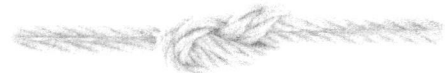

16 YEARS OLD

The heat of the shower matches the burn of tears running down my cheeks. My hands tremble as I clutch the shower bar to hold myself upright. Who knew a broken heart could feel so endless? I'm going to die right here in the shower. My vision narrows. I blink hard to get rid of the dark haze. My legs give out. Pain explodes in my knees as I crumple to all fours, struggling for oxygen between dry heaves. I'm suffocating. How will I live? I cannot survive. Please, God, just let me die.

The razor blade gleams from its place on the tub ledge.

Something my friend Jamie once said plays through my mind. "People don't do it right, you know? To do it right, you cut from the wrist to the elbow, and you cut deep."

I

I will the razor to move on its own. It doesn't. I bite my tongue hard to keep myself from maniacal laughter. Metallic blood seeps into my mouth; it tastes delicious. I look up and open my eyes. The hard water stings. *At least I can still feel that.* I haven't felt anything since Dad showed up in the Fine Arts hallway and yanked me from Michael's lap. Why did I write the note? They are going to arrest Michael for rape.

It wasn't rape. It was my idea. I can't live with myself if they send him to jail. I love him.

Death will make the pain stop. Death will bring silence. Death is the only way to hurt Dad, the only way to make him see.

Just do it.

Fast.

Deep.

No one will check on me. Not for hours. They are too busy screaming at each other.

As if in confirmation, Mom's voice screeches over the sound of the shower.

"No right... tell her... why... promised..."

I'm so familiar with their fighting that I can fill in the blanks. "You had no right to tell her about *your* first time! Why would you do that? We promised to keep it a secret."

Big fucking deal. So, Dad had sex before they got married, so did his parents, so did her parents, so does half the world, probably more. Once again, Mom is focusing on what people are going to think of *her.*

Typical.

My body shudders at the thought of Michael being slammed into a cop car and my Dad's grin at his "success." No one wins against Dad, not ever. I start dry heaving again. Death is the only way to make this nightmare end. I reach for the razor. Everything seems to move in slow motion. My vision clears as I focus on the pink handle of the three-bladed Gillette. A burst of anxious, almost excited energy flows through my body. Like someone flipped a switch to turn on the light; my limbs seem to buzz with electricity.

STOP!

The baby!

I jerk my hand away from the razor.

It's too soon to know if I'm pregnant. Most likely I'm not, since Michael came all over my stomach, but I want there to be a baby. Not because I want to have a baby, but because having a baby would be my ticket out of this hellhole disguised as a perfect Mormon family. I'm not allowed to "mess up." A baby is the only way, the only hope of ever seeing Michael again.

The water begins to run cold, but I don't care. The goosebumps on my arms are the only thing that feels real. I play the scene from the last two hours over again and again.

"If you are pregnant, you *will* place that baby for adoption," my father had yelled, his scarlet face inches from mine. I stayed silent, but inside I knew I would *never* let that happen.

If I am pregnant, Michael and I will love the baby like no one has ever loved a baby before.

A scream of anguish rips from my soul. It takes me aback. Had I actually made that sound? I roll to my side, curl into the fetal position, and continue to sob.

Please, God, I'll live for a baby. I need you to make sure Dad won't take my baby from me. If you don't let him take my baby, I promise to live and to make sure the baby knows it is loved no matter what. We can find a way. Michael's grandma in Tennessee will keep us safe. We just need to make it to her.

Despite the cold water, warmth washes over me. I welcome the ensuing peace and wonder if it is a witness from the Holy Spirit.

Pounding shakes the bathroom door and jolts me from sleep. "Sarah! Get out of that shower. You've been in there over an hour," Mom yells.

I sit up slowly on the tub floor. I don't remember turning the water off.

More pounding on the door. "Sarah? Did you hear me? Get. Out. Now." She emphasizes with another bang to the door. "You have five minutes. Dad wants to talk to you again."

Dread consumes me. My jaw trembles. I have no tears left. My head throbs. I need Motrin. "Okay."

I pull myself up, still weak and dizzy, my legs seizing beneath me. I stand still to steady myself. I grab a towel to dry off. As I step out of the tub, my foot knocks the Gillette to the floor.

I missed my chance.

PART ONE

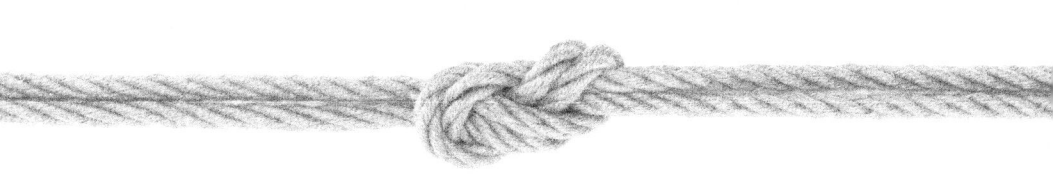

STORIES OR LIES

1985–1988

4–7 YEARS OLD

The afternoon sun of Snowflake, Arizona, warms my four-year-old cheeks. My younger brother, Joey, and I play next door at Sister Cafer's home with the helium-filled balloons the dentist gave us that morning for being cavity-free. Our neighbor's name isn't Sister. That's just what people in the Mormon Church call the grown-up women. They call the men Brother. The swings in her yard make squeaking noises as they move in the wind.

I gaze up at my cherry-red balloon and revel in the sensation of my dress spinning out full around my legs twirling over and over again. The ribbon, clutched tightly in my sweaty fist, twists around my small frame. My bare feet skim across the cool grass. Mom hates it when I don't wear shoes. I hate it when I do. I hide my shoes from Mom whenever I can. How can I be a barefoot princess when I grow up if I can't practice being barefoot?

My dream of rescuing swans and dancing with them is interrupted when Joey lets out a piercing scream. In his attempt to climb into the swing, his blue balloon has escaped his grasp. Racing over, I jump as high as I can. Without my shoes, I'm sure I can jump higher than a goat. My fingers brush the yellow ribbon, but I'm too late. I leap again, willing all of my superpowers to force me high enough to fly. It's no use. The balloon has been carried off. It will probably blow away to Disneyland for their big parade.

His tears leave tracks on his dusty round cheeks. A flash of annoyance and fear causes my heart to pulse deep within my ears.

"Here, you can have mine. Just stop crying. Shh, shh."

He shakes his head and refuses to take the string in my outstretched hand, instead crying louder. Mom and Sister Cafer step out of her red brick house onto the front porch. Sister Cafer's face is pinched in concern as she hurries our way. Mom's face isn't concerned… it's mad. Mom always looks mad when someone is crying.

A mad mom usually means trouble for me. I'm out in the open, and there's nowhere to go. I should have taken off when Joey started crying or hidden myself like my shoes. It's too late. Mom will probably paddle my butt again with the wooden spoon.

"Sarah Elizabeth Lee," Mom yells. "What did you do this time?"

"It wasn't me. He let go of his balloon. See?" I point to the barely visible blue speck high above our heads.

Mom squints up at the balloon and then glances at Joey who is pointing to the sky, his screams getting louder. His hair is brown as dirt, like mine, except mine is clean and his has pieces of dried grass in it.

Mom's pursed lips soften with her heavy sigh. Maybe I'm safe from the wooden spoon this time. I watch Mom's face closely. I'm not sure if she's still mad. I decide to tell her a story, just to make sure I'm out of the dog-house. At least, that's what Dad calls it when he's in trouble with Mom. We don't even own a doghouse. We don't even own a dog, not since Puppers got hit by a car.

"Mom, I tried really hard to get Joey's balloon. I saw him climbing into the swing all by himself, and I knew he was going to let go of his balloon." I pinch the rough grass between my toes and begin to talk faster. "So then, I ran to get the ladder from the carport, just in case. I climbed up the ladder when he let go of his string and jumped off to catch it, but I barely missed, so I climbed up the ladder again. Then I super-jumped, but the wind blew the balloon and me like five feet away. I landed on my knee. See?" I lift my dress to show her the grass-stained dirty spot permanently etched onto my bony joint.

The space between Mom's eyebrows wrinkles up, and her face turns redder than the balloon bobbing at the end of the ribbon still clutched in my fist.

"Where is the ladder now, Sarah?" Sister Cafer asks. Her blond, heavily hair-sprayed hair barely moves with the bounce of her head.

Heat crawls up my face as I shrug and break eye contact.

"Sarah, Joey, go home." Mom's voice is terse, her lips pulled thin again. Maybe I will get the spoon after all.

Joey and I obey like soldiers.

"You need to break that nasty lying habit she has, Emma," Sister Cafer says to Mom.

"She's worse than her father." Mom sighs loudly.

She has been sighing a lot lately.

I don't wait around to hear more about how horrible Mom and Sister Cafer think my Dad is. They always talk about how bad Dad is. I'm expected to keep my mouth shut. I'm not good at that part. God forgot to give me a filter when he made me.

They're wrong. Daddy is a hero. He does all kinds of superhero things. He's the favorite teacher at his school. When students other than his are bad, he tells them how they're messing up and they listen to him. He's the best teacher in the world. Sister Cafer is just too stupid to know how good Daddy is. If he is so awful, why do his students love him and do what he says? If he is awful, he'd have bad students like some of the other teachers do, but he doesn't have bad students because his students like him so, so much. I don't even know why Mom likes Sister Cafer.

Why does Mom let that lady say mean things about my Daddy? She should tell her to shut her mouth. Why does Mom say mean things about Daddy? He's always nice to me. His spankings don't even hurt 'cause he only pretend spanks. Not like the wooden spoon.

Maybe he embellishes his life stories like Mom and others say he does when he talks about growing up in Burbank, California (when it was cool to live in Burbank). Tales of riding around town shirtless and wearing flip-flops and shorts on his Honda Hawk motorcycle. Dad always creates a world of wonder that entertains my three younger siblings and me. His stories have us dreaming of getting paid to clap or laugh for television shows or hanging out around the stables where Hollywood animals are trained. He brings to life all types of adventures as he reminisces about his personal hero and role model, my Great-Grandpa James.

In most of Dad's stories he's an innocent troublemaker. His Grandpa James is a hero, and his Grandma James is the soft place to land. Dad especially enjoys relating crazy, off-the-wall teenage shenanigans for which he narrowly escaped serious discipline. Some of his stories are harmless, like putting rock salt in the sacrament water during

Mormon services. Others are criminal, like setting off small explosives in the local pool hall.

Everyone knows that the best stories have an element of truth, so I'm sure there is some truth in Dad's stories. They are a haven for him to experience the reality he wished he lived because his reality wasn't pleasant. Due to his mother's multiple affairs, his father insisted on a divorce when Dad was nine. Dad blamed himself because his father left right after an argument his parents had about him "digging holes to China" in their backyard.

After the divorce, his mother invited her multiple boyfriends to their home. Many of them were straight-up abusive assholes and victimized Dad and his four siblings. Dad refuses to talk much about it. Pieces of his nightmare will come out as weapons, however, especially when he's angry. Dad doesn't use his fists like Grandma's boyfriends did, but his words will knock the wind out of you all the same.

It wasn't until I studied counseling that I learned my father's stories were an escape from reality. As a child, I wanted to be a hero like my Dad was in his stories.

When Joey and I get to our house, Joey stops by the front porch to look at a bug. I'm smarter than that. Mom is going to yell when she gets here, and I don't want to be around when she does. I walk around our tiny white brick house and hide in my bush fort where Mom can't see me.

The branches of the lilac bush tug at my hair as I push my way to its center. The bush is taller than Dad and fatter than an elephant. Dad cut away some of the bush's inside branches, creating a sort of cave so that Susan Davis, my best friend, and I could have enough room to play cards. I curl up on the packed dirt floor next to the cardboard fireplace Susan and I built. I'll stay here until it's safe. With the leaves for cover, I lay down on the magazine bed and stretch my feet out, tickling the trunk with my bare toes. Mom usually forgets about being mad when Dad gets home… and she has something new to yell about.

Growing up as an orthodox Mormon, I never questioned our religion; it was simply my reality. From a young age, the wrongness of lying was drummed into my head. At the time of the balloon incident, I didn't think of what I said as a lie. To me, it was just a story, like one of the "big whoppers" Dad created.

In the Lee home, we were expected to be better and smarter than everyone else at everything we did. Failure was not an option, and outsiders weren't allowed to know we had flaws, lest we be judged and gossiped about.

The balloon story was not the first lie I told in the pretense of perfection, nor would it be the last.

Susan's family and the Cafer's live on either side of our tiny white brick home on Stinson Street in Snowflake, Arizona.

Even though Susan is a year older than I am, we've been best friends since before I started kindergarten. We love our bush fort. In the years since Dad cut the inside branches away, the bush has grown over eight feet tall and is just as wide. Susan and I spent last summer braiding some of the branches above our heads to create a ceiling. The bush grows across the four-foot chain-link fence into both of our yards, and we spend hours creating cardboard furniture for it. The big boxes from refrigerators and other large appliances are the best for propping up branches to make the cave even bigger and for making furniture.

Among other things, Susan and I have made a fireplace, a toilet, a dresser, a couch, and a bed. We even repurpose old *The Friend* magazines (children's literature published by the Mormon Church) into blankets. We could rock the homeless life for sure.

When we're grounded from each other, we meet inside the bush fort and play where our moms can't see us. With only a fence between us, that overgrown lilac bush provides endless hours of fun and adventure.

Even though I'm younger and smaller than Susan, I'm better than she is at almost everything except camping. On their camping trips, her dad lets her help build the fire, so one day during summer break before my second-grade year, I decide to hone a new skill.

"This one will fit you, and it's our favorite color," I announce as I hand Susan a blue scarf from the depths of my bedroom closet. "You don't want to get cold on our camping trip."

She wraps it around her chubby neck. "It's not really cold, and we're only pretending, so I'm not bringing your blanket to the fort this time, okay?"

I glance at the blanket stuffed in the corner and shrug. I'm not going to bring it either because my shoes are hiding under it.

We sneak out the front door. Mom is reading a book on the couch, and we know better than to interrupt her. We race up the hill to the shed at the top of Susan's driveway. Susan glances over her shoulder to make sure her mom isn't looking out the window. We are not allowed in the shed where her dad's tools are, but we need matches if I'm going to learn how to light a campfire. Susan's strong arms flex as she pulls herself onto the tall workbench to reach the matchbox while I stand watch.

"Run!" I yell, as we sprint back down her driveway and scurry into the bush fort. The blue scarf has come loose and gets caught on the fence as Susan and I climb over to my side of the fort.

"Wait," Susan says as she climbs back again. "I'm gonna go get plates to put our cooked food on."

While she's gone, I examine the matches. I've never lit one before, but I've seen Dad do it a lot on our family camping trips. I open the cut-out door to our cardboard fireplace then slip out of the fort to gather some small sticks from the backyard. Sticks in hand, I construct a teepee in the fireplace just like I've seen my Dad do. Susan is taking forever. She better hurry up, or we won't get this done before Dad gets home. I slide out the insert of the match-box and remove a match. I glance over my shoulder and practice running the match across the rough red strip on the side of the box.

Nothing.

I hear the rumble of Dad's motorcycle from a block or two away. He'll be home from work soon. What if he catches us? I wipe sweat away from my forehead. My hair sticks like glue to my temples in the summer heat. I grab a copy of *The Friend* from the pile we have stashed in the fort's "bathroom" cubby.

Susan's footsteps finally approach as I rip out pages and make paper wads for the inside of my kindling teepee.

Susan tosses a box of pink and white frosted animal crackers over the fence at me along with her plastic teapot and matching blue plates. She ignores the scarf, still caught on the fence. It's way too hot to put it back on. Our bare feet are covered in dust and muddy sweat streaks. I've spit-painted the word "Hi" in the dust on my feet above my pinky toe.

"You ready to cook our food and get warm?" I ask.

Susan's eyebrows pinch together as she focuses on opening the cracker box. "I'm hungry," she huffs. "We are eating this first."

I shrug. My stomach feels weird. I hate that feeling, like frogs jumping around. I don't know why my stomach gets all knotted up and jumpy, but it does it a lot.

I put a pink cracker on top of the dried mud pie we made a few days ago. The red clay of Arizona's White Mountain has dried hard like an adobe brick. I pretend the cracks in the pie are like the cracks on top of a chocolate chip cookie. I spit in my hand and draw some polka dots with one finger while I suck the frosting off my cracker.

"Whatcha doin'?" Susan asks, her mouth full of cracker mush.

"My mud pie looks like a cookie so I'm adding chocolate chips," I explain.

It's her turn to shrug. "Mine is still a chocolate pie, and *no*, it's not a poop pie. That's gross."

I shoot her my impish grin, and she scowls back. Susan doesn't like to be teased. She's the only other member of my secret-sister gang, and she's very obedient, which is all that's required in my friend group.

I grab a match and try to light it again. The smell of the phosphorus on the strike plate reminds me of camping.

Nothing. I try again. Still nothing.

"You're doing it wrong," Susan says. "You aren't holding it right." She reaches out to show me, and I brush her hand away.

"I've done this a million times," I say. "I make all the fires for our family when we camp. Even my Dad can't light the matches. It's just windy right now, so it's harder."

Susan looks doubtful, but she knows better than to question me.

Heat rises into my cheeks as match after match fails to light. "These matches must be old," I finally snap.

"Mom just bought them yesterday," Susan reassures me.

"Did she get them from Ed's? Ed's sells bad matches. Everyone knows that." My gaslighting skills are epic for an almost second grader. "It's too windy to do it this way anyway." I grab the magnifying glass from under our cardboard dresser. We use the magnifying glass to roast roly-poly bugs and feed them to Joey when Mom isn't looking.

I grab three matches and place them on the ground. I angle the magnifying glass and wait for the smoke to rise.

Still nothing.

The frogs in my stomach jump around again. It never looks this difficult when Dad makes a fire. I have to get this to work. I'm the hero. I prop a match upright between two rocks in front of the cardboard fireplace hearth and angle the magnifying glass so it catches the sunlight just right through the branches of our fort. Thin, wispy smoke rises from the tip, and to my relief the match ignites with a soft pop.

"Wow," Susan says. "That was neat!"

I nod, as certainty replaces my frustration. "Told you I could do it."

I carefully lift the match from the side and hold it next to the wadded-up magazine pages. A thin white tendril of smoke rises. Fire licks its way up the match and burns my fingers. I immediately drop it. Then, Susan and I reach our hands forward and hover over the fire.

"It's soooooo warm," we say in unison.

Susan rubs her hands on her upper arms as if to banish the pretend chill. More melted chocolate mud streaks appear as she does it.

"Your pie will be ready in five more minutes," I proclaim with a smile as the small teepee I've made catches fire. I knew I could start a fire. Too easy!

Susan lets out a startled yipe as our cardboard fireplace bursts into flames. We scramble out of our bush fort, and the smell of melting plastic nips at the back of my sinuses. My eyes water and sting as the dried tumbleweed wall that has gathered for months along the fence line behind our fort in our backyard is devoured by the red-orange flames. Thick black smoke fills the air, and soon the top end of my backyard campground is on fire.

Susan bursts into tears.

I'm frozen in place as the last remnants of our lilac bush ignites.

"Fire!" Sister Davis screams. "Dave, Emma, fire, fire!" She's taller than Mom, but she's a little fat, so she looks like a frantic chicken squawking around the yard with her flour-covered apron flapping in the wind. She finally notices Susan and me.

"Sarah, go get your Dad," she screams.

Dad emerges from the back of the carport, towering over me, armed with our garden hose. I stop, rooted to the spot. He's as tall and strong as Superman.

Sister Davis has run back to her house and is wrestling with their garden hose. Susan has disappeared and is nowhere to be found.

Dad has a slight smirk on his face as he sprays our lawn, not the fire.

"Sarah, go inside please," he instructs. The gentleness of his voice confuses and reassures me.

I move slowly, cautiously toward the house, but I stall. I need to know what Dad is going to do.

"It's okay, Cindy," Dad calls to Sister Davis. "It'll burn out once the weeds are gone. Looks like our girls did me a huge favor."

Sister Davis shoots me a sharp look.

Her hose is too short to touch the flames, so she's watering the driveway on her side of the fence. Then she turns and starts watering the shed with her hose.

"Sarah," Dad's voice startles me.

When I turn to him, he is smiling.

The tension, which has ratcheted my shoulders up until they almost touch my ears, releases, and I relax. "Yeah?"

He holds the hose out to me. "You wanna water the grass so it doesn't catch on fire, too." He explains as he shows me how to aim the water low to the ground in a sweeping motion.

"What about the garden?" I ask.

"Well, everything was mostly dead, so it'll be fertilizer for the ground. I was planning on burning the weeds off next week anyway. You just saved me a huge chore."

A smile spreads across my face. I helped Dad. I'm a hero too.

"Dead, dry things burn fast, Sarah. I once saw a trailer house burn to the ground in less than five minutes. That's why we will never live in one. People who live in mobile homes and trailers aren't very smart."

I look over to Susan's house, a large four-bedroom double-wide I had been jealous of for a long time. They live in a double-wide *and* they water their shed. Dumb-o-dumb. When I glance at our tiny two-bedroom, one-bathroom, white brick home, I've never been prouder to live here. My Dad is smart. Brick won't burn.

"Sarah," Mom says as she pulls my pajama shirt over my head. My clothes stick to my still wet body. "Dad and I aren't mad," she says softly. I shift uncomfortably, not sure if I believe her. She and Dad have been yelling about the fire since Dad and I came inside. First at each other, then at Sister Davis. "Can you tell me again what happened?"

I'm good at this part. Stick to the story, and no one will ever know. "Susan said she was cold, so she took my blue scarf. Then she was still cold, so she got matches out of her dad's work shed. She lit them. I don't even know how to light them." This is an important detail.

Earlier that evening, Dad had handed me a box of matches and told me to light one in order to prove to Mom that I was incapable of doing so. Just like earlier, I tried several times to get that match to light to no avail—okay, maybe I didn't try as hard as I had earlier, but it was obvious to my parents that matches still outsmarted me.

"Susan wanted to cook her mud pie. I told her not to because our fireplace was a cardboard box, but she didn't listen. She told me I was being a wimp, and she lit the fire. She knows how to," I end. That last detail is gonna seal the deal.

Sister Davis had confessed to Mom that Susan lit matches for her dad all the time on family campouts. She also had insisted that Susan knew how to be safe around matches because her dad had taught her all the safety rules.

"See," Dad said, "I never liked that Susan anyway. She can't even speak right. She's the reason Sarah has to take speech. Susan knows how to light matches, and she ran away crying because she knew Ted was going to beat her butt with his belt. Sarah is smart enough to know you don't light a fire in a cardboard box."

I look up at Mom with my practiced innocent face and nod. Mom gives a heavy sigh, looks at me and says, "Either way, Sarah, you are grounded from Susan for a week."

Victory is sweet, until it backfires. Once the week is over, Susan tells me she doesn't want to be in my secret-sister gang anymore because I'm a liar. I call her stupid for living in a double-wide and speaking funny. She runs home, crying to her mommy. We never play together again. I don't want stupid friends anyway. My Dad says I'm smart to be more careful in picking my friends.

"You don't want to be friends with a liar, Sarah," becomes his practiced response whenever I lament about being lonely. I don't tell him I know he lies to be the hero, because then he won't like me anymore either. At least no one knows I'm the bad girl.

FRIENDSHIP IS HARD, SINNING IS EASY

1988–1989

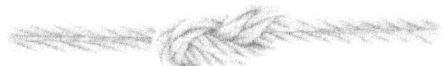

7–8 YEARS OLD

By the middle of second grade, I have burned through quite a few friends. They don't seem to like my stories, and they usually stop asking me to come over and play after I show them how to feel better by rubbing their own private parts. I don't touch them, I just show them how to touch themselves.

Dad says I'm better off on my own, and Mom won't talk about it at all. She just tells me I'm smart and beautiful. If I'm so smart and beautiful, why don't I have friends?

I'll get baptized soon, though, on my eighth birthday in March. I've learned that once I get baptized, I'll get a gift from Jesus, called the Holy Ghost. The Holy Ghost will help me know what to do and what to say. Maybe after I have Him to guide me, my friends will like playing with me again.

After Christmas break, I meet Jared. He's new and he's good looking with straight blond hair and a dimple in one cheek. Jared does backflips off the brick wall in front of the elementary school, and he loves motorcycles just like Dad does. Jared chases me every day on the playground, and when he catches me, he kisses me on the cheek, releases me, and chases me again. I love the attention.

Our teacher, Mrs. Dimes, is a yeller, and most kids hate her because she's so scary. I don't mind. I'm used to the yelling. I often volunteer to help her grade papers. I leave little hearts and notes on Jared's homework.

One day in front of the entire class, Mrs. Dimes holds up Jared's graded paper and says, "Jared, we all love you. Class, repeat after me... I will *not* profess my love for my classmates when I help Mrs. Dimes grade papers." She looks right at me. I get the point and stop volunteering to help her grade papers.

Maybe the other kids are right about her being mean because she yells at me again a few days later for lying about living in the White House. I'm so confused because I do live in the white brick house. Mrs. Dimes tells the entire class I'm lying about living in Washington, D.C., but I don't think I ever said the house wasn't in Snowflake. She gives me lunch detention anyway. Just like at home, I get in trouble even when I tell the truth.

Jared has detention too, and we're both mad at her for embarrassing us. Mrs. Dimes leaves us alone for a few minutes to run to the bathroom, and we get our revenge. Taking the stack of homework that she told us to grade, we rip it into tiny pieces and drop the paper shreds into the heater under the window. We drop several of her sharpened pencils in there too, just for fun. When she returns from the bathroom, we tell her we finished grading the papers and placed them upside down on the right desks with the papers she had graded earlier.

She thinks we're wonderful and tells us we can enjoy the last few minutes of recess. We run out of her classroom high-fiving each other and laughing.

Later that afternoon, the heater kicks on.

It rattles and cracks like it usually does. However, a few minutes later, smoke starts pouring out of the grate. The fire alarm screams overhead.

In unison, the class jumps up and hurries to line up at the door as we've rehearsed several times this year. Mrs. Dimes leads us out of the classroom as usual, except this time, she leads us across the street instead of to the flagpole.

Sirens wailing, four fire engines pull up to the school soon after our exit. They put the fire out quickly, and within minutes we're cleared to go back to class. The blackened heater, the burned wall above it, and the acrid smell of melted art projects are the only signs there has been a fire. The firemen relay that there appeared to be a lot of paper inside the unit that caused it to ignite. The school alerts the custodial staff and insists they check all the school's heating units to prevent another accident.

Not long after we return to class, Jared claims the smoke made him sick, and he goes home. As for me, I'm shocked that the custodial staff doesn't clean the heating units regularly. Fire is dangerous; they should know better.

When we return to school after the weekend, the heater has been replaced and the walls repainted. I say hi to Jared, but he glares at me and walks away. I decide to corner him at lunch and ask him what's wrong.

"We almost burned the entire school down, stupid," he says. "I don't want to go to jail like my dad did."

I frown. "What are you talking about? We didn't light any matches."

He stares at me like I've got two heads or something. "The heater, dummy. God, you can be so fucking stupid."

I flinch at his use of the "F" word because it's a bad word. And then it clicks. Revenge… detention… shredded homework in the heating unit… this *is* our fault. We caused the fire. I turn and flee to the office and call my Mom. It's my turn to go home sick.

I can't tell Mom I almost burned down the school. If Mom finds out about this, maybe they won't let me get baptized because burning things down is a serious sin, like masturbating. People who masturbate can't go to heaven because they aren't obeying the law of chastity. I need to get baptized so I can get the Holy Ghost so I can stop doing that.

Turning eight is a huge deal in the Mormon Church. You can't get baptized or become an official church member until you turn eight. Usually the dad does the baptizing, but if he's not a good church member, or he's dead or something, a grandfather or someone else's dad will do it.

The day after Christmas before my eighth birthday, I overhear Dad arguing with Mom. "No one but me is going to baptize my daughter!"

After that he starts attending church with us. For as long as I can remember, attending church meant the kids went with Mom, and Dad stayed home. He said he doesn't like Bishop Cafer. Neither do I since Bishop's wife and Mom always say mean things about Dad.

Even though he goes to church with us, his rebelliousness toward Mormon traditions doesn't change much. He refuses to wear a white shirt to meetings and wears one of his colored button-up shirts instead with a funny tie. It's fun to have him there with us because he likes to tickle us and play games during the boring talks (sermons). Mom ignores our muffled giggles. She isn't going to say anything to stop Dad from joining us. Mom doesn't even say anything when Dad pinches my youngest sister, Charlie, to make her cry out so he can walk the hallways with her to "calm her down" and "keep her reverent."

In the days leading up to my baptism, Dad and I rehearse the motions we'll need to perform when the time comes. Mormons baptize by immersion, meaning the person being baptized has to go completely under the water. No toe or elbow or other body part can be out of the water, or it doesn't count. They even have "witnesses" to make sure it's a proper dunking.

Dad and I practice how I'll grasp one of his arms and with my other hand plug my nose. He holds onto my wrist with one of his hands and raises the other high into the air to wave at Jesus while he says the same old prayer they always say when they baptize people. When he says "Amen," I'm to bend at the knees and keep my feet flat on the bottom of the font (the huge bathtub thing where I'll be baptized). It's hard to practice without water, but we're pretty confident we'll do it better than anyone else ever has.

Dad used to go to church, and he married Mom in the Washington, D.C., temple, so he already has the priesthood he needs in order to perform my baptism. I asked him what the priesthood was, and he said it was just permission from God to make decisions in His name. In Primary we learned that you have to get baptized and even married by a man who has the priesthood, otherwise it won't count.

Another part of the baptism ceremony is the clothing. Dad and I both have to wear all white jumpers. Jesus must not like color very much because Mom and Dad wear all white clothes when they go inside the temple too. Dad borrows his baptism outfit from the church, but Mom sews mine. Mom is well known throughout our community for being the best seamstress. During prom and homecoming seasons, she makes hundreds of dollars sewing formal gowns for lots of girls in our community.

A baptism in the family also means an influx of relatives. Mom's parents, Grandma and Grandpa Thomas (lovingly known as Grandma and Grandpa T), can be counted on to show up for all the important life events. Turning eight and "choosing" to be baptized is a big one. It's not really a choice though. It's not like my parents take me to other churches and ask if I want to be Mormon or something else.

They've taken me to a different church only a couple of times. Once we went to the Catholic Church with Great-Uncle Don and Aunt Val. Most of their service isn't even in English, and you stand up and kneel down a lot. It was so boring. The other time was for a funeral at a Baptist Church for Black people.

Dad's student, Orelia, was the same age as me and black as soot. She was the only Black student Dad had ever had in his class, and he bragged a lot about treating her the same way that he treated his White students, which seemed weird since he never bragged about treating a White student the same as a Black one.

As soon as they moved in, they became our family's new project.

"We don't want them to feel different," Mom had said to me. "Treat them just like you would anybody else."

"But they are different. Won't they feel different because they are different?" I asked.

"Don't be rude, Sarah." Mom answered so firmly I knew I needed to save my questions for someone else.

Orelia liked being outside like I do. While the adults were talking about boring stuff, she and I would "run away" so we could talk about interesting stuff. We never went far, but in our make-believe land, I was allowed to ask her why her skin and hair looked different. She let me braid her hair, and I let her braid mine. We weren't very good at it, but she said that was okay.

Orelia loved my stories. She would laugh in all the right places, and she would help me grow them even bigger. She drew pictures of fantasy animals for me, and I would write stories for them in my notebook. We decided that when we grew up, after I quit my job swimming with the dolphins at SeaWorld, I would write stories and she would draw all the pictures.

One day, before my baptism, Dad came home really sad. Orelia's mom had died in a car accident. Orelia was going to move away to go live with her grandma after the funeral.

"Why can't she just live here with us? Please, please, please can we adopt her?" I begged.

"I wish we could adopt her, Sarah," Dad comforted, "but she needs to be with her family."

Mom and Dad said that the funeral would be different from a Mormon funeral. I hoped that meant it wouldn't be boring.

My wish came true. For the first time in my life, I was the minority at a church function. We had to drive a long way to Holbrook to find the funeral house, and we were the *only* White family in the building. I'm not even sure where all the Black people came from because there were only a handful of Black families in the White Mountains of Arizona. For a long time, I thought the area was called the White Mountains because only White people and Native Americans were allowed to live there. I was in kindergarten when I learned the mountains were called that because of the white granite rocks.

Mormon funerals are somber, sad, and a missionary opportunity. Not the Black Baptist funeral. I had so much fun. I sat squished between the abundant hips of two Black grandmas. When it was time to sing, they sang louder than the high school marching band, and my little body swayed back and forth with them as they rocked to the music with their hands raised in the air.

The pastor mopped moisture from his brow with a white handkerchief as he passionately bellowed his sermon. "Amen" and "Praise Jesus" were shouted out more in that one-hour service than I'd heard in my entire life. I didn't know you were allowed to shout in church. If there had been a chandelier in that shanty of a church building, I know it would have shaken. After the sermon, they prayed together, and everyone hugged and clapped and shouted more "Amens" anytime anyone said something they all agreed with.

That's why if my parents had bothered to ask which church I wanted to join when I turned eight, I'd have chosen Southern Baptist with the Black grandmas.

But they didn't ask. And I didn't protest being baptized Mormon, because good girls don't complain, and they don't masturbate.

Thanks to Sister Cafer, everyone in our ward knew I wasn't a good girl in that regard. They said I was dangerous. I never hurt anyone, and I mostly touched myself. It felt good, and it helped me feel better when the frogs started jumping around in my stomach.

I don't understand why I liked it so much, but I did. I rubbed my pubic bone against anything and everything. My parents tried redirection, spanking, yelling, screaming, and shaming, but it didn't stop me. In fact, the more they yelled and spanked, the more I dry humped. I masturbated like an Olympian. I rubbed myself against furniture and my toys. I even tried rubbing against my Dad, but he pushed me down and said I was a filthy whore.

Sometimes I forgot where I was and would masturbate in the grocery store, at the homes of babysitters—you name it, I humped it. I even taught Susan Davis how to masturbate one night at a sleepover before we burned our fort down and she stopped liking me.

Sister Cafer expressed concern to Mom that maybe I had been sexually abused. Mom swore no one had ever hurt me in that way. When I asked her what "abused" meant, Mom told me not to ask those types of questions.

One day, Sister Cafer caught me pooping behind the lilac bushes in our yard. I don't think she knew I was pooping, just that my pants were down. Joey and I were playing Indians. Pooping in the "forest" and wiping with leaves was one of our favorite games. It also kept us out of Mom's hair since we didn't go inside to go potty. I made sure Joey and I turned around and didn't look at each other's privates, but that didn't matter to Sister Cafer. She went straight to my Mom who responded by spanking us both with a wooden spoon. I suppose it didn't help matters that Sister Cafer's husband was the bishop of our ward (the church's congregation, organized by geographical location). That meant he was our leader and oversaw the spiritual and social needs of our neighborhood.

Mom and Dad were furious that I had literally been caught with my pants down, and by the bishop's wife, no less. Their interventions on *my* behalf intensified immensely. I learned very early that embarrassing my parents brought the worst punishments, and there seemed to be something wrong with me because I couldn't stop touching my vagina.

I didn't know what a vagina was supposed to look like. I tried to look at mine to figure it out and see if something was there that made me touch it, like a sliver you can't leave alone. My head wouldn't bend far enough to see what was past my tiny penis. I couldn't ask to see someone else's either because it's forbidden for anyone to see a vagina after you've been potty-trained.

I masturbated myself to sleep every night, even though I tried really hard not to, but my brain was always "on" in the dark unless I was humping my blanket. Mom caught me one night, and in a fit of rage she tied my hands together with one of Dad's ties. Mom wasn't a good knot tier, even though she was a Boy Scout leader. I slipped right out of that tie and kept on humpin'. Dad came in later. I looked up guiltily.

He shook his head and picked up the tie and headed out of the room saying nothing.

The morning of my baptism, Mom asks to speak to me in her bedroom.

"Once you're baptized, you'll come up out of the water clean and pure. You'll be perfect. All the sins you've committed up to this point will be washed away. Any wrong you do after your baptism will count against you, Sarah. That means you'll have to stop masturbating. It's wrong."

I don't understand why God would make it feel so good and then say it's wrong, and I'm not sure I'll be able to stop, but I nod because that's what Mom expects.

After the talk with Mom, one of the teenage girls from church comes over and French braids my hair. It's tight and gives me a headache. Later, we gather at the church for the ceremony. The waistline of the white jumper Mom sewed for me itches just above my belly button. My jumper is a little more see-through than Mom expected, and she is mad when she realizes I'm wearing my favorite pair of pink underwear. Mom drives home and brings me some of my boring white ones since everything I wore needed to be white to represent purity. I'm not sure how she found them, but I obediently put them on after Mom explains pink is not suitable because once my jumper is wet, everyone will see my underwear.

"We don't want grown-up men seeing your panties. It will give them bad thoughts. You don't want all your friend's dads to have bad thoughts about you, do you?" she warns. I wonder if they already think bad things about me since most of them don't like me very much anyway. I will have to try harder to help them think good things and make Mom proud of me.

With the panty fiasco averted, the outlined service proceeds. Mormon services are *boring*! First, we sing a hymn, then someone gives a dreadfully long prayer that we are supposed to keep our eyes closed and head bowed for, then someone gives a talk about baptism that we've heard a million times before. I'm tired of pretending to listen, so I pinch Joey, who is sitting next to me. In return, he punches me in the leg. Grandma T shoots us a warning look, and we become silent statues after that. Grandma T looks like an older version of Mom but with dark brown and gray hair, which make her scary looking when she's mad.

When the talk is finally over, we move to the font. I go through a special door that leads to the font and find Dad is already waiting for me in the water. I take the few steps down into the baptismal font and move toward him. Dad and I love the water, and I have to fight back the urge to splash him. One look at Grandma T's stern face, and I decide to keep things in check.

Dad puts one hand in front of me, and I grab on just like we practiced. He raises his other arm and begins the baptismal ordinance.

Bishop Cafer interrupts. "No, Dave, stop, you're doing it wrong."

Dad finishes the prayer anyway and looks up; annoyance clouds his round face.

"You're backward," Bishop Cafer says. "You raise your right hand, not your left."

Dad spins me around, and puts his left arm out for me to grab so he can raise his right arm as Bishop Cafer instructed.

Dad repeats the prayer and dunks me so fast that I don't have time to get my hand to my face and plug my nose. I emerge from the water sputtering a bit only to hear Bishop Cafer tell my Dad he has to do it again. My feet came up out of the water.

At this point, Dad's face is red. He repeats the prayer for the third time, and just before he shoves me under the water, he stomps on my toes.

"Ouch," I say as he shoves me under, and my mouth fills with water. Dad pulls me up, makes eye contact with the two men acting as witnesses, gets the nod saying all is well, and then pats me on the back like he's proud that *I* finally got it right.

Standing in the water and coughing, I wait for the warm feeling that everyone says will come over me after the baptism. I'm supposed to feel clean and pure. The love of Jesus should fill my soul. I've been led to believe some extraordinary event will happen, and I'll feel different from when I went into the water.

I do feel different.

I feel... wet.

"Sarah?" Mom's voice pulls me out of my waiting to feel pure. I climb out of the font and cover my private area with my hands so the men don't have bad thoughts.

"How do you feel?" Mom asks me as she wraps a towel around me, her voice expectant.

"The water was cold," I lie. And just like that, I'm not perfect anymore. But Mom wanted me to say something, and since she told me the water wouldn't be very warm and she's always cold, I thought that would be the best thing to say.

"I'm sure it was, honey," she says with a smile as she helps me peel off the now very see-through jumpsuit.

I feel bad for lying, and I learned in Primary that repentance is how you fix your mistakes, so maybe telling Mom the truth will help. "Mom?" I begin in a questioning tone.

"Yes?" my Mom asks as she tries to pull my now acceptable pink panties up over my wet thighs.

How do I tell Mom that I feel the same way I did before I got dunked? How do I explain that I don't feel clean, or pure, or warm, or loved more by Jesus? There must be something wrong with me because Lucas, a boy from Scouts, said he felt all warm inside. So did Susan. I just feel wet and worried that I'm going to mess everything up like I always do, so I can't tell Mom the truth. She'll be mad at me.

"Nothing," I sigh, feeling defeated and small. Of course, I don't feel warm like Luke or Susan. I do everything wrong. I touch my privates too much, I give grown-up men bad thoughts, and I tell stories. I probably need to get dunked at least two more times to erase all of those sins.

Why did Jesus make me so broken?

I begin to cry, not loudly because I don't want Mom to notice, but a tear escapes my eye and runs down my cheek anyway.

Mom gives me a big hug. "Sarah, the feeling you are having right now, the one that's making you cry a little. That's the Spirit of God speaking to you."

I swallow hard. "Really?"

Mom nods.

I guess Jesus isn't perfect then because he made a mistake when he made me. That's why no one believes me, not even when I tell the truth. That's why my friends decide to play with the other kids. That's why all the grown-ups talk bad about me. That's why I tell a lie right after my sins are washed away.

"I'm really proud of you today, Sarah," Mom says. "You made the right choice getting baptized."

Mom doesn't know I'm not clean. She thinks that one baptism is enough. She thinks it fixed me.

"Thanks, Mom," I say. I give her a tentative smile. The day isn't over yet. Maybe getting the Holy Ghost will give me the warm feeling I'm supposed to have.

Back in the meeting room, someone gives a familiar speech about the Holy Ghost feeling like a warm blanket wrapping me in a big hug. Once the talk is over, I sit in a chair positioned with enough space around it so that all the men in the room who hold the same kind of priesthood Dad does can gather around me in a big circle and place their hands on my head. Priesthood is only given to the men.

Dad gives an eloquent prayer and tells me to receive the Holy Ghost. Then he finishes the blessing he had been writing out that morning, even though Mom told him you aren't supposed to prepare the prayer like that. I hear his confident voice, but I'm not paying much attention to what he's saying because I'm focusing really hard, waiting intently for the warm fuzzy feeling to wrap me up like a blanket.

The only thing I feel is… uncomfortable.

My small head is heavy from all the men's hands piled on top of it. Dad says something about my golden heart. He's always saying God gave me a golden heart. Then it's over. The men all say "Amen," and I feel lighter. It's not from any warm blanket or holy manifestation from heaven. It's because there aren't hands on my head anymore.

I don't think Dad's prayer worked. I don't feel warm like a blanket is hugging me. The Holy Ghost doesn't want to live in me because He knows I'm a bad girl. I can't help it.

Bishop Cafer gets up and welcomes me as the newest member of the church. He gives me a silver dollar, a dime, and a penny. That means I have one dollar and eleven cents. The dime and penny are so I can pay my 10% tithe on the money he gave me. I can put that 11 cents into one of the special tithing envelopes and give it back to Bishop Cafer next time we go to church. But Bishop gave me the money as a present, and giving back a present is rude.

The meeting is almost over. Normally, the Primary president would get up and say something to me, but she's not here, so Sister Cafer gets up and confirms what Mom said earlier. "Sarah, that feeling you have inside of you, that's the Holy Ghost. Always listen for His voice. He will help you choose the right and tell the truth."

Then it's over. We pile in the van and head home. I'm an official member of the Church of Jesus Christ of Latter-Day Saints. I was only perfect for about five seconds before I lied, and I want to spend my tithing money on tootsie rolls, so I'm not much different than I was before the whole thing.

Mom is scolding Dad for embarrassing all of us for baptizing me backward. Ordinances (baptism, getting the priesthood, temple covenants, marriage) are rituals in the Mormon Church that have to be done exactly the same for everyone in order for them to count. They'll stop arguing as soon as we get home because Grandma and Grandpa T will be there, and they don't want to look bad in front of Mom's parents.

The rest of the day is pretty normal. Grandma reads us stories. Grandpa and Dad talk about sports. We play, Joey and I argue, we eat dinner, and we get ready for bed. Nothing special. No new feelings. Just normal.

Mom comes into the room that I share with my three siblings. "Goodnight, Sarah," she whispers as she leans over me. "Listen for the Holy Ghost. He will help you be a good girl."

I nod sleepily as she pulls the covers under my chin and kisses my forehead. Normally, it's Dad who tucks us in, but I'm too tired to ask about the change in routine. Mom turns out the bedroom light and leaves the room.

I roll onto my stomach and thrust myself to sleep.

I guess the Holy Ghost is too busy helping someone else feel good to stop me from masturbating.

DOUGHNUTS AND A MASTER'S DEGREE

SUMMER 1989

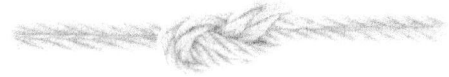

8 YEARS OLD

The summer before third grade, Dad announces that he is going back to college so he can get a master's degree and a pay raise. We move into a small apartment in Flagstaff, near Northern Arizona University, and Mom works at a doughnut shop with a guy who hates Mormons. Even though he says mean things about our church, he and Mom are friends, which makes Dad jealous. Mom and Dad yell at each other a lot more than normal, which makes my stomach get "froggy" more than ever, so my already hypersexual behavior kicks into overdrive.

Since Dad has morning classes and Mom works early on the weekdays at the doughnut shop, they have to hire a babysitter. My parents have always been too poor to hire someone, but somehow they make it work. Before now, Joey, Evelyn, Charlie, and I have never been left alone with a teenager.

They hire Greggory, the boy in the apartment across the hall from us, to come over and babysit for a few hours every weekday morning after Dad leaves for class. Gregg seems nice, and he's cute. His brown curly hair sticks out funny around his ears, and he has big arm muscles.

Gregg doesn't do much other than just hang out at our house. We don't have cable television because Mom and Dad can't afford it, so we watch recordings of *Sesame Street* and *Mr. Rogers' Neighborhood* on VHS over and over again. The episodes get boring really fast, so we find other ways to entertain ourselves. Dad has taught us how to use our imaginations to create games, and we kids are good at it. Even though Gregg is a teenager, he still plays games with us since there's nothing else to do. Sometimes Gregg tickles us. One time, he accidentally touches my vulva. He apologizes immediately and stops tickling us after that. He won't even look me in the eyes anymore.

His accidental touch triggers something in me, and I spend the rest of the summer trying to get him to do it again. When we play hide-and-seek, I leave him notes saying, "If you want me, you have to come and get me." I hide in the bedroom, hoping he'll come find me and touch me. He does come find me, but when I try to get him to lay down and play mommy and daddy with me, he says to stop hiding in the bedroom and walks away. I need to get him to like me. I know touching makes boys like girls, so I keep trying. I need him to want me more than a dehydrated hiker in the Arizona desert needs water.

Gregg's younger sister, Nancy, and I are friends. She has the same curly brown hair as Gregg and has freckles just like mine, so the three of us look like we could be siblings. Nancy whispers in my ear that sometimes Gregg tickles her too, so maybe we can get him to tickle us on our frequent weekend sleepovers at her house. Her parents don't watch us much. Nancy's family has an intercom system in their apartment so their parents can announce bedtime over the speakers without having to take a break from the television shows we aren't allowed to watch. Nancy and I often join Gregg in his bed and beg him to touch us. He never comes to her room, so we use the intercom system to talk to each other from her room to his.

Gregg says, "If you want something you have to come here to get it."

We always go.

My memory gets really fuzzy around this time, and I have lots of gaps. I remember going to Gregg's bed. I remember dry humping his leg, and I remember waking up in Nancy's room on the floor where we crashed for the night. Everything from Gregg's leg to Nancy's floor is gone.

Mom finds one of my notes to Gregg and confronts me about it. I tell her it's just our hide-and-seek game. She doesn't believe me and tells Dad.

"Emma," he says, "we have to believe our kids. All of them say it's just hide-and-seek."

Nothing changes. Gregg keeps babysitting us, Mom and Dad keep fighting, I keep spending weekends at Nancy's, and we keep going to Gregg's room at night. The gaps in my memory get longer.

Part of me knows getting Gregg to touch us is wrong, but it also feels good. I convince myself that as long as I keep quiet and no one talks about it, it's okay. But the frogs in my stomach jump around a lot more, I startle at the slightest noises, and I can't stay focused on things for very long. Keeping the secret is messing me up, and the gaps in my memory freak me out. I can't tell Mom and Dad because they'll say I'm just lying for attention.

Dad says that girls lie about getting touched on their privates because girls are crazy. Maybe I'm crazy, since I keep forgetting things. My friend

Melody wasn't allowed to come play with me anymore because someone had touched her on her privates and ruined her. Dad said Melody lied about a man touching her and that a good man had to go to jail because of her, which is why you can't trust girls or women who say those things about men.

Dad's adult cousin would go to his local high school and take all his clothes off. He got arrested and had to go to jail. His mom, my Great-Aunt May, said he had a mental illness. Dad says mental illness is just a made-up excuse to get attention. Dad said his big sister was a little crazy too. I didn't remember her because she died when I was two, but her daughter, Beatrice, had a "mental illness" that Dad said she was probably faking to get attention. He said she was crazy too, and wouldn't let us be alone around her either. He said Beatrice was the type of person who would lie about being touched by a man to get him in trouble.

Dad doesn't love people who are crazy, so I can't tell him or Mom about Gregg 'cause now that I've been touched, I'm crazy too. I don't want him to stop loving me, so I smile and agree with him that Bea is dangerous. I even help him grow his stories about her, just so he knows I'm on his side.

Dad graduates from NAU at the end of the summer and we move back to Snowflake and away from Gregg. Our new house is huge. Mom says the yellow paint makes it look happy from the outside. I think she's trying to convince herself that she likes the new house, because it's full of mice. I get my own room in the new house.

Even though the tension between my parents is better, things are getting harder for me. I had graduated from elementary school before we moved to Flagstaff. Snowflake Intermediate School is a few blocks away from our new house, so I get to walk to and from school every day. I can't make eye contact with any of the boys, or else they'll know I'm dirty. I'm pretty sure that the girls know my secret. I don't know how they would have found out because I hadn't told anyone, but they were always whispering with each other. I just know they are talking about me, so I try to avoid them too.

I didn't know that fourth grade would be so hard. I squint at the chalkboard because all the numbers and letters are blurry. I get my eyes checked, but the doctor said my vision is perfect. I try to listen to my teacher, but my mind wanders, and I daydream through the entire lesson. I catch myself thinking about Gregg and then my stomach gets all wonky, and I feel like I'm going to throw up. I get in trouble for asking to get a drink of water too many times during class. I'm just trying to get the nausea to go away.

I'm afraid to go to the bathroom 'cause I don't want to pull my pants down at school. I'm afraid someone is going to look through the crack in the door and then they'll know I'm a dangerous girl, just like Bea. If I need to pee, I hold it until I can run the five blocks home from school. My bladder gets used to the new schedule so usually it's no big deal. Except for that one day when I got home and the front door was locked.

I prance in place and ring the doorbell over and over again, my bladder begging for relief. Finally, Grandpa T opens the door. I'm so surprised to see him that I pee my pants right there on the front porch.

Grandpa T looks over his shoulder and says, "Quick, go change your clothes, and no one will ever know." I don't know how he pulled it off, but Mom never even mentions my soiled pants. Grandpa is my hero. Mom and I got our short genes from him. His dark hair and gentle smile feel safe. He always has my back, and he never gets mad at me, ever. Grandpa also loves all people, even when they are crazy. I know because my cousin Jay is gay, which means he's got the mental illness, and Grandpa loves him and treats him the same as me. I like Jay, even though Dad hates him. Dad says gay people are dangerous too.

Even though I'm terrified of being watched in the school bathroom, my habit of masturbating in public gets worse. In grade school, I had been too busy moving from one task to another to masturbate in my classroom. The few times it did happen, my teachers reminded me to go to the bathroom, but I was never shamed in front of the class for my behavior.

Intermediate school is different. We spend less time running and playing on the playground, which increases the jumping frogs in my stomach. Dry humping helps sooth my nerves, but my friends don't want to hang out with me because I'm "embarrassing." Everyone in class thinks there is something wrong with me. I hope it's not a mental illness.

A few weeks into the school year, Mr. Jackson welcomes us to class. He looks like he's been crying.

"Boys and girls, Ammon was hit by a car this morning on his way to school. He's alive, and the doctors are working hard to fix his broken bones."

I look around as some of the other kids gasp. I realize that I don't know who Ammon is, and yet, I'm suddenly terrified for him.

"I would like for our class to say a prayer together, asking God to guide the doctor's hands so that Ammon will be okay." Mr. Jackson's voice soothes my nerves.

We fold our arms across our chests and bow our heads, waiting for the familiar cadence of a Mormon prayer.

The next day, Mr. Jackson announces that Ammon will live because he got a priesthood blessing in time.

Several weeks after our prayer, Ammon came back to school in a full body cast and a wheelchair. He needed help with everything, and no one was willing to give up lunch recess to help. I decided right then and there that I could be Ammon's hero. Dad had blessed me with a golden heart when he gave me the Holy Ghost. The Holy Ghost might have skipped over me, but my heart wouldn't. I was destined to be Ammon's new best friend.

The next day, I volunteered to push Ammon to the playground. Soon after, I started eating lunch with him. He needed a lot of help, so I helped him reach his food. He was a good listener, and he laughed at all my jokes. One day, I asked him how he went to the bathroom. He told me there was a hole with a door down there that he could go potty with. Gratefully I didn't have to help him with that.

Ammon and I developed a strong friendship that year. Once his cast came off, he and I would play good guys and bad guys on the playground. Ammon never touched me in a way that made me uncomfortable. Lots of kids in the class didn't like him much because he smelled funny. Once the cast came off, he stopped smelling weird, but people had already decided he was the stinky kid in class. That was okay with me because it meant I had Ammon all to myself.

The summer after fourth grade, Ammon and I joined the band. I started playing the flute, and he started playing the clarinet. Band was where I found my social feet, and where I started to comprehend social rules and make more long-term friends. I started lying for my friends to keep them out of trouble instead of turning against them to get them into trouble.

Music also helped me soothe the anxiety I felt almost constantly. I would play for hours, losing myself in the music. Music is what my feelings sound like. I learned to trust the notes and rhythms to tell my story, since words failed me.

I quickly rose to the top of my section. My parents paid for private flute lessons, and Dad bragged to anyone who would listen about how I was the best. I practiced a lot, because once I earned first chair, I couldn't lose it. I would always be the best in my section for the rest of forever. That way Dad would always love me the best.

Dad loved being the best. I inherited his competitive nature, as did Joey. Dad encouraged sibling competition. Joey and I had at-home wrestling matches. Dad called it "wrastling" because it was girl against boy. Joey didn't like wrastling as much as I did. Despite being two years younger than me, most strangers thought we were twins with our freckled noses and chestnut hair. He may have been bigger than I was, but he was much gentler. I was willing to fight dirty, especially as Joey grew stronger and it became harder for me to win. Losing wasn't an option. Not only was I the best flute player, but I needed to be the best at everything—a trait that would both serve me well and destroy relationships for years to come. Dad only loved the superstar.

Sunday wrastling matches always started out friendly. Joey and I would face off, then I would shoot at his legs and knock him to the floor. With a sharp twist, I would roll Joey over and punch him in the shoulders.

"Go, Sarah. You got him," Dad would yell. "Come on, Joey. It's your turn now."

Joey worked hard to sit up and tried to push me over. He finally shoved me off of him, and I landed hard on my butt. A puff of air escaped from my mouth, and I felt a thunk in my stomach. I blinked back tears. I am not a crybaby.

"You got her, Joey," Dad hollered.

I was pissed! Joey wasn't allowed to win this game, or any other for that matter. I needed Dad to know that I was the best. I looked up. Joey stood above me, smirking. I rolled to all fours and pretended I couldn't catch my breath. Joey leaned down to make sure I was okay. As soon as he let his guard down, I swiped at his legs, knocking him, once again, to his back.

I scrambled to my feet and jumped on him. In my rage, I wasn't aware of where I was or what I was doing, but I knew I was going to win this match once and for all. I landed on his head.

"Whoa, good job, Sarah! You got him," Dad cheered.

I'd done it. Dad was proud of me again.

Joey's cries pulled Mom out of her latest sewing project. She glared at Dad as I scrambled off of Joey's bloody face.

"Dave!" Mom screeched. "What on earth are you letting these two do?"

"Oh, Emma. They were just wrestling, and Sarah got a bit carried away," Dad growled. "Come here, Joey. Let me see that nose. Stop crying like a girl."

Mom huffed and turned on her heels. Dad never seemed affected by her frustrations, at least not in front of us kids.

"Good move, Sarah, but remember, no heads or faces," Dad reminded me.

I was shaking… my knees trembling so hard I thought I might trip if I moved. The sight of Joey's blood extinguished my anger like a blown-out birthday candle. I was shocked that I had hurt my brother. We fought like crazy, but I loved him. I didn't want to hurt him, not for real anyway.

Standing in our living room watching his nose pour blood after I had jumped on him shifted something in me. I wasn't proud of myself for winning like I usually was. I felt… bad, sad, and angry at myself all at the same time. I bit my lip and swallowed hard to keep myself from crying. That was the last wrastling match Joey and I ever had. He claimed I stopped because he got too strong for me. I told him he was a crybaby, and we would start arguing about something, but we never let it progress beyond angry words. It was like an unspoken contract between us.

Now that we're adults, Joey makes sure my kids know that I never fought fair and that I would jump on his head. My kids are shocked that I was ever that mean. When they ask me about it, I confirm the story and then tell them that I learned that day that winning is never important enough to hurt someone else.

AUTHOR'S NOTE

Looking back on these early years of my life makes my heart ache for my small self. It's clear that I was confused about my sexual development. Snowflake was a very small community with a high population of ortho-dox Mormons. Inside Bubbleville (Snowflake), no one talked about sex, as the expectation was "that's the parents' job." I never received any formal sex-ed in school, no "stranger danger." The only message I was taught was that sex was a serious sin before marriage. If you did anything other than holding hands, hugging, and kissing, you needed to tell the bishop in order to repent.

Studies on human development have demonstrated that children rely on external sources, such as their parents, caregivers, or teachers, to define their reality.[1] Openly discussing *anything* having to do with sex, puberty, good touch/bad touch was considered wrong or evil in my household. It's pretty normal for a child who isn't allowed to ask *any* questions about what is going on inside their body to internalize the message that they are bad because of what is happening to them.

I'm fairly certain Greggory never touched my body underneath my clothing. Mom had sent a clear message to me early in life that sex meant touching naked body parts, and I never viewed the sexualized play between Gregg, Nancy, and I to mean I had had sex. Looking back on that part

---

1   Joan E. Grusec and Tanya Danyliuk, "Parents' Attitudes and Beliefs: Their Impact on Children's Development" *Encyclopedia on Early Childhood Development*. December 2014. https://www. child-encyclopedia.com/pdf/expert/parenting-skills/according-experts/parents-attitudes-and-beliefs-their-impact-childrens-development. (Accessed Jan. 15, 2023).

of my life with a "professional lens" leads me to believe the blackouts or lost time had more to do with the fear that if my parents knew how bad I was they would stop loving me. After our summer in Flagstaff, I felt an increased need to please my parents and be a good girl in order to maintain the status quo and hide how evil I was. Keep in mind, the lesson I learned in life was that a girl was responsible for a man's failures in all aspects of his life.

SIXTH GRADE

1992–1993

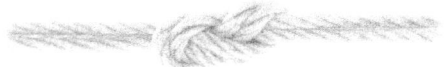

11–12 YEARS OLD

Despite doing incredibly well with the flute, my anxiety is still really bad. I'm constantly worrying that the wet stuff coming from my vagina is leaking through the back of my pants. I haven't started my period yet and it's sixth grade, but no one has talked to me about what will happen. I can tell my body is changing. When I ask Mom about my nipples being sore, she just says, "I don't remember" and changes the subject.

I annoy my friends by constantly asking them if it looks like I have peed my pants. One day, someone tells me to just go to the bathroom and check if my period has started, because she's tired of looking at the back of my pants with my butt in the air.

I also discover that masturbating feels good in a very different way. As well as masturbating to soothe my anxiety, I do it for pleasure. Sometimes the urge is so strong I rub my fingers over my pubic mound under my school desk. I look around at my classmates to see if anyone is looking at me, but no one seems to notice. Eventually it becomes something I just do without thinking about it.

One day in early fall, a couple of boys notice me grinding against the corner of Ammon's desk while listening to the teacher give directions on our group project. As soon as Mr. Franklin turns the time over to the class, the boys make fun of me. They call me "slut." They tell me I'm a nasty hooker. They say they need to take the desk out of the classroom and burn it. I'm utterly humiliated, but I stop masturbating in public.

In the late fall, my body decides to sprout breasts overnight. For months and months, the hard little nubs forming under my nipples throb, and I avoid touching them. The next thing I know, I'm a C cup, and the boys won't keep their hands to themselves. I wear front-clasp bras because they're easier to put on. Several boys make it a game to grab my bra from the front, right between my breasts, pull back hard, and release it to give me a "front snap," as they call it.

I used to enjoy and seek out attention from boys, but now I hate it. The gauntlet of grabbing hands makes it impossible for me to concentrate in school, and my grades suffer. One of those "front snaps" makes the clasp come undone, and I attempt to slide underneath my desk to put it back together. The boys catcall and whistle, and I wish I could vanish. Ammon tells them to stop, but no one will listen to him because he's not "popular."

One boy passes me a note that says, "Look at slutty Sarah, playing with her boobs now!"

I'm tired of being victimized. I don't even know what victimized means, but I know how dehumanizing this is, and I hate it. I develop asthma—at least that's what the doctor thinks it is. It makes sense since my Dad has asthma, except mine only happens when I have to walk by the boys who constantly grab at my body. The prescribed inhaler doesn't help, and it tastes gross, so I stop using it.

I'm the second shortest kid in my grade and am tiny and curvy. Like the other girls, I'm insecure and nervous about my changing body. Unlike the other girls, I try to hide my changes by donning my Dad's extra-large T-shirts. I decide not to talk to anyone about the changes in my body because I'm afraid they'll laugh at me or tell me to go to the bathroom and check for myself. I don't even know what I'm supposed to be looking for. I can't ask Mom or Dad, because we aren't allowed to ask them questions about our body or we'll get in trouble.

Dad loves that I wear his shirts to conceal my changing body. Our relationship has changed with my body. I'm not allowed to sit on his lap anymore. He's stopped giving me hugs. In fact, he avoids touching me at all. I don't understand why, but I know it's my fault.

My sister, Charlie, is small like me and seven years younger. One of our favorite family games is Baby Monster. My Dad gets onto his hands and knees, and Charlie hides underneath him. Evelyn, Joey, and I try to kidnap Charlie by pulling her free without Dad pulling us off our feet or tossing us onto the nearby couch.

Bucking Bronco is another favorite game. Dad gets on his hands and knees, we climb onto his back, and he tries to buck us off. I'm the best at hanging on. I hook my feet together under his belly and thread one arm over his shoulder and the other arm under his other shoulder. I interlace my fingers and lock the palms of my hands closed. The only way I'm going to come off is if Dad does a near headstand. Even then, I squeeze my thighs and arms together and affix like a leech. The truth is, I'm afraid of getting hurt from flying off his back like Joey often does.

One day I'm allowed to play those games, and the next, I'm not. I'm not sure what I did wrong, and I'm scared I'm going to get yelled at, or worse, spanked with the wooden spoon if I ask. I'm supposed to just know and then not do whatever it is ever again.

My confidence takes a nosedive, and I wonder if I'm ugly. My parents hound me about washing my face. I pick at my acne trying to keep it clean. No one teaches me how to do my hair or apply makeup. No one teaches me how to use deodorant. Mom takes me to a lady who sells Mary Kay. She helps me wash my face, but when we don't buy anything, she doesn't want to help me anymore. I have to learn these things from Jamie, whose thick bangs cover any breakouts on her forehead.

Jamie is my best friend. We don't share many of our classes, but we are the same age and in the same ward, so we are in the same classes at church. Jamie is an expert on how to be a popular girl because she has a subscription to *Teen Magazine*. I go to her house and read the magazine while she plays *Mario Brothers* on her Nintendo 64. I borrow her razor and learn how to shave my legs. Jamie knows how to apply makeup to best accentuate her angular features. I learn how to apply makeup for my heart-shape face; hell, I even learn that Maybelline is the best kind to use from looking at all the ads in *Teen Magazine*.

Jamie is also an expert secret keeper. She hardly ever talks to anyone other than me. Jamie and I talk about everything—well, almost everything. I don't talk about masturbation, but we talk about everything else and we never worry about the other sharing our vulnerabilities with the world. We spend hours together talking about everything from toenail polish to which boys we think are cute.

When I complain to Jamie about not being able to play rough-housing games with Dad anymore, she fixes me with an incredulous look and declares, "Those games sound completely stupid. Why would you want to play like that in the first place?"

She's right. When Joey, Evelyn, and Charlie play with Dad, I sit on the couch. When I start feeling left out, I remind myself that the games are stupid. I remind myself that I don't care. I still feel left out, though.

At least I'm still allowed to participate in paper-wad fights. Dad keeps an empty box in his classroom where his students can return their graded papers if they don't want to keep them. Dad brings that box home on the weekends for paper-wad fights. We rearrange the living room furniture to make hideouts. Then we wrinkle the graded papers into hundreds of balls.

It's always Joey and me against Dad, Evelyn, and "Baby Monster" Charlie. We throw our paper wads at each other. If you get hit, you have to "die" until one team runs out of ammunition. Joey has a good arm, and I'm a good dodger. I'm almost always the last person out in dodgeball at school. It's probably all that practice dodging groping boys that keeps my body contorting in all different ways, so I won't get hit. At least it's good for something.

Since Evelyn is normally "dead" within the first volley, Dad waits until Joey and I run out of ammunition. Then he provides backup for Charlie to gather all the paper wads in the center of the room to replenish his stash. Charlie doesn't play dead very well, and since she's the youngest she's allowed to cheat, especially if it helps Dad win. With his stores refilled, he launches a frenzied attack at Joey and me while we scramble to recover some of our ammo.

No matter how many times Joey and I lose due to this strategy, we still tell Dad how many paper wads we have left when he asks us. We played paper-wad fight for years before Joey and I decide to lie about how much ammo we have so that we can win for a change.

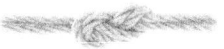

I turn 12 in the spring. Turning 12 is a big deal for Mormon youth. It means I graduate from Primary and get to attend the Young Women's and

Youth Sunday School class, where I will learn everything I need to know to be a good wife and mother someday. It's a good thing since Primary is boring. I've been taught the same lessons on repeat since I was three. The only good part about Primary was singing time and only because I love music. Even though I'm in Young Women's now, I still love many of the Primary songs.

Dad makes a big deal about my turning 12. Mom made Dad a Superman costume complete with leotards that he uses during assemblies and other fun events at his school. On my birthday, in the middle of completing my sixth-grade writing assignment, my classroom door bursts open, and in walks Superman. Dad and Mr. Franklin's wife teach together at Taylor Intermediate, so Mr. Franklin is probably in on Dad's surprise visit since he doesn't seem very surprised at all. My classmates roar with laughter as my Dad calls out, "Mr. Franklin, is there a birthday girl in this classroom?"

Heat flushes my face. I'm not sure whether to be excited or embarrassed or flattered or ashamed—my stomach feels froggy. I release an uncomfortable chuckle while wringing my hands under my desk in anticipation for the next joke.

"Well, Superman, let me see," Mr. Franklin says, pretending to search the science homework he'd just collected but hadn't put down yet. "Why, it's Sarah Lee's birthday today, sir."

"Mr. Franklin," Dad/Superman says, "I am here to rescue Sarah from more of your useless busy work. Where is she?"

My classmates point at me as if on cue.

Dad grins and steps toward me. "Are you Sarah Lee?"

I roll my eyes at him, just like Mom does when she doesn't appreciate his jokes, then glare at him. He extends his hand with the flowers in them.

"These are for you," he exclaims.

I take the flowers and reach my hand expectantly toward the vase.

Dad/Superman looks into the empty vase, shrugs, and says, "I'm not sure what this is for. I think it's in case you can't make it to the bathroom."

My classmates either whistle, catcall, or groan.

My smirk vanishes. Hot, shameful tears sting my eyes. I don't want to cry. I will not cry! How could Dad do this to me? He and Mom know I'm afraid to use the bathroom at school, even though they don't know why. I always rush home and head straight for the toilet to relieve my aching bladder.

"Sarah definitely needs that," a boy at the front of the room calls.

Dad and Mr. Franklin chuckle at what they think is just a silly joke. I swallow the lump in my throat, then step toward Dad and snag the vase from his hands.

"Goodbye, Mr. Franklin, and goodbye lowly students," Dad trumpets.

He grabs my hand and playfully pulls me from the room.

"Hang on tight, Princess, prepare yourself for flight," he says as the classroom door closes behind us.

As soon as the door closes Dad looks at me and laughs.

I know I'll mess everything up if I act like a crybaby, so I laugh along with him even though I'm shrinking inside. I don't want Mom to yell at me for embarrassing Dad in public again.

"Where do you want to go for lunch?" Dad asks.

The knot in my stomach will make it hard to eat anything, but I can't ruin this day.

"That hamburger place," I say. There aren't many options in Snowflake, and that's his favorite diner.

"Great choice. I always knew you had great taste in food."

Putting aside my anger and embarrassment, I enjoy lunch with Dad, and we talk about all the things I've held in for weeks—except the trouble with the boys touching me or how it feels to be excluded from games at home. I know better than to bring that up.

After lunch, it's time to go back to school.

"Can I wear your cape?" I ask.

"Absolutely," Dad says. "I'll even let you stand up in the back of the truck as I pass the playground, so that it looks like you are flying."

A smile breaks across my face. Dad can be so cool. Maybe I was just overreacting. I'm the luckiest girl *ever*!

Dad pulls over his sky-blue 1966 Ford pickup truck just before turning onto the street below Snowflake Intermediate School's playground. I tug his cape over my head, stand up in the bed of his truck, and hang on to the top of the cab as he drives slowly up the street. The cape billows in the wind behind me. This is turning into the best birthday. Jamie is right: It's weird for dads to hug their daughters once they are in Young Women. Dads just show their love in other ways.

AUTHOR'S NOTE

Ughhh, sixth grade was a rough year for me. As I became more consciously aware of how the outside world might view me, the fractures in my sexual development exploded in my face. Combine that with my Dad's discomfort of my growing body and… gut punch.

Dad really struggled with the idea that women were simple-minded or dangerous. His mother had multiple affairs and multiple live-in boyfriends who traumatized him. I suspect Grandma Hansen struggled with borderline personality disorder, though she was never formally diagnosed. Personality-disorder traits are common companions to those who have been traumatized and not allowed to process it. My theory is that Dad felt comfortable with Mom because Mom hated sex, refused to talk about it, and avoided it at all costs. While her apathy left him sexually frustrated, it was also a direct contrast to how his mother felt about sex. When I began to act out sexually and develop, it almost felt like Dad began to punish me for the mistakes of my grandmother. Her borderline behaviors made it impossible for Dad to work through his feelings, and I became the target of his anger.

UNDERWEAR IS DANGEROUS

1993–1994

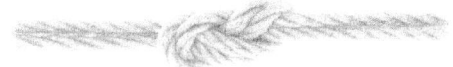

12–13 YEARS OLD

Junior high is amazing! Half the kids know Dad from his fifth-grade class at Taylor Intermediate School. They want to be my friend because of how awesome they think he is. I'm like a celebrity. Good thing they don't know what he says about them at the dinner table, or that he doesn't really love me anymore.

Since they combine Snowflake and Taylor into one school starting in junior high, it's like everyone gets a fresh start. No one even seems to remember how slutty I was in sixth grade.

I make the cheer team, and Mom tells me I'm still not allowed to shave my legs until high school. She thinks I'm too young for grown-up stuff like shaving and makeup. I've been shaving for almost a year already. Jamie and I laugh about it all through lunch. Cassidy and Brent join our friend group, and they think Mom is way too strict. Well, not Brent. Brent is a goodie-goodie and walks away every time we talk about girl stuff, his cheeks flushed.

Mom never really notices me anyway. She only pays attention when I'm doing something loud, and she tells me to be quiet. She's even stopped reading bedtime stories to me because I'm too old. Dad won't stop picking on me. I don't know what changed, but he's always telling me that my body is tempting, and I need to cover it up more.

"Don't sit cross-legged," Dad says during early morning family scripture study. "The boys will be able to see right up your dress. It's not their fault if they touch you when you are showing them your underwear."

I stop wearing nightshirts after his admonition and start wearing sweatpants instead.

Shorts are against the dress code in Snowflake/Taylor Unified School District, and I hate dresses and skirts. I only want to wear outfits that might discourage the boys from touching me. I had enough of them groping me last year, so anything I can do to lessen the possibility is good by me. I figure the cheerleading uniform is okay because the entire squad wears them, so I won't stand out. There is safety in numbers, and I am thrilled to be making and keeping friends outside the music department.

Besides, I'm not the only one with boobs anymore. Most of my friends are starting to look more grown up. There are more teachers around, too, so it's harder for the boys to get away with grabbing me all the time. I stop wearing Dad's T-shirts and dress like everyone else in jeans and a normal size T-shirt.

Then comes the "bad girl" issue again. Dad isn't pleased that I need to buy a pair of blue bikini panties for cheer. Mom says I need two pairs in case I have games two days in a row. They argue about it while I practice my flute; their voices carry over the screeching of notes written three lines above the scale.

"If we buy her colored panties, she'll think it's okay for the boys to see them," Dad towers over Mom and bellows.

"If we don't, the boys will see the white lines of her underwear sticking outside of her bloomers," Mom retorts.

"We need to petition the school board. The girls can wear shorts under the cheer uniform so the color of underwear is not an issue," he demands.

"Dave, we told her she could try out for cheer, and she's good. Much better than I ever was; she's small like me but more flexible and she's stronger."

"Doesn't mean she can start running around like she's on the beach."

"Stop being ridiculous. When she high-kicks, it's just a flash, you can't see anything. It's part of the sport."

"Boys only need a flash to get the wrong idea, Emma."

"You said just the other day that boys won't like her until her acne clears up and she learns how to calm her frizzy hair."

"Men can get around acne and frizzy hair."

On and on they go. I blow with more force into my mouthpiece, raising the pitch of my warm-up one octave.

"Sarah! Stop playing your stupid flute," Joey says as he purposefully bumps the end of the foot joint, slamming the mouthpiece against my braces.

"That hurt, jerk." I try to kick him, but he slides his shins out of the way just in time.

"Missed me, missed me, now you gotta kiss me."

His sing-song voice grates my nerves.

"You're disgusting," I snarl.

"No, you're the disgusting one. Why don't you go pop a zit, Frizz Head?"

I set my flute down gently on top of the piano where I've been practicing and turn slowly to him with fake tears in my eyes.

"I'm gonna tell Mom you called me Frizz Head again," my voice a fake whimper.

He steps forward with a pleading look on his face. I punch him hard in the stomach, and he doubles over.

"No one would ever want to kiss you, Dog Breath," I hiss.

Evelyn walks in from the living room, trying to get as far away from Mom and Dad as possible. She looks at Joey and me and smiles triumphantly.

"Joey and Sarah are fighting! Joey and Sarah are fighting!" she calls.

"You walk like a boy," Joey says to her. "Are you gay?"

Her wails pierce our ears. I know better than to make eye contact. I stare intently at my music and listen while moving my fingers across the keys as if I'm practicing the correct fingering patterns. I listen intently to the cacophony of yelling voices now directed at Joey for teasing Evelyn.

"Joey, stop calling your sister gay. She isn't gay," Mom scolds.

"Yes, Joey. Evelyn is gay. Look at how happy she is," Dad counters.

Dad's doublespeak infuriates Mom even more. "Dave, you can't say things like that. She's going to get ideas in her head that being gay is okay or something."

My shoulders loosen as my nerves calm down. They aren't talking about me anymore. I decide I'm tired of practicing, so I pull one of Dad's threadbare white handkerchiefs out of my flute case and thread it through the metal needle in preparation for removing spit from the inside of my instrument.

"What's gay?" Evelyn manages to croak out between sobs.

"Gay means you're happy," Dad tries to reassure her. "Aren't you happy, Evelyn?"

I picture her shaking her eight-year-old head back and forth, her jet-black hair swishing against her shoulders.

"Boys are tough. It's good to be like boys. They don't cry when people call them happy." I roll my eyes at Dad's "encouraging" statement.

"Dave," Mom says, her firm lecturing tone indicates she's nearing the end of her tolerance for Dad's reasoning. "You can't teach her that. She's going to repeat what you are saying at my parents' house this weekend. Eddie—I mean Dallas—and his boyfriend will hear her and think we don't like them."

"No one is going to call him Dallas," Dad says. "And changing your name doesn't make kissing boys okay."

I zone out into memories of Eddie. It wasn't until I saw Eddie and Linus, his boyfriend, holding hands that I began to understand what made Mom and Dad act so weird. Mom had asked Eddie not to kiss Linus in front of us because it might give us "the wrong idea." Eddie didn't look happy when Mom told him that, but he didn't argue either. Dad warned us to be careful around him now because men like him were child molesters. I didn't know what a child molester was, but if Uncle Eddie was one, he was the coolest one around.

Uncle Eddie is my favorite uncle. I'm excited he'll be at Grandma T's house when we go visit them in Payson tomorrow. Uncle Eddie and his friend Linus live in California and are really fun to hang out with. They're relaxed and let me say things without telling me I'm dumb, and they laugh at my jokes.

Last year when we visited Grandma Hansen in California, we went to see Uncle Eddie. He invited me to spend the night at their apartment. Dad was furious, but Mom had already said I could go.

I climbed into Eddie's Jeep Wrangler, and we were off.

"What do you want to do, Sarah?" he asked as he turned down the radio.

"I want to stay up late and watch grown-up movies."

He laughed and said, "An eleven-year-old watching grown-up movies... I won't tell if you don't."

Anything rated above G was strictly off limits. I hated that family rule because I hadn't seen half the cool movies my friends had, like *Who Framed Roger Rabbit.* In junior high the rating I was allowed to watch got bumped up to PG and some PG-13, but never R. Even Mormon grown-ups are discouraged from watching R-rated movies because it invites evil into your house and makes you more susceptible to Satan's powers.

I have no recollection of what movie we watched that night. Eddie, Linus, and I squished together on their couch and ate popcorn and Skittles. Both of them rested their arms across the back of the couch above my head.

I gave my purple Skittles to Eddie because I think they are gross. After the movie, the three of us compared the color of our tongues in the bathroom mirror.

When it was finally time for bed, Linus went into his room while Eddie made up the hide-a-bed for him and me to sleep in.

"Where's your room?" I asked.

"I sleep in Linus's room, usually," he responded, sounding dejected.

"Like on bunk beds? I didn't know grown-ups slept on bunk beds."

"Only in the military, Kiddo."

"You don't have to sleep with me, that's weird. I'm not afraid of the dark anymore, Eddie."

"I know you're not. You're really brave. Don't worry about it. We'll sleep together here, and in the morning, I'll show you how to fix your hair so it's less poofy."

"Eddie, I can sleep on the floor. I don't want to sleep with a grown-up boy."

For the first time since the movie had ended, Eddie looked me straight in the eyes.

"You are one of the kindest people I know, Sarah. Your Mom is afraid you won't like it if I sleep in my bed in Linus's room. She thinks it will make you uncomfortable."

"Why would that be uncomfortable? If that's your bed, you should sleep in it."

Eddie's shoulders tremble a bit, and a tear forms in the corner of his eyes. He clears his throat and wipes it away really fast. I pretend not to see it.

"If only the world could see it as simply as you do, beautiful."

"Why do you want people to call you Dallas? That's not even a name. It's a big city in Texas, at least that's what Dad says."

A flash of anger crosses Eddie's face for an instant. He furrows his brow and huffs.

"Hard things happened to me when I was named Eddie. I wanted a new name to go with my new life."

"I'll call you Dallas if you sleep in your own bed," I say matter-of-factly.

"I promised your Mom I would sleep next to you to make sure no one hurt you or touched you wrong." He looks so sad.

"Lock the door then. No one is gonna do that here."

Dallas nodded. "How about I stay with you 'til you fall asleep?"

I shift uncomfortably. Mom and Dad said I'm not supposed to have a boy in my bed until I'm married unless it's my siblings, cousins, or friends for a sleepover. They never said anything about my uncle. I feel like I'm going to be in trouble no matter what Dallas and I do. I look up at him and see the pleading in his eyes.

"I won't tell Mom you slept in your bedroom with Linus, I'll call you Dallas from now on, and you can lock the door. If someone tries to touch me while I sleep, I'll scream really loud, and you and Linus can come beat up the bad guy."

Dallas looks at me for a long time.

"Sounds like a good plan to me. I love you, Sarah. Thank you for being you."

I didn't know what that meant, but Dallas tucked me in, kissed my forehead and said, "Sweet dreams, beautiful, beautiful girl."

"Goodnight Ed—I mean, Dallas. Blow a kiss to Linus and tell him it's from me."

"I will," Dallas says as he turns off the light.

The sound of Mom slamming the door pulls me out of my memories. The house is quiet for the first time all day. I rise from my bed slowly, listening just in case.

Nothing.

The fight must be over. I move carefully in my room, afraid of making too much noise. I don't want to be noticed. I reach under my desk and very slowly drag my backpack to my feet. I hold my breath and listen again.

Silence.

I grasp the zipper pull and cough as I tug it open. The blue bikini underwear Cassidy bought for me to wear under my bloomers is still there. I pull the blue cotton panties from their hiding place and examine them, expecting to figure out what the problem is. They look the same as my white panties, and I wore colored underwear when I was in grade school. How are these supposed to make boys or men get the wrong idea? What is the wrong idea?

I give up. Coach said we all had to have blue underwear to wear under our blue bloomers, and since Dad won't let Mom get me any, I'm grateful to Cassidy. I pull the tags off the panties and bury them in my dirty laundry basket.

Mom doesn't seem to mind that I need blue underwear, and Dad never does the laundry. If Mom asks about them, I'll just tell her they aren't mine and must have gotten mixed up in my stuff after a game or something.

I never heard my parents say a word about my blue underwear again, and I wore those same blue panties with my cheer uniform for the rest of high school.

AUTHOR'S NOTE

Saying my parents struggled to accept my uncle's sexual orientation is a gross understatement. Dallas's homosexuality changed all the normal rules for engagement in ways that were confusing to me then and infuriating for me now. My parents felt the need to go out of their way to make sure Dallas didn't contaminate their children with his gay-ness.

I wasn't allowed to go into a grown-up's room at all, so I never would have known that Dallas and Linus shared a bed. I had no concept of the mechanics of intercourse for either sexual orientation. My parents' fear that homosexuality was contagious led them to be okay with my sleeping in the same bed with my uncle, just to control his interactions with his partner.

This shift in rules due to some unidentified threat was a common occurrence in my childhood. Children need predictable structure in their lives with emotional connection from their caregivers. This acts like a framework that helps them navigate their physical and emotional world safely for healthy human development.[2] For me, the structure kept shifting with the wind, leaving me confused about which rule needed to be applied in any given situation.

---

2   Gottman, J. M., & DeClaire, J. (1997). *Raising an Emotionally Intelligent Child* (pp. 19-41). New York, N.Y., Simon & Schuster Paperbacks.

THE BIRDS AND THE BEES

WINTER 1994

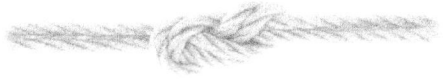

13 YEARS OLD

The warm wetness of my underwear feels strange. I don't think I peed my pants. I pull my pants down, and my white underwear is stained crimson. I even have blood stains on my favorite white pants. I scream, then gag and yank my underwear off. Hot tears slip from my eyes as I pull my pants back on and bolt from the bathroom, yelling and gasping for Mom.

Mom bursts from her bedroom door looking frantic. I show her my underwear.

"Calm down, Sarah," she says. "It's just your period. Your body is turning into a grown-up."

"So, now that I bled in my underwear, I'm a grown-up?"

"No, just that your body is preparing to be a mother." Mom shifts her weight to her other foot, then turns away and calls back to me over her shoulder. "Hang on."

She goes into her bathroom and comes out with a square thing wrapped in light-pink packaging.

"Here."

"What is this?"

"It's a pad. You unfold it and stick it in your underwear to catch the blood."

I frown. "Why do you have these?" I'm still not sure what's going on.

Mom looks incredulously at me. "For when I have my period."

"Oh, right," I say too quickly. I don't want to look stupid, so I grab the square and head back to my bathroom.

"Bring me your stained pants and underwear," Mom calls after me.

I drop the bloody underwear into the sink so that I can focus on the pad Mom gave me. I carefully remove it from the pink wrapping, peel off the paper on the top sticker and open the "wing." I stick it to the bathroom counter so I can peel my pants away from my wet thighs. When I peel the pad off the vanity, the wing tears off. I look down at my underwear in the sink, then to my pants in a tangled knot on the floor near the tub. This is gross. I flip over the pad and examine the longer sticker. I peel this one off as well.

Warmth trickles down my upper inner thigh. I scratch at it, and my fingertips come back covered in bright-red blood. It dawns on me that the pad is supposed to catch the blood, kind of like a big Band-Aid for my vagina, except the sticky side must go in the underwear.

I grab my underwear from the sink and put the long sticky side on the spot of blood, then turn the panties right side out and step into them. The remaining wing sticks to my leg. I unstick it, and pull my panties back into place, but the wing sticks to the crevice where my thigh and labia meet. I can feel it tugging on my curly fuzz.

Shit. Mom told me to bring her my stained underwear and pants. I pull my underwear back down and yank the pad out of it. Shit, shit, shit. I don't have clean clothes in here. I try to put the pad back in the underwear. The sticky strip is covered in white cotton fuzz and tiny blood streaks; it's not very sticky anymore.

I can't ask Mom for a new pad. She'll know I'm stupid. I put the not-so-sticky pad back in my underwear, pull the wing back out straight and pull my panties back up. At least the wing thing is still sort of sticky.

I crack open the bathroom door; no one is there so I sprint to my bedroom in my underpants, leaving the pants on the bathroom floor.

The pad feels sideways in my underwear. I tug at the crotch of my wet panties, trying to situate the thing so it stops pulling on my pubic hair. I give up on being comfortable in this thing and grab a dark pair of paint-stained sweatpants.

A sharp yipe echoes from the bathroom.

"Ewwww," Joey squeals. "What is this?"

I step out of the bedroom, warmth rising to my face.

"Shut up, Dog Breath!"

"Why are your pants all bloody?"

"I crashed my bike."

He glances over to the toilet. It's then I realize I forgot to flush.

67

"Why are you peeing blood?"

"I'm not peeing blood, stupid. I crashed my bike, and my leg is bleeding. Go away."

"Sarah's peeing blood, Sarah's peeing blood! Frizzy Head is peeing blood."

I want to punch his mouth to make him stop teasing me.

"Joey," Mom's warning voice calls from the kitchen. "Go outside before I find a chore for you to do."

Joey shuts up and sprints outside. Relieved, I go clean up the bathroom. As the pad shifts with my movement, a rush of shame consumes me. I feel like I'm being punished even though I didn't do anything. I flush the toilet, fold my white jeans to hide the scarlet stains and meet Mom in the laundry room. Gratefully, she doesn't notice I didn't give her my underwear.

She gets to work spraying 409 on the crotch of my pants.

"You probably don't want to wear white pants anymore."

"Like, ever again?"

"You're going to bleed for a few days once a month from now on," Mom clarifies, irritation at the edge of her voice.

"Wait, this isn't a one-time thing?"

"Of course not. Don't you know what a period is?"

"No. Why would I know that?"

"I told you about it when we lived in the yellow house, remember? We talked about how a girl gets pregnant?"

"Yes, you said the boy puts his sperm in a girl's belly so it can get to the egg and then a baby is born later."

Mom's startled expression makes me feel uncomfortable.

I was 11 the night Mom decided to explain the birds and the bees to me. She had given up on preventing me from masturbating once I had my own room, then she just quit coming into my room at night. If she didn't see it, it wasn't happening, which worked out well for me because I didn't get yelled at for it as often.

Then one night, Mom walked into my room holding one of the children's encyclopedias from our home library. I lowered my book and looked up at her when she sat down on my mattress. I folded the corner of the page I was on to make sure I didn't lose my spot.

"Sarah, do you know how a girl becomes pregnant?"

"Yes."

Her surprised expression scared me. I braced myself for the inevitable scolding.

"How do you know?" she asked.

"Well, I watched you get pregnant with Charlie. You lay on the couch with a heating pad on your back and your belly gets bigger while the baby cooks in there. But I haven't laid on your heating pad. I'm not pregnant, I promise."

Actually, I had laid on her heating pad. It was Joey who told me that's how Mom had gotten pregnant, and I quickly got off it because being pregnant before you are married is a sin, and Dad would get really, really mad, and Mom would cry a lot. I had used her heating pad for my Barbies, though.

Mom's face finally relaxed into a smile.

"No, Sarah. You can't get pregnant with a heating pad. I used the heating pad because your back can sometimes hurt when you are pregnant."

Mom was making me uncomfortable. I was afraid I'd get in trouble if I said the wrong thing.

"It's time to teach you about the birds and the bees."

"The what?"

"That's what we say when we mean having babies."

I ran my thumb along my book, wanting to get back to it. I knew better than to ignore her, though. I'd learned how to dance on the precarious tightrope between when to engage and when to vanish.

"Well, girls have an egg inside their stomach," Mom continued.

"Like a chicken?"

"Yes, but much smaller, so small you can't see it."

Mom opened up the encyclopedia about the body. I'd looked at the book many times before, but it was boring. Mom showed me a picture of a speck with a blurry red/brown background.

"This is what an egg looks like, and this," she paused as she flipped the page to show me another speck with a tail, "is the sperm."

"What's sperm?"

"That's what boys have."

"Where is their sperm at?"

"What?"

"You said the egg is inside the mommy's belly, so where is the sperm?"

"Oh, it's in their private parts."

"That's weird."

"Sarah, are you paying attention?"

I was now. Mom said it's not okay to talk about private parts unless they were sick and even then, only with a doctor. Our doctor, Dr. Kline, is Cassidy's dad, and I'm not about to discuss my private parts with him. Mom talking about private parts, especially a boy's private parts, is unfamiliar territory.

I nodded quickly and sucked on my upper lip to keep myself from asking too many questions. The sooner this is over, the sooner I can quit being uncomfortable and get back to reading my book.

"Well, the sperm gets into the girl's belly…" Mom's words come out slow, like she's thinking really hard about what she wants to say.

"How?"

Mom scowls and clenches her jaw. "Please, just listen."

I bit my bottom lip and stared at Mom's forehead. If I asked too many questions, she'd get mad at me and then I'd never find out how the sperm got into the girl's belly.

"The boy and the girl love each other a lot. They lay down in bed together and then the sperm goes into her belly. When the sperm and the egg meet in the girl's belly and…" She flipped the pages, until I was staring at a black-and-white photo with a white bean-looking thing in the middle, "…a baby starts to grow."

"That doesn't look like a baby."

"Not yet, but it will grow into a baby. Nine months later a baby will come out of the mommy's belly and that's how babies are born."

I felt a heavy dread grow inside me. I loved Joey, and we laid down by each other when we went camping. What if he got me pregnant?

"What if the girl doesn't want the sperm to get in her belly?"

"That's called rape."

"What if the boy doesn't want the girl to share her egg with him?"

"That's also called rape, but that doesn't happen. Anyway, it's time for you to go to sleep now. Goodnight, Sarah."

She snapped the encyclopedia closed and sprang up from my bed. I wasn't sure I understood everything, but she turned around sharply and swatted the bedroom light off as she walked out the door.

I replay the memory of that night once or twice, trying to remember her saying something about a period.

I come up blank.

Mom sighs loudly, which she does a lot when she doesn't feel like she has time, and Mom never has time. She drops my pants into the washing machine and pulls out the start switch. The lid closes with a loud thump.

She grabs my wrist and leads me into the kitchen where a calendar is hung on the corkboard next to our telephone.

"Today is day one of your period," she explains as she circles the date. "Twenty-eight days after your 'day one,' your period will start again and that will become your new day one." She counts down the four weeks and underlines the next date. "Does that make sense?"

I nod like I understand, but I don't.

"You need to keep track of the day your period starts. That's how you know whether or not you are pregnant. If you *don't* have a period, it means you're pregnant."

"Okay, can I have this calendar?"

"Sure," Mom says.

I take the calendar to my room, and I start circling dates. If today is day one, then... one, two, three, four, ...28 becomes the new day one. I plan out my periods and head back to the kitchen.

Mom is wiping up the peanut butter mess that one of the little kids abandoned after lunch. She looks up at me. "I thought you wanted to keep that calendar."

"No, I just wanted to make sure I don't miss any periods, see?" I point at the calendar and lift the pages. I have circled every fourth Saturday for the rest of the year.

"No, Sarah, that's not how this works. Sometimes you might start a day or two early or a day or two late. You don't start counting over until the first day of your next period."

"But if I miss it... I don't want to get pregnant."

Mom's exasperated voice turns angry. "Then don't have sex."

DEATH BY PERIOD

WINTER 1994

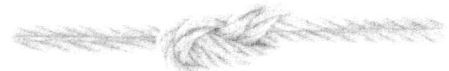

13 YEARS OLD

Several days passed before I ran out of the pads that Mom had given me. My abdomen is hurting so bad, I had asked to stay home from school almost every day. The answer is always no, but that doesn't stop me from asking again.

I need more pads, but Mom is too busy fulfilling her church callings. A calling is a job you don't get paid for; they claim it's volunteer, but it's more like voluntold. God inspires the bishop to offer you the job, and if you say no to the bishop, you're really saying no to God. Mom would never say no to God.

"Dave, I need you to take Sarah to Ed's and buy pads tonight," Mom says, drying her hands on the kitchen towel hanging from the oven door handle. "She went through all of my pads, and I don't have time to get more."

Dad sets the red pen on top of the stack of ungraded papers on the kitchen table in front of him.

"Are you sure you can't take her, Emma?"

"Yes, I'm sure, I have a scouting meeting tonight." The edge in her voice is unmistakable.

After dinner, Dad and I climb into his sky-blue 1966 Ford Pickup and drive the four blocks to Ed's.

He checks Mom's note and reads, "Pink and white package, size regular, Always." His voice trails off. He looks at me and asks, "You ready?"

I shrug, and we head into the store. I go past the cash registers and to the left, but Dad gets a shopping cart and walks toward the produce section.

I turn around and follow him. "Dad, you're going the wrong way."

He stops walking and just stares at the note. "I'm, uhhh, going to grab a few other things before we, uhhh, get your… supplies."

I'm not sure who is more uncomfortable with this arrangement.

"Are you okay?" I finally ask when he stops again.

"What? Oh, yeah, I'm fine. I just don't want to mess it up. Your Mom usually buys these things."

The front wheel of the shopping cart is squeaking like my hamster's exercise wheel and it keeps veering to the right, but he doesn't exchange it for a different one.

"Let's get some Pepsi while we are here."

Good Mormons quit drinking it because our prophet, Gordon B. Hinckley, told Mike Wallace from *60 Minutes* that faithful Mormons don't drink caffeinated soda.[3] Dad pretends like he didn't hear that message. He's good at reasoning his way out of church messages he doesn't want to obey. "It wasn't said over the pulpit during General Conference. Therefore, it was spoken by the man, not the prophet," he proclaims.

That's how I learned that prophets can say the wrong thing, unless they're speaking in General Conference, in which case it's gospel truth and directly from God. I figure God must be a pretty boring dude because the prophets and apostles always talk about the same stuff, twice a year, every year in General Conference. And it's the same things I've been taught in Primary and Young Women's every Sunday. As far as I can tell, the scripture stating God is the same yesterday, today, and tomorrow seems pretty legit.

"We probably need more milk," Dad says. "And go grab some bananas, Sarah."

Mom's "list" was only the packaging description for the pads, and she's in charge of grocery shopping, but I know better than to point that out. In the beverage section, Dad hefts a case of Pepsi into the cart. I trail after him to the candy aisle, and Dad grabs some Boston Baked Beans, another one of his favorite treats. We keep wandering and stop at beef jerky.

My lower abdomen has started to ache again, and the way Dad keeps shifting his weight from foot to foot and meandering around is putting me on edge.

When Dad gets uncomfortable, he starts calling me Frizz Ball or other mean names and then he'll slap me on the shoulder and say, "Just teasing."

I wish he would stop that kind of teasing.

Other times he rants about my clothes. "You are responsible to keep the men in line. You don't want them thinking about you in *that* way."

---

3   "60 Minutes." Episode. *"The Mormons"* 28, no. 30. New York, New York: CBS News, April 7, 1996.

Guys must be so weak when it comes to girls. Apparently, "guys can't help themselves."

The only time getting his attention doesn't feel bad is when we are competing. Dad and I are both competitive, so this is the one place where we still have common ground. I let my mind wander to the last time we competed.

"I bet I can read ten books before you can," Dad had taunted during the summer between seventh and eighth grade.

"What do I get if I win?" I asked.

He thought for a minute. "I'll do your dishes for one month."

Mom snorted in the background.

Dad ignored her. "And if you lose, you have to do them for a month."

I imagined one blissful month without being yelled at for doing the dishes wrong.

"You've got a deal." I leapt off the couch and headed for our small in-home library.

No one liked to do the dishes at our house. Mom wanted them done a certain way, and none of us could meet her expectations.

"Sarah, you never get the grease off," she complained as she tossed half the dishes I had just finished back into my soapy water. "And look at this," she extended a plate to me and pointed to a stained area. "There is still a gritty spot."

"I've already tried to get that off three times," I answer.

"No one in this house cares if we live like disgusting pigs. There are streaks on the bathroom mirrors, no one ever does the dishes right. I'm so sick and tired of the water spots on the bathroom faucets." Everything she'd been holding onto since her last meltdown comes blasting out.

In a way, I understood. The house on Fourth Street was the nicest we'd ever owned. When we moved in, Mom's temper intensified about keeping it that way; we could rarely clean to her expectations because her expectations were unreasonable.

Before we moved in, we had a massive cleaning session. We spent hours washing the disgusting boogers off the wall left by the children of the previous owners.

"I will not paint over snot," Mom demanded.

And so we scrubbed and scrubbed for days.

Once the boogers were gone to her satisfaction, I got paid two dollars to scrub the grout in the music room/library.

Mom oohed and aahed, she was so pleased she told me to do it again. Even doing a great job resulted in more work.

After my bet with Dad, I got busy reading. When we were allowed to watch television, I read books instead. I brought books on car rides, read books outside, and when I wanted to go hang out with my friends, I reminded myself that every time Dad was doing the dishes, he'd think about how smart his daughter is and smile. I finished my 10 books in two weeks. Dad lost the bet. Mom ended up doing the dishes for a month.

Losing that bet didn't deter him. One night at dinner, I declared, "I'm the fastest runner in P.E., but I hate it. I think I'll stick with cheer. Cassidy can do cross-country by herself."

I could see from the smirk that spread across Dad's face that he saw an easy bet. Mom saw it, too. She put her fork down and looked at Dad with anticipation.

"I bet I can run a mile faster than you," Dad said. "I'll even give you a head start."

Joey, Ev, and Charlie stopped eating, too. They all watched Mom.

"What do I get if I beat you?" I asked.

"I'll do the dishes for you for one month. And if I win, you'll do them."

Mom's nostrils flare. "No, Dave, I am not going to do dishes for a month again."

"Emma," Dad said, "she's never going to beat me. I referee football and basketball. I'm in excellent shape."

"You better win." Mom stood up from the table abruptly and slammed her plate on the counter, making Charlie jump.

Dad gave me a 25-yard head start that weekend on the junior high's running track. He blew his whistle, and we ran.

There was no way I was going to let him win. Ever since I stopped wrestling with Joey, Dad acted like I just couldn't handle a physical challenge. I was going to prove to him that this *girl* was still strong and fast. I started off at a sprint and put half a lap between us before I slowed into my pace. I glanced over my shoulder every few steps to make sure he didn't catch up. I could do anything to get out of dishes for another month.

After Dad's second lap, he slowed to a walk and inhaled a puff from his inhaler. I was determined not to give him a reason to gloat, but I needed a break, too, so I slowed to a walk. As soon as he started running again, I started running. We continued in this way, with my finishing a half a lap ahead of Dad. Later that evening Joey talked back to Mom, and Joey got grounded to the dishes for a month.

The squeaking wheel of the shopping cart pulls me from my memory. It feels like we've visited every aisle in the entire grocery store, except for the feminine hygiene one.

"Do you need a new hairbrush?" Dad asks.

"No," I say.

"Well, I guess there's only one more thing we need." He clears his throat, and we walk to the feminine hygiene products.

A young female employee is stocking shelves. Dad's demeanor changes.

"Oh, look what we have here," he says, making eye contact with her. "My daughter is all grown up. She's a woman now."

My face burns hot. I elbow Dad. "Shh, that's not funny."

Dad seems not to have heard me. Or he's ignoring me. "Yup, just a dad with his daughter buying a catcher's mitt for her womanhood."

I start to chew on my lower lip. My right knee starts bouncing up and down to some internal beat that paces itself based on my moods.

"Ma'am, she's just a young thing, can you help us find the regular size?" Dad asks. "She's not grown up enough yet for heavy." He thrusts Mom's note at her. She reads it, then hands it back to him.

"Sure," the young girl says. She glances at me out of the corner of her eye, pity etched on her face.

I look up as though the store's ceiling is the most fascinating thing in the world and hum the Christmas music from last semester's band concert, even though Christmas is long over.

"Thanks, young lady," Dad says and smiles. "I'm sure you wish you had a dad who would buy your girly stuff for you, don't ya'?"

Her eyebrows hit her hairline as her head tilts forward. "Yes sir," she says politely and turns her back to us.

"I wonder what got her so upset?" Dad says.

Is he really that oblivious? I grab the cart and make a beeline for the checkout. Ignoring Dad usually makes his taunting end faster.

I begin to unload the groceries, slamming the Pepsi and other items harder than necessary, causing the conveyor belt to quake.

"Did you find everything okay?" the cashier asks in a robotic, uninterested tone.

"Yes ma'am, we did. I got me some snacks and this," he says loudly, handing the package of pads to her. "This is the treat I got for my daughter who passed into womanhood recently."

I cover my face with both hands and mindlessly kick at the loose wheel on the shopping cart.

She stops scanning and looks down at me. "Are you okay, sweetheart?"

I nod and wipe away the tear that escapes my eye.

"I'm just a dad doing all the fatherly stuff," Dad continues in his hero voice.

The cashier purses her lips and picks up the pace.

I fight the urge to bolt from the store.

Dad shoots the cashier a knowing grin as he counts out the cash to pay for our things. I refuse to make eye contact until we are out the door.

"That wasn't too bad now, was it?" Dad asks as he takes the bags and milk from me and loads them into his truck. "Good thing we drove the truck. I wasn't planning on buying all this stuff."

When we arrive home, I grab clean underwear from my room and head straight to the bathroom.

The pad that Mom gave me earlier has somehow escaped my underwear and slid down my leg. Blood stains my sweatpants, but it's hard to see against the dark fabric, so hopefully no one at the store noticed.

I sit on the toilet, and the cold rim of the seat sends goosebumps down my naked legs. This day sucks. I blink away tears. The package of pads has pictures on the back demonstrating how to apply it. Finally, I know how to do it correctly.

My first cycle only lasted a few days. Joey made a huge fuss about the remnant bloody spots in the toilet bowl that first cycle, which I got in trouble for. Apparently, I'm going to bleed every month, and Joey isn't allowed to know about it, which means there can't be any evidence of my period in the bathroom that Joey and I share.

It doesn't take long for me to question Mom's wisdom regarding periods, because two weeks later my period starts again. I do my best to keep it contained, but there is blood everywhere. The toilet looks like I've beheaded a small animal.

"Mom, my period started again, and it's a lot of blood," I say. "I'm going to need more pads."

"That's really early, are you sure? Sometimes you might have a little brownish discharge, but your period won't start again for at least two more weeks," Mom assures me.

"Well, I don't know what's wrong with me, because I'm bleeding again. I only have two pads left." I brace myself for the lecture.

"It's not *blood*, Sarah, it's just a little discharge and you don't need to keep going through pads for that. They aren't free, and I'm not paying for you to use pads when you don't need to."

I bring her my bloodstained sheets to prove I'm not lying, and she examines the fresh stains.

"Sometimes it takes the body a bit to figure things out," she concedes.

"Please don't make me go buy pads with Dad this time," I beg.

"I'm sorry about your Dad. He makes jokes when he's nervous."

She hands me another package of pads after dinner that evening. The next morning, I bring her my bloodstained sheets again.

"I don't feel well. I feel really dizzy, and my stomach hurts," I complain.

"You have to go to school, Sarah," Mom says. "You can't be absent every time you are on your period. It's only a few days."

I drag myself to the bus stop. I rest my head on my desk during homeroom.

"What's up?" Cassidy asks as she slides into the desk behind me.

"I'm on my period."

"Didn't you just finish your period like last week?"

"Yes, but Mom says sometimes it takes a couple of months for the body to figure things out."

"I'll have to ask my dad about that," Cassidy says. He *is* a doctor, so he'll probably know what's wrong. Not that I'm thrilled with the idea of her talking to him, but I'm too worn out to argue.

By lunch I have to call my Mom.

"I bled through my pants."

Mom brings me new pants. I call her again before cheer because I bled through those pants. She comes back to the school and gives me a package of pads marked "heavy" in the lower corner.

The next morning, I bring her my sheets again.

"Sarah, you must be using the pads wrong."

She follows me to the bathroom, and I show her the pad on my underwear.

"Well, you're doing that right," Mom says. "Use the heavy pads and bring extra clothing to school today."

I excuse myself several times during classes to change my pad.

The following day, I ignore the bloodstained sheets and figure I'll just wait to have them washed until the bleeding stops.

I feel awful. I'm too nauseous to eat breakfast, and I'm light-headed every time I stand.

I fall asleep on the bus that morning. Another student shakes me awake when we arrive at the junior high.

"Thanks," I manage to mutter. I stand and grab the back of the seat in front of me in order to stop myself from falling backward. It takes a moment to steady myself. The wave of dizziness dissipates, and I trudge slowly down the aisle.

By noon, the nurse calls me to her office.

"Sarah, we've called your Mom. She wants us to talk to you about using the restroom to tend to your feminine needs between classes. Your teachers have let me know you are excusing yourself in the middle of instruction time."

"I am changing my pad between classes, too." I'm too tired and dizzy to be embarrassed. "If I wait the entire class period, I'll bleed through."

The school nurse looks doubtful. My tendency to exaggerate hasn't escaped her.

"I swear," I say. "I'm bleeding so much. I'm changing my pad every 30 minutes, and it's still getting on my underwear. I'm afraid I'm going to bleed through onto the chair."

The nurse takes my temperature and sends me back to class.

The next day, I'm assigned detention for leaving class too often.

The day after that, I run out of pads.

"Mom, I need more pads again."

She startles at the sound of my voice. She's making dinner, and I can tell I've interrupted her thoughts.

"No, Sarah. You do not need more pads. You aren't letting them get full enough before you change them." Her tone rises as she pounds the wooden spoon against the side of the pot. Bits of potato slide back into the soup she has been stirring.

"I don't have any left, Mom."

She sets the spoon down and turns to face me. Her lips are pursed and she's tapping her toe. I can tell she's trying not to yell. I take a step back.

"There are forty-two in each package. I bought you two packages. How have you gone through eighty-four pads in less than five days?"

Tears slide down my cheeks. "I don't know, I change them when the blood gets on my panties."

"Bring me your underwear, right now."

I stumble on my way out of the kitchen. My legs wobble beneath me, like I'm going to collapse at any moment.

"Stop being so dramatic," Mom yells.

I dig through my dirty laundry basket, separating all of my blood-stained pants and underwear from the rest of my clothing. I grab the pile of stained jeans and underwear and head to the laundry room. Mom meets me there and rips the pile from my hands. She tears at my clothes frantically, turning my pants inside out and scrubbing the crotch points with an old toothbrush.

"You need to pretreat these pants or they'll stain permanently."

I lean against the door frame for support. She continues her furious scrubbing.

When she gets to the third pair, she stops. She picks up a pair of my underwear that has fallen to the floor, then another one.

"This is a lot of blood. I'll call the doctor tomorrow."

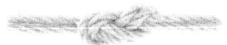

Mom forgets to call Dr. Kline the next morning, which isn't surprising. My parents almost never take us to the doctor. They can't afford the copay.

Month after month, the bleeding lasts anywhere from three to six weeks with only a short break between cycles. I stop tracking my period on the calendar. Mom buys tampons for me, saying it should stop me from bleeding through my pants at school. The tampons with the pads buy me a little more time between bathroom trips, which keeps me out of detention for the frequent bathroom breaks. I still have to change my tampon and pad between every class and halfway through cheer practice.

Dad says I'm making things up. He and Mom keep fighting about whether or not it's time to take me to the doctor. I try to function through the constant haze, but staying awake gets harder and harder.

I spend the summer before high school watching the 1985–1987 version of *Anne of Green Gables* and *Anne of Avonlea* on repeat. I barely spend any time with my friends. It's getting hard to go anywhere too far from a toilet, and frankly, I'd rather not leave a bloody mess in anyone else's bathroom, or worse, on their furniture.

I struggle to stay upright in marching band camp during the two weeks before the start of highschool. I have to put my head between my knees to fight the light-headedness when we play too long.

About a month into my freshman year, Mom pounds on my bedroom door.

"Sarah, I've called you four times! You are going to be late for school."

I hear her, but it feels like a dream. I can't seem to open my eyes. My arms and legs feel like lead. I don't have the strength to lift them off my bed.

Mom opens my bedroom door and shakes my shoulder. I groan, but don't move.

"Are you sick?" In my semi-conscious state, I feel her press the back of her hand against my forehead. "You don't have a fever. Come on Sarah, Zoe will be here any minute. You need to get up."

Zoe is my new best friend. She plays the clarinet. We met during marching band camp, and we connected in a way I never had before. Zoe is 16 and has her own car. She picks me up every day for early morning band practice.

Mom rips my comforter and sheets back trying to rouse me.

"Sarah, oh goodness, that's a lot of blood. Sarah, wake up!" her voice desperate.

Her tone alarms me. I open my eyes and struggle to focus on her.

"Did you forget to wear a pad last night?"

I shake my head. Then fall back to sleep.

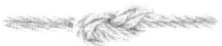

Yelling wakes me from a deep sleep. I think I've slept all day. I feel the pangs of hunger crawl up my stomach. A wave of cramps matches the growling of my stomach, and nausea sweeps over me. I clamp my mouth shut and breathe slowly through my nose.

"No, Emma! She does not need to see the doctor!"

"Dave, she's bleeding for weeks on end. She couldn't wake up this morning. She was sleeping in a pool of blood. She's always pale and tired. This isn't normal."

"No, she's making it up, Emma, just like she makes everything else up."

I hear her slam the dishes into the sink.

"Well, I wonder where she learned that from, Dave?"

Mom's never stuck up for me before. I brace myself for the worst, but he just says, "Emma, you are going to check *every* pad before she throws it away to make sure she really *is* bleeding. We can't afford to keep buying her all these pads."

"Fine, Dave."

For the next three weeks I bring my soiled pad to Mom for her inspection and then go bury it underneath clean toilet paper in the trash bin so Joey won't see it. When Dad accuses me of bringing her the same full pad every time, Mom starts taking them away from me to dispose of them herself. When I pass a fist-sized bloody clump, I bring it to her, sitting on top of a pad like a gelatinous, shiny mound. Mom gags and drops the pad on the floor. Her face is pale, her jaw trembling.

She washes her hands in the sink, then picks up the phone and calls Dr. Kline's office.

PELVIC EXAM

FALL 1995

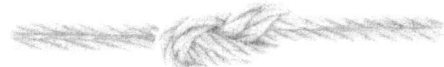

14 YEARS OLD

Mom taps her foot nervously on the linoleum floor in Dr. Kline's exam room. The nurse removes the blood pressure cuff from my arm.

"She's a little low, probably just dehydrated." The nurse sticks the thermometer in my mouth. "No fever."

"She's been having really heavy periods," Mom says, the concern in her voice is unfamiliar to me. "And they last for a few weeks at a time."

"How many days?" the nurse asks.

Mom looks at me.

I shrug. I've lost count.

"Over three weeks." Mom's voice trembles a bit.

"How long has this been going on?"

"Since her first period, over a year ago."

"And you're just bringing her in now?" Judgment seeps from the nurse's voice.

Mom shrinks in her chair. "Well, at first, Dave thought she was faking it. It's been getting a lot worse, though. I've been scrubbing the blood stains out of her pants and sheets for months. Then yesterday, she passed a huge clot."

The nurse huffs and shakes her head as she writes stuff down.

"The doctor needs to do an exam. Have you talked to her about it?"

I'm watching this exchange with curiosity, unable to decipher their code.

"She's only fourteen. I didn't have my first one until after I was pregnant with her." Mom's words tumble out of her mouth like she's trying to win a race.

"Emma, the doctor needs to make sure she only has one uterus. He needs to make sure he doesn't feel anything growing that shouldn't be there. He's going to need to do an exam. It's better if you tell her, but I will if you can't."

Mom deflates. "Okay, give me a few minutes."

When the nurse closes the door behind her, Mom looks up at me from her chair. The paper under my butt crinkles as I shift to focus on what my Mom is about to tell me.

"Sarah, you're bleeding too much so the doctor has to take a quick peek at your vagina in order to make sure it looks normal, okay?"

Silently I scream to myself no, it's not okay! Cassidy is going to know that her dad looked at my private parts.

"Why can't the nurse do it?"

"Because only the doctor knows what he is looking for."

"What is he looking for?"

"I don't know, Sarah. All women have to do it. Usually not until after they are married, but it's okay because I'm here."

It doesn't feel okay. I picture Dr. Kline, sitting down to dinner with his family, telling them about his day, just like my Dad does. Unlike my hearing about some kid farting during Dad's presentation, Dr. Kline will be telling Cassidy about looking at my messed-up vagina. And who knows what Cassidy will say at school. In our small Mormon community, gossip tends to make big whoppers out of even small stories. It'll be months before people find something bigger to whisper about.

Mom hands me a paper sheet and tells me to take off my pants and underwear. It's awful enough that Dr. Kline is going to look down there, but I'm going to be sitting in a mess.

"I'm going to bleed on the exam table."

"Just do it, Sarah."

I can tell from her tone that I don't have a choice. She doesn't care if I'm gross, sitting in a mess, as long as I don't embarrass her. With trembling hands, I remove my pants, fold my wet pad and underwear in on itself and tuck them inside the pants so no one will see all the blood. I can already feel the wet stickiness escaping when Mom helps me climb back onto the table and tucks the paper sheet under my hips. I can feel the warm liquid seeping out under me.

We stay in silence as we wait for the doctor to return. I hoped that maybe he would get lost and never come back, but a few minutes later Dr. Kline knocks softly before he opens the door. "Good morning, ladies." His voice is gentle.

My stomach knots and the jumping frogs return with a vengeance. I sit up tall on the table and avoid eye contact.

Dr. Kline rolls his stool over to me as his nurse wheels the tray over. His voice is very direct. "Emma, did you tell Sarah what we need to do today?"

Mom nods.

He pulls a hidden metal arm from each side of the table. I stare at them. "Sarah, do you have any questions?"

I have a million questions, but the words don't come. I shake my head.

As he instructs me on what to do, I feel like I am floating. The image of a horse's saddle comes to mind, the metal arm doesn't look like a stirrup. I look over at Mom, whose face is blank and pale as I follow his instructions, and she nods.

Dr. Kline turns his back to me as he washes his hands and puts on rubber gloves.

"Slide your bottom down to the end of the table, Sarah," his nurse instructs. The wet paper is stuck to my butt and tears as I slide my body forward. "Slide down just a bit more."

A cool rush of air hits my vagina as the nurse peels the stuck paper away. Mom grabs the paper sheet and pulls it over my knees so no one can see, which seems weird since everyone I don't want to see is standing on the exposed side. I'm freezing, but I'm sweating like I've been running.

"Squeeze my hand if it hurts," Mom whispers in my ear.

Hurt? What does she mean?

"Okay, Sarah, you are going to feel my fingers tap down your leg, then I'm going to spread your vagina open and insert the speculum," Dr. Kline says.

What the hell is a speculum, and why the fuck is he touching my leg?

I freeze when gloved fingers tap my knee. This isn't just a quick look, and Mom isn't doing anything to stop him.

My heart is pounding so hard I'm sure they can hear it.

His gloved fingers touch my vagina. I close my eyes and start to cry. I press my heels into the stirrup holes, but I'm pasted in place as Mom's words comes to my mind. *A person isn't a virgin anymore once someone touches their vagina underneath their underwear.* Why is she letting him touch me? Why doesn't she make him stop? I try to move away to get his hand off of me.

"Try to hold still," a voice says.

Mom isn't helping me. I want to disappear. If I can just disappear, then it will be like this isn't happening.

A searing pain splits my body in half. I scream and kick my leg out. My foot makes contact with something soft and hairy. I hear the metal tray clatter to the floor. Maybe now that everything is dirty, he'll stop.

"Jodi, I think my nose is bleeding."

I feel the vinyl peel away from my hips as I scoot my butt away from Dr. Kline and sit up.

Blood drips down Dr. Kline's handlebar mustache. His nurse grabs a tissue and pinches his nose.

"Emma, did you explain to her what the exam would entail?" he asks.

I look over at Mom, whose face is redder than her hair.

"I didn't know you were going to do a full pelvic, I... I... I didn't know what to tell her."

"How about the truth?" he growls.

Jodi finishes wiping his face. She slips a plastic duckbill-looking thing from its package and hands it to the doctor. She moves quickly, replacing small foil pouches and long Q-tips on a new metal tray.

"Sarah, I need to access your cervix," Dr. Kline says, looking directly at me. "I'm going to put this speculum into your vaginal canal so that I can open it up to get a good look and make sure your cervix looks okay. Then I'm going to gather a sample using a really long Q-tip. You need to hold still so it doesn't hurt as much."

Tears trickle down my cheeks. Mom pushes against my chest signaling that I need to lay back down. Jodi puts my feet back into the stirrups and has me slide my hips back in place. It feels like I'm about to drop off the end of the table. Mom holds my shoulders down so I can't sit up again. Jodi has hold of one of my knees.

"Take a deep breath, Sarah. Try to relax." I can't tell who is talking to me.

Something inside of me burns and tears. I can hear my body rip open. I let out a small cry as the fire reaches past my breasts and into my throat.

I'm not a virgin anymore. No one will love me.

"I'm pulling the speculum out now. Are you okay?"

I don't move.

"She's okay," Mom says.

I'm not okay.

"I'm going to start the exam now."

I stiffen as Dr. Kline twists two fingers inside of me. This is worse than the speculum. It doesn't hurt as bad, but Cassidy's dad is touching the inside of me. He pushes on my belly. The cramping in my lower abdomen explodes.

When he is done, he says, "Everything looks and feels normal, Emma. There's no anatomical cause of her menorrhagia. I'm going to prescribe birth control to help regulate her menstrual cycle. She needs to take two Flintstone vitamins with iron once a day for the anemia until her periods are more regular."

He peels the blood-smeared latex gloves off and washes his hands with soap and water. He leans into the mirror, then wipes the rest of his blood off his nose with a wet paper towel.

"Do you have any questions for me?" He scratches something out on a little white pad then looks to my Mom, who is not saying anything, then to me.

Mom chokes out, "Dave won't like her taking birth control."

I don't move. I'm not really in the room anymore. I'm floating somewhere above myself.

I look out the window and what did I see... The Primary song echoes from somewhere in my brain. I blink.

Popcorn popping on the apricot tree!

Hot tears slip out of my eyes. I blink again.

Spring has brought me such a nice surprise…

Blink.

Blossoms popping right before my eyes.

"Sarah," Mom touches my shoulder. I turn but don't really see her. "Are you okay?"

I can take an armful and make a treat.

Blink.

A popcorn ball that would smell so sweet.

Blink.

"Sarah, here. Use this to clean yourself up and then put your clothes back on. Look, they left you a new pad."

It wasn't really so…

Blink.

But it seemed to me.

Blink.

Popcorn popping on the apricot tree.[4]

My stomach contracts, and I barely have time to say "throw up" before vomit spills from my mouth and splatters on the floor next to Mom. She jumps back. I retch again and again, until there is nothing left in me.

Nothing.

---

4   Georgia W. Bello, "Popcorn Popping on the Apricot Tree" Magna, Utah, 1957

I need to run, but I'm stuck in the van. Mom pulls into the high school parking lot after my doctor's appointment. Students are walking around the last few minutes before the end of lunch hour. I feel the need to hit something but can't seem to move.

"Are you going to be okay?" Mom is acting like I can go from no longer being a virgin and slip right back into my classes at school like nothing even happened.

I glare at her. She let it happen. She just gives me a blank expression and waits for me to get out. We stay that way for at least 30 seconds before I relent and push the van door open and climb out. My feet crunch across the asphalt. I'm on a mission to find a place to hide.

People bump into me in the hall. I clench and unclench my fists, fingernails digging into the palms of my hands. I really need to hit something.

"Hey, Sarah," Cassidy calls out from across the hall. She pushes her way toward my locker. "Where were you this morning? You totally missed it. Brent started—"

"Shut the fuck up, you slutty bitch!" Spittle splatters her face as I scream at her. "I don't ever want to see your ugly face again. Go to fucking hell."

I punch my locker. My knuckles crack and hot blood drips down my fingers.

Cassidy just stands there, frozen, looking at me.

I shove her.

"Get the fuck away from me, stupid ass bitch!"

She bursts into tears and runs past me.

The knot in my stomach loosens. I head for the Fine Arts hallway, where the bathrooms aren't monitored. I sink into the corner stall, pull my knees to my chest and cry. My cramps intensify as my body convulses from the tears. I shift on the floor trying to avoid the burning between my legs. I stay there the rest of the school day. When the final bell rings, I walk out to Zoe's car.

"Sarah! You look awful, are you okay? Why did you yell at Cassidy?"

"Hey, Zoe, can you just take me home?"

"What about cheer practice?"

"I can't. I don't…"

Zoe squints at me. "Do you need to talk?"

"No, I just want to go home."

"Okay, you probably need to apologize to Cassidy. She said you called her a slut."

I slide into the passenger seat of her Dodge Colt and stare at a dirty speck on the side window and tune her out. Zoe gives up trying to get me to tell her what happened. My house is only a few blocks from the high school. I open the door of the car and begin to climb out. I feel a tug at the back of my shirt. I swing around hard and jump away, my heart racing. I feel trapped.

"What the hell are you doing?" I screech at Zoe.

She pulls her hand away quickly.

"Geez, sorry, Sarah. You seriously need to chill. I don't know what is up with you today, but you need to pull yourself together before you lose all your friends."

None of that matters now.

AUTHOR'S NOTE

This chapter was hard to relive as I wrote it. I was never "raped" in the criminal sense. As a clinician, I've heard multiple stories of women and girls being held down for a gynecological exam and have seen that the effects of this type of exam on long-term mental health are similar to those of criminal rape.

At the time of the exam, I knew very little about the mechanics of sex. I had been told that a girl is no longer a virgin as soon as a man touches her on her naked vagina. I also knew that my mother hated sex. In my young mind, I understood why she hated it if it was anything like that pelvic exam.

I am deeply grateful that informed consent and gentle exams are the new standard of care. Dr. Kline trusted my Mom to inform me of what was about to happen, which wasn't uncommon in the '90s. Knowledge of experiences like mine, combined with a better understanding of mental health, has changed the landscape so this type of medical trauma occurs less often. The men and women (especially the women) who advocated for this change are unsung heroes. I find comfort knowing that because of them, my daughters will never have this type of experience in the name of health care.

BIRTH CONTROL

FALL 1995

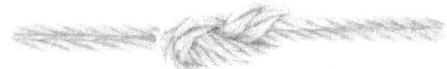

14 YEARS OLD

I slam Zoe's car door, then the front door as I enter my house. I listen intently for a few moments and hear nothing. The house is unusually quiet. No one appears to be home.

Good.

I storm into my bedroom and slam that door, too, before throwing my backpack at the wall. A bloodcurdling scream rips from my throat. I punch the walls and kick my desk chair.

I crumble to my hands and knees. It feels like I'm being smothered.

I am dirty.

I am exposed.

I am small.

My Mom held me down and let that happen to me. She didn't protect me. How could she do that? Aren't moms supposed to protect you? I trusted her.

I roll to my side, waiting for the tears that refuse to come.

I can't trust her. Ever again.

She always told me that protecting my virginity was of the upmost importance and yet she allowed the doctor to just take it. Now I'm a chewed-up piece of gum that no man will ever want to marry, just like they taught me in Young Women's.

I pull myself up, grab an old T-shirt and my "period sweatpants," and stomp into the bathroom. I turn the knob in the bathtub and yank on the shower pull. The plumbing sputters to life. I thrust my hand into the water, shifting from foot to foot, waiting for it to turn hot. With my other hand, I scratch at my crawling skin.

Steam finally billows above the shower curtain. The seam in my shirt tears as I yank it off, and I bump into the sink. In a tangle of pants, I stumble and accidentally pull one side of the towel rack from the wall. I yank it the rest of the way out, towels and all, and throw it against the bathtub's outside wall.

"Fuck you!" I screech.

I step over the pile of clothing and towels into the shower and let the hot water burn the filth off my skin. I pull the shower curtain closed and punch the tiled wall over and over.

"Fuck. Fuck. Fuck."

The cream tile turns pink as the cuts on my knuckles open back up.

I kick the drain lever, tearing the toenail away from my big toe. The pain feels good.

I scrub furiously between my legs, raking the goo from Dr. Kline's gloved fingers out of me. The water at my feet darkens as the period blood mixes with the toe blood. I gag on the metallic smell. The bloody water escapes down the drain.

My vision darkens.

I reach out, grasping for anything.

"Sarah," Mom's voice echoes from far away. "Sarah?"

My cheek explodes, and I open my eyes, finding myself on the floor of the bathtub. Did Mom just slap me? I stare up at the ceiling. It takes a few seconds before I realize I'm naked. I'm hot and wet, but the water isn't on. I don't remember why I'm in the bathroom.

"I think you passed out, Sarah. Sit up slowly."

I wipe at my throbbing forehead with my fingertips and examine my hand, expecting to see blood, but the wet is from the shower. Mom throws a towel over my naked body, then slides her icy hand under my shoulder blades, making me flinch.

She extends her other hand in front of me to hold onto for support.

"Your shower water was way too hot. Your skin looks burned. Go slow, sweetheart."

The walls bend inward as Mom pulls me into a sitting position. I pull my feet close to my bottom and rest my aching forehead on my knees. My limbs are trembling.

Mom grabs another bath towel and dries my skin.

"We should have taken you to the doctor weeks ago. You've lost so much blood. I picked up your medicine at the pharmacy."

I pull my forehead off my knees and squint at Mom. She has gathered the bottom of my T-shirt up to the neck hole and holds it out for me the way she used to when I was little. She pulls the shirt over my head and feeds my arm through the sleeve.

"I can do it," I mumble when she reaches for my other hand.

With my shirt pulled down, Mom places her hand between my shoulder blades again. I grab the side of the tub and the washcloth bar and pull myself up slowly. Mom holds me steady. I wait for the wave of dizziness to subside, carefully step out of the tub, and sit down hard on the toilet.

"Don't worry about the towel rack," Mom says as she digs under the sink. She opens the old tampon box that hides my stained but clean underwear. "Good idea, Sarah, keeping extra underwear in here." She reaches deeper into the cupboard and pulls a pad from its plastic casing. She affixes it to the crotch of my stained underwear before squatting in front of me.

I lift one foot at a time, and she guides them into place before pulling my underwear up to my knees. She continues to dress me, moving with slow intent, ensuring I don't fall again. Then she wraps her arms around my back and pulls me into a standing position so I can pull my pants over my hips.

I place one arm around her shoulder. We shuffle carefully into my bedroom. Mom helps me into my bed, then pulls the covers over me. She hasn't been this gentle with me in years.

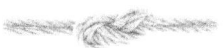

Something heavy is on my chest, pinning me down. I try to shove it off, but it won't budge. My legs are butterflied open; my ankles feel tied to something. I'm suffocating.

Dr. Kline's laughing face hovers inches above mine. "I ruined you. Now you belong to me."

I scream myself awake. The early morning light peeks around the curtains in my bedroom. I'm hyperventilating and my face is tingling; my body won't calm down. I hurt everywhere. My hand grazes a lump above my right eyebrow. Why am I so sore?

Memories of the previous day flood in. I clasp my hands over my open mouth; hot tears pour over my fingers.

I can't go to school today. I can't leave my bedroom. People will know I'm dirty and used.

I hear Mom's quiet knock. "Sarah, are you okay?" She cracks the door open. "May I come in?"

"I can't go to school today," I sob. "Everyone is going to know what Dr. Kline did."

"Don't be silly, Sarah. He's not going to tell anyone." She flips the light on, and I reach up to shield my eyes, wincing when my hand brushes the lump over my eye.

"Mom, please," I beg. "Don't make me go to school."

Her gentle concern fades. She huffs with her hands on her hips, her left foot tapping the carpet beneath in quick rhythmic motions. "You need to go to school. Besides, you can't miss cheer practice again. There's a game tomorrow."

"Please, Mom, can you just homeschool me? Karen is homeschooled, and she's really smart."

"You're being dramatic. Get up and eat something. You'll feel better."

How can she brush off something this serious?

Mom lifts my comforter and sheets away from my body and heaves a resigned sigh at the sight of blood. "Get dressed. I'm going to get these sheets and your soiled clothes in the washer before your siblings wake up."

I stand up slowly, fighting the familiar dizziness.

Mom strips my bed sheets. The permanent brown stain on my mattress is crimson again from the fresh blood.

"You have five minutes to be at the table for breakfast. Bring me your soiled clothes when you've finished getting dressed."

She closes my bedroom door behind her. The latch doesn't catch. I push the door closed again and lift the knob until I hear the click.

It takes a lot for me to get dressed. It's hard for me to move. I meet Mom in the hallway and hand the soiled clothing off to her, fighting the familiar dizzy spell, and cross the hall into the kitchen. I need water. My hand trembles as I fill the glass. I chug the water, then put both hands on the sink's edges to steady myself. The water sloshes in my stomach, making me feel nauseous. I fight back a gag. I'm starving but don't want to eat anything. My stomach churns in protest at the smell of pancakes and bacon.

Mom hands me a small envelope. I open it and squint at the small pills encased in the foil package.

"Take one every morning to stop the bleeding."

Even though I'm 14, I still can't swallow pills whole. I can't even get through a dental exam without gagging and choking. I push the pill out of the foil and slip it under my tongue to let it dissolve. It's disgusting. I drink more water to stop myself from retching.

"Sarah, you're white as a ghost," Mom says. "Sit back down and eat. I'll finish setting the table."

I slide back into my chair just as Dad joins me at the table. "Wow, Sarah, looks like you hit your head hard last night. Just tell everyone you got jumped by a biker gang."

"Dave," Mom's voice warns. "Not this morning."

She slides the envelope of birth control pills under the towel on the counter as my friend Zoe joins us for breakfast.

The moment she sees me she asks, "What happened to you?"

"She fell in the shower and knocked herself out," Mom answers before Dad can tell one of his whoppers.

"Ouch. I hope you are feeling better than yesterday," Zoe says. "I was on the phone with Cassidy for hours last night. She's willing to talk to you this morning, but we have to leave early." I shoot Zoe a panicked, wide-eyed warning look.

"What's up with Cassidy?" Mom asks.

I shrug. "No idea."

"She just had a rough day yesterday. Sarah and I are going to try to talk to her today to help her feel better," Zoe covers.

Shame consumes me as I think about the shock and sadness on Cassidy's face.

"What did Cassidy say?" I ask Zoe once we are safely inside her Dodge Colt.

"That you yelled at her, and she didn't know why. She said her mom and dad told her you hadn't been feeling well and to give you a second chance. You were obviously having a bad day. You never yell at anyone… except Joey."

"I didn't yell at her," I lie again. I can trust Zoe with almost everything, but I'm too ashamed to be honest about this.

"What else did Cassidy's dad tell her about me?" I ask.

Zoe raises an eyebrow. "Nothing that I know of."

I shrug again. "I've been bleeding so much, I passed out in the shower last night. I don't remember much of anything that happened yesterday."

Another lie.

"Mom won't let me stay home. She says I'm not sick. Lees only stay home when we are dying."

"Bleeding to death doesn't count as 'dying?'" Zoe huffs. "It's crazy."

I rest my head against the passenger window.

Zoe glances over at me as she slows to a four-way stop.

"Zoe, can you tell her I passed out and don't remember yelling at her," I plead.

At school I'm hyperalert listening to all the conversations around me, waiting for the first sign that someone knows what Dr. Kline did.

No one knows. Maybe I am safe.

When I get home that day, Mom hands me my envelope of birth control pills and a large bottle of Flintstones vitamins. "Keep these in your bedroom," she instructs. "Take them right before you come to the table for breakfast every morning."

"Okay."

The next morning, I chew the birth control pill with the vitamin. It helps with the taste. I buy a Dr. Pepper at lunch and store it in my backpack so I have something better than water to wash down the pills with tomorrow morning. At least my new routine is tolerable.

Dr. Kline might have ruined me, but he's right about the pills. Within 48 hours, the bleeding slows, and I'm only changing my pad four times a day. I'm no longer rushing to the bathroom several times a day, worried about bleeding through. After the first week, the bleeding stops completely. Between the vitamins and starting the second envelope of birth control pills, I notice my energy coming back. My stress level is lower, making me less anxious, and school becomes fun again.

Cassidy is still nervous around me, but not as much.

"I'm glad you are feeling better, Sarah," she comments one day during lunch. "You're more like you used to be. I missed you."

"I missed me too. I was just so tired and crabby all of the time. Sorry." I concede and we hug. I can feel the unspoken forgiveness and silently thank God for fixing our friendship as much as possible.

My sense of safety increases as the weeks pass rumor free, well no rumors about me, anyway. And then, John Wright asks me to be his girlfriend.

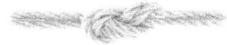

Now that the pills are working and I haven't been running off to the bathroom all the time or falling asleep in class, my grades are better and people seem to think I'm fun. It's been three months since John Wright asked me to be his girlfriend, and he likes me so much that he asked me to call him Johnny even though only his family calls him that. It feels amazing to be wanted, not just by Johnny, but I have more friends than I've ever had before. When I'm home, I have to remind myself to stop smiling all the time so that my parents don't suspect something.

Then one evening, everything comes crashing down.

"Birth control?" Dad yells, shaking the entire house. "Dr. Kline prescribed her birth control?"

I lick my lips. They are talking about *me*.

"Yes, Dave, and it's working," Mom says. "Her periods are normal now, and she obviously feels better. She looks better, too. Even her acne is clearing up."

"Giving a kid birth control is like giving them permission to have sex!" He waits for his declaration to land then adds, "She's going to feel like she can sleep with every boy she thinks is good looking."

"Stop being ridiculous, Dave. People take birth control all the time for lots of different reasons. If you want him to change it, you take her back," Mom retorts.

Mom is finally standing up to Dad!

Fifteen minutes later, the engine of Dad's 1966 pickup truck roars to life. I hear the crunch of the gravel as he pulls out of his parking spot.

FIRST LOVE

OCTOBER 1995

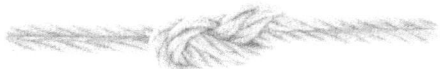

14 YEARS OLD

Despite the purple scar that runs down the side of his face, Johnny's smile is infectious. He was nine when his family vacationed in Zion National Park. Johnny fell over a large boulder. Gratefully, he only had a couple of broken bones and a gash that ran from the corner of his eye to his jawbone. The scar on his face pulled his eye to the side in a funny angle, which made it look like he was winking at me all the time.

"Good morning, beautiful," Johnny calls from across the band room. He sets his mellow horn back in its case and walks toward me, lighting me up with warmth.

I love how excited he always is to see me. The last eight weeks have been the best two months of my entire life.

Lots of kids tease him about his face. I know it bothers him, but he doesn't show it. One day I told some of them off. Johnny thanked me, and then he kissed me for the first time ever.

"Good morning," I reply. I slide my flute together as fast as I can so I can steal the seat next to Johnny until the rest of his section arrives.

"What did you eat for breakfast?" Johnny asks me with a sly smile.

"Why do you want to know?"

"I'm curious how you might taste this morning."

Heat rises to my cheeks. "Pancakes with syrup again."

"Delicious," he proclaims as he leans in for a quick kiss. "Mmm."

I push him away playfully. "Whatever. I brushed my teeth, dork."

"I love syrup and toothpaste in the morning."

I roll my eyes. "You would love kissing me no matter what I eat."

"For sure, for sure."

I go back to my seat when Mrs. Patterson enters the band room. Mrs. Patterson does not allow public displays of affection other than holding hands. On road trips, she kneels backward in her seat at the front of the bus to make sure no one is making out in the back. Students usually find a way around her watchful eye, so her uncomfortable seat position isn't very effective.

I'm on the junior varsity cheer line, which means Johnny and I travel on the bus together with the band for all the varsity football games. When the team qualifies for the playoffs, the JV cheerleaders join the varsity squad on the sidelines. I decide to travel with the band instead of with the cheerleaders so that I can sit with Johnny. When I'm cheering, he makes funny faces at me, and I mess up. Then he laughs at me and catcalls when I high-kick.

During halftime, I go sit next to Johnny in the stands. We snuggle up in a blanket to keep warm.

"You look great out there, beautiful," Johnny says after a playoff game. Just hearing him say it makes me feel beautiful.

"Thanks, you look goofy with all your funny faces."

"Are you making fun of my scar again?"

I shake my head nervously, and he laughs and hugs me hard against his side, the mouthpiece of his horn clonking my ear.

I love that he calls me "beautiful" or "princess." I love that he notices the little things I do, like when I change my hairstyle, or when I help the flute section work through a difficult riff. I love the way he talks about his mother.

On the dark bus rides home, Johnny and I hide under a blanket while we kiss. He keeps his hands north of my belly button. He slips his hand under my shirt, and my heart skips a beat as his hand cups my breast; his fingers fondle my nipple.

He shows me how to touch him so his penis grows and hardens in my hand. We are oblivious to our peers, too engrossed in making out to care who is watching. The darkness and blanket keep us covered. Besides, we aren't the only ones exploring in the dark.

He's into me for more than just the physical stuff. Johnny introduces me to his little sister, Jessica, shortly after we start going out. Soon, Jessica is my friend and like a little sister to me. Johnny is one of three boys. All of their names start with the letter *J*. No one messes with the Wright siblings, unless they want the entire crew on their back. I've never seen a family so close and so happy, and I want to be one of them, too.

Johnny loves to tell me stories about his older brother, Jacob, who is serving a mission for the Mormon Church. He even asks me to write Jacob a letter introducing myself. I'm excited to get to know Jacob, even though I have no idea what to say to him. I don't know anything about him, except that Johnny looks up to him and wants to be like him. I wish my siblings admired me the way Johnny does Jacob.

I sit at my bedroom desk that night trying to figure out what I should say to a total stranger.

So far, I have:

Dear Jacob,

I'm Johnny's girlfriend. I like him a lot. How do you like your mission? What is your favorite part? What is the hardest part? I can't wait to meet you.

Love, Sarah.

Dad knocks on my door and asks me what I'm doing. I shift in my chair. I'm not sure what version of him I'm going to get. He comes in and looks over my shoulder. I hesitate too long.

"Who are you writing to?"

He knows I have a crush on Johnny, but he doesn't know we are boyfriend and girlfriend. I quickly slide my hand over the words on my paper.

"Bishop asked us to write letters to the missionaries from our stake. He said they love to receive mail, so I'm writing to Johnny's older brother, Jacob."

A stake is a group of wards in a geographical area.

"Why would a boy you have never met ever want to get mail from you? You should be writing to your Grandma Hansen. You haven't written to her in a long time."

"I wrote to Grandma two Sundays ago."

Dad is a believer in handwritten letters. He has organized family letter-writing day every Sunday. He says they take more effort and thought and are more valuable to the receiver. I alternate my letters between Grandma and Grandpa Hansen and Grandma and Grandpa T.

"What does your letter say?"

I'm not sure I want to share that information, but I can't say "it's private" without getting into trouble.

Dad folds his arms in front of his chest expectantly. There is no way out of this, so I read him my letter, but replace the word "girlfriend" with "friend."

"That's a dumb letter, Sarah. He's going to think you want to marry him since you ended it with 'love.'"

I hadn't thought of that. I don't want Jacob to think I'm hitting on him. I love Johnny. Dad's right, this is a dumb letter.

Dad doesn't let it go, even when I tear the letter in half then crumple it up and throw it away.

"You shouldn't be writing letters to missionaries while they are on their mission anyway. Their families should be doing that, not you. Girls are just a distraction to boys on missions. You don't want him to be sent home early, do you?" His tone is a mixture of triumph and accusation, his face smug.

"No!" I cry. "I don't ever want a missionary sent home early."

"Well then, you better not write to Jacob Wright, or it'll be your fault he gets sent home early." Dad turns around sharply. "Mom says dinner's ready, by the way." He closes my door behind him.

Being sent home early from your mission is almost as bad as not being a virgin before marriage. I heard Mom and Dad talking about a boy I never met who got sent home early because he was depressed. Mom said no one will want to marry him now. Dad said he faked his depression because he was a homesick wimp.

When you serve the full two years and come home honorably, you're a hero for Jesus and the prettiest girls will date you. Especially if you served a foreign mission and can speak another language. The most righteous boys go on foreign missions. But if you come home early, the entire town talks about the shameful thing you must have done to get sent back, and you become a dark stain on your family forever.

I decide I will never write to Jacob, no matter how much Johnny encourages me to. I don't want to send Jacob the wrong idea, and I don't want to lose Johnny or be the cause of hardship for the Wright family if Jacob gets sent home because of me.

After dinner, I practice my flute before trying to finish my algebra homework. I hate math and have a hard time focusing. I dream of marrying Johnny, instead.

In my daydream, I glide down the aisle in my white dress. He lifts my veil, and we kiss for a really long time. I imagine fireflies sparkling like glitter in the grass… even though fireflies don't frequent Arizona's summer nights.

Johnny and I will have to get married in the Washington, D.C., temple so that I can have fireflies at my wedding. That's where Mom and Dad got married. Then we can have the reception at Grandma and Grandpa T's cabin on Otter Lake in upstate New York. We'll dance barefoot on the dock, and the fireflies will light up the late summer forest like magic. Johnny and I will take the orange canoe to the general store on the other side of the lake, climb into a limo, and go to Paris or Rome for our honeymoon.

My daydream is perfect. Johnny never finds out I'm not a virgin, and my parents are happy I get married in the temple. Johnny has to serve a mission first, and they're happy about that, too. While I wait for him, I'll get my teaching degree so that I can work while he goes to school. Then I'll quit my job once we have our first baby so I can be a stay-at-home mother the way the prophet says all women should. The most righteous women stay home and raise children, while the most righteous men go to work and support the family.

After an hour, I give up on the homework and go to bed where my daydreams turn into night dreams. I roll over and pleasure myself as I fall asleep to images of Johnny kissing me.

I talk to Johnny on the phone for hours every day during Christmas break. I never knew a person could miss someone as much as I miss him. Over spring break, my parents go to Mesa to attend the temple. I make Joey, Evelyn, and Charlie play in the backyard so that Johnny can sneak into the house. We make out on the floor in my bedroom.

"I love you, Sarah," he whispers.

"I love you, too."

"I want to spend the rest of my life with you."

My heart surges. I'm so happy. I want to give him whatever he asks for. I reach up and slowly unbutton my shirt from my neck to just below my bra line while he watches. He leans forward and kisses me on the neck, then my collar bone and down toward my chest. I continue to unbutton my shirt. His breathing comes faster.

He stands up abruptly. "I can't do this with you. I don't want to mess things up." He grabs his keys and rushes out of my bedroom.

I lay on the floor, startled. Did I do something wrong? I replay our conversation over and over in my mind. I'm confused. First, he tells me he wants to spend his entire life with me, and then he leaves.

"Sarah, I'm hungry," Charlie's voice calls to me from the other side of my bedroom door. "Can I stay inside now and eat some lunch?"

I forgot they were out there.

"Yes, Charlie." I pull myself off the floor and button my shirt closed. I run a brush through my hair before exiting my bedroom. I take Charlie by the hand and guide her into the kitchen to make Kraft macaroni and cheese with cut up hot dogs in it. It's disgusting, but the younger kids love it.

"How much longer 'til Mom is home?" Evelyn asks with her mouth full.

"Remember to chew with your mouth closed, Ev," I say. I'm trying to be a good sister, but I can't stop thinking about Johnny; I don't know what his leaving meant.

The telephone's shrill ringing makes us all jump.

Joey bounds out of his seat and yells, "I'll get it." A moment later he's smirking. "Sarah, it's your *boyfriend*. Sarah and Johnny sitting in a tree. K-I-S-S-I-N-G."

"Shut up, Joey," I hiss, relieved that Johnny's calling, but I wish the little kids weren't here watching and listening.

"What do you think you'll name your kids?" Joey asks. "I think your first baby should be named Always, so they can be Always Wright."

Joey ducks when I swipe at him. I yank the telephone out of his hand.

"Johnny? Is everything okay?" I ask.

"Sorry I took off like that."

I'm nervously wrapping the cord around my finger, waiting for him to tell me that it's over. "That's okay."

"I just wanted to say I still love you."

"Me, too." My voice is eager, and I promise myself I'll calm down and try not to sound so desperate.

"I just don't want to go too far and mess things up for us. I need to stay worthy in order to go on my mission and get married in the temple. I'm making you a tape. I'll give it to you tomorrow before band. Please, don't be mad at me for leaving, okay?"

"Yeah, okay, I get it. I want to get married in the temple too… someday." I swallow the hope rising in my throat, trying not to sound too obvious. My hand cups the receiver to cover my mouth. "I love you, too," I whisper, with a silent plea that Joey doesn't hear me since he is still harassing me about talking to Johnny on the phone. I can't risk Mom or Dad finding out about any of this later when they get home.

The next morning, Zoe and I are late for school. We arrive in the middle of warm-ups. Johnny appears behind me, drops a cassette tape onto my lap, and then heads to the drinking fountain and pretends to get a drink. He watches me over his shoulder.

I slide the tape into my backpack and mouth, "I love you."

I have to wait all day to hear what is on the tape. I run all the way home, pop the cassette into my boom box, and hit play. Johnny's voice fills my room. I lean close to the speakers. I don't want Mom or Dad to overhear.

"I love you, Sarah. You make me happier than any man alive. I'm a better person when I'm with you. I like the country version of this song better than the All-4-One version. The words are different, so pay attention, especially to the second verse. I want this to be our song so that you know I will always be there for you."

John Michael Montgomery's voice is barely audible. I turn the volume up and rewind just a bit to make sure I don't miss the words. I close my eyes and sway to the music. I've never heard John Michael Montgomery's version before. I hum along to the familiar tune *"I Swear"* and try hard not to flinch at the country twang of the opening lines. The nasally tone "is the wrong way to sing," at least that's what Dad says.

I lip-sync along with the lyrics and soon Montgomery's deep syrupy voice isn't bothering me as much as I thought it would, even with the southern drawl. As the first chorus comes to a close, I lean closer to the speaker for the second verse, turning the volume up a little bit more. I close my eyes and grit my teeth in focus, listening for the change Johnny had mentioned.

I gasp and sit back. Building dreams, and silver hair? Is Johnny telling me he wants to be with me forever, till I'm old and gray? I rewind the tape and play it again.

He really does want to marry me! I feel like I'm floating. Tears form behind my eyes. I've never felt so important in all my life. Through the song, he's promising to make my dreams come true and decorate our future home with picture memories.

I lean back against the wall in my room and let the rest of the song carry me back into my daydreams. New York, Otter Lake, my white gown, the fireflies. It will be perfect.

Johnny's voice fills the room again. I jump and unplug the boom box in my haste. I turn the volume almost all the way down and plug it back in.

"Just remember, Sarah, I want to take you to the temple. Our marriage won't be 'till *death do us part,'* it will be for time and all eternity. This second song can be our secret backup song. Just know we have to wait until after we are married. I promise to always honor your virtue, no matter how hard it is."

There's some rustling in the background and then a click. I recognize the intro to *I'll Make Love to You* by Boyz II Men. I lean back against the wall again and continue to dream. As the song comes to a close, Johnny's voice repeats, "I'll love you forever." Then the sounds of whale calls and the ocean replace Johnny's proclamation of love and songs. I wince. What the hell is this?

I pull the tape out and read *Songs of the Whale.* Johnny must have recorded over the first part of an hour of whale sounds. I like it. I don't have to hide this from my parents. No way anyone is going to steal a tape of whale sounds.

AUTHOR'S NOTE

Johnny was the first male to give me the type of attention I was craving from my father. As my body began to change due to puberty, my father stopped showing affection, withheld his love, and began to criticize my body, the way I looked, and most of my actions. Johnny's admiration and friendship were like a drug. I loved him completely and would have done anything to keep him from breaking up with me. I required constant reassurance that he would not withhold his love and affection for me.

Like my father, I was obsessive and needed to control the environment in order to protect myself from abandonment. If left unchecked, these characteristics could have evolved into borderline personality traits.

I have come to learn that borderline and narcissistic traits are often associated with severe trauma and emotional neglect in childhood or adolescence.[5,6] I am forever grateful to Jim, the first counselor I saw as an adult, who helped me identify the behavioral tendencies I used to control my environment, as well as his help in learning how to regulate my emotional responses, especially during acute anxiety. With his guidance, I have learned how to manage the fear of abandonment that comes with attachment trauma.

---

5   Diana Kwon, "Borderline Personality Disorder May Be Rooted in Trauma," *Scientific American*, Jan. 1, 2022. https://www.scientificamerican.com/article/borderline-personality-disorder-may-be-rooted-in-trauma/.

6   Nina Bertele and Anat Talmon and James J. Gross, "Childhood Maltreatment and Narcissism: The Mediating Role of Dissociation," *Journal of Interpersonal Violence* 37, no. 11-12 (December 2020). https://doi.org/10.1177/0886260520984404.

CRACK IN THE DOOR

OCTOBER 1995

14 YEARS OLD

"Someone seems happy," Mom says as she sets the meatloaf on the table in front of Dad.

I flash her my happiest smile. "Yeah, I had a good day today." I glide toward the cupboard with the cups in it, thinking about Johnny's tape while humming "I Swear," my feet falling naturally into the foxtrot Dad had taught me years ago.

"I'm glad to see you feeling so much better, Sarah."

"Thanks, Mom, I feel much better, that's for sure." I count out six cups and begin to set the table without her asking me.

Mom has been more attentive toward me since that day in Dr. Kline's office. She probably wants to make sure that I'm not mad at her, or that I don't tell anyone that she held me down while Dr. Kline took my virginity. Even though I like her more gentle approach, I can't trust it.

Throughout dinner, I say "uh-huh" in the right places in the family conversation, but I'm not paying close attention to anything. I am full of joy, like light is bursting from my breastbone. Johnny's tape had erased all my fear from our weekend make-out session.

After dinner, I claim I have homework and float back to my bedroom. I close the door behind me and decide to memorize the country version of "I Swear" because it's Johnny's promise to me even though I like the All-4-One version better.

I pull my blouse off over my head and undo my bra clasp, pulling my arms out of the shoulder straps. As I feed my hands through the arm holes of my pajama top, Dad bursts into my room.

"How dare you, Sarah?"

I stare at him, not knowing why he is here or what to say.

"Do you have any idea what this does to a man?" He waved at my body; his scarlet face is inches from mine. "It is not a man's fault when he is aroused by a woman's body."

He grabs my upper arm and drags me from my room into the library.

Mom rushes in. "What did she do?"

"I didn't do anything!" Hot tears spill over my cheeks. I'm panicked, wondering if he knows about Johnny, Dr. Kline, or both.

"She took her shirt and bra off with her door open," Dad snarls.

I shake my head. "It was closed when you barged in and started screaming at me."

He shoves me so hard that I tumble into the piano bench behind me.

"Stop lying! Your door was cracked open. Do you want someone to touch you?"

Images of Dr. Kline's gloved hands flash through my mind.

"No, I don't want to be touched!" I scream back. I stand and take a daring step toward him. "Why were you even watching me?"

Crack!

His hand slaps my cheek so fast I don't have time to duck.

My head whips to the side. Something pulls painfully in my neck.

"Dave!" Mom yells.

"She's always showing off her body!" Dad screams. "The teachers at the school tell me that she's hanging on all the boys. She's probably rubbing her vagina on them between classes. She's promiscuous, Emma, and now she's blaming me for her laziness."

Warm embarrassment rises to my cheeks.

What teachers are calling Dad? Why would they say that about me? Johnny is the only boy I'm with, and we mostly just hold hands. We only make out on the bus, or we go somewhere private, never any place that teachers would see us. Other than the bus, we've been careful to not be seen so that we wouldn't get caught.

"I didn't leave the door open on purpose. Sometimes it doesn't latch unless I lift up on the doorknob." I glance over to Mom, who makes eye contact with me. She knows my door doesn't shut right, but she doesn't say anything, she's just frozen in place. "I didn't do anything wrong," I say again. A sharp pinching sensation in my neck won't subside.

"No, Sarah, your door closes just fine," Dad growls. "You left it open on purpose. What if Joey had seen you changing? You're lucky it was me this time."

I can't look him in the eyes as I wonder how long he had been standing there staring at me. Heat crawls up the back of my neck. I feel ashamed even though I didn't do anything.

"If Joey had seen you, he'd want to see it again and again. Once a boy sees breasts, he wants to see them again, right Emma?"

Mom continues to ignore my pleading looks. In fact, she doesn't move or make a sound.

"It will be your fault if he starts looking at *Playboy* magazines."

Dad lifts his hand like he's going to slap me again.

I recoil and step backward, with my arm protecting my head. His right hand hovers high above my face. I squeeze my eyes shut and brace myself.

Nothing.

I open my eyes just enough to peek through my lashes.

Dad has dropped his hands, and he's trembling. His face is still bright red, and he's panting. "Never let me catch you changing with that door open again."

Mom still hasn't moved.

I escape back to my bedroom and lift the knob to make sure the door latches. I let out the sob I've been holding in. Dad has never hit me before. Even his spankings are purposefully gentle. It's been a long time since he paid much attention to me at all.

Why can't boys control themselves? I can't be perfect all the time.

Johnny has sort of seen my breasts. Does that mean he looks at porn now?

I pull my pillow to my mouth and scream into it. It feels like my chest is going to split open. My head throbs.

Why doesn't Mom ever help me? She pinned me down while Dr. Kline crammed his fingers into me, and she just stood there while Dad screamed at me and slapped me. She knows my door is hard to latch. I hate her, I hate him, I hate being in this family. I get in trouble for telling the truth, I get in trouble for lying, I'm never good enough. No one gives half a shit about me until something dramatic happens. Even then it's not like they care about me, they just care about how it makes them look.

I wish I could call Johnny or Zoe, but the family telephone is in the kitchen. I hate feeling alone at times like this. I need someone to tell me I'm not crazy.

It's been a week since Dad slapped me. Most of the time he avoids me, but when we are in the same place, he won't look me in the eye. At dinner, he asks Joey, Ev, and Charlie about their days, as usual, but he acts like I'm not there. When I try to talk to Mom, she acts like it wasn't a big deal.

"Dad was just trying to make you more aware so you don't accidentally expose yourself. You don't want to give boys the wrong ideas."

I sleep, but it's not restful. I usually wake up in a cold sweat, screaming just before Dr. Kline twists his fingers inside of me. No wonder Mom doesn't like sex.

Since I'm up early for band, I take extra time on my hair and makeup, and greet Zoe at the door. Breakfast is the one meal a day that isn't awkward and uncomfortable for me; Dad pretends to be normal with Zoe there. Zoe asks me if pancakes are my Mom's favorite breakfast to make, because we eat them at least twice a week. She is shocked that we never have cereal. Mom diligently cooks all our meals from scratch; Dad says all good Mormon women do.

Zoe and I are walking out the front door when I realize I've forgotten to take my birth control pill and Flintstones vitamin. I race back into my room, wrestle the child-safe lid off the Flintstone vitamin container, and slide the birth control envelope out of its hiding place. After I race back out to Zoe's car, she backs out of our driveway, shifts too quickly, and the tires slip as she moves forward.

Then it hits me.

I'm three days into a brand-new envelope of birth control pills.

I didn't have a period last week.

I scan the back of the band room for Johnny when I arrive, but he isn't there.

Mrs. Patterson snaps at me for messing up a flute solo that I've nailed a hundred times before. "You're first chair, Sarah, I expect better out of you."

"I'm sorry, I lost count. I'm having a hard time focusing today."

"You got this," Deckland calls from the percussion section.

Mrs. Patterson shoots him a warning look, and he twirls his drumstick in his hand.

Show off.

I relax a little when I see Deckland. I love Deckland. Not like I love Johnny, more like a big brother. Deckland sticks up for me when the boys swat my butt or whistle at me. He'll tell me if I say something stupid, but without making me feel like I am stupid. I don't know how many times Deckland has loaned me his hoodie so I can hide my bloodstained pants.

After three failures at my solo, Mrs. Patterson sends me to a rehearsal room behind the percussion section to practice alone. I shoot Deckland a pleading look as I pass, and he slips into the room behind me and closes the door. He slides to the floor so Mrs. Patterson can't see him. I hold my flute to my mouth but don't play. She can't hear me over the rest of the band, so I sway my body to make it appear like I'm practicing.

"Are you okay? That's like the easiest solo of all time," Deckland asks. He looks ridiculous laying on the floor, but it works, Mrs. Patterson doesn't even look my way.

"I can't focus or count." I lower my flute and lean forward, pretending to squint at my sheet music on the stand in front of me. "I missed my period; I think I'm pregnant. Johnny's not here today so I can't talk to him. What do I do?"

"Whoa, Sarah, that's huge. Your Dad is gonna kill Johnny. I didn't even know you guys were having sex."

"We didn't. I don't think we did. I haven't taken off my clothes. I'm not sure how his sperm got through my clothes."

"Wait, what the fuck? Is this your idea of a joke?"

"No, I'm serious. We make out all the time, but we keep our clothes on."

"Did he put his dick inside you?"

"Ewww, no. I wouldn't let anyone put anything in there. That would hurt, like a lot." My palms get sweaty, thinking of the pain with Dr. Kline.

"Yes, it's painful for the girl the first few times. Did he get his cum on his hand and then put his fingers inside of you?"

"No."

"You can't be serious, Sarah. Stop joking. This isn't funny. Are you really pregnant? Have you, like, peed on a stick to find out?"

I stop pretending to practice and join Deckland on the floor. Hopefully Mrs. Patterson will forget I'm in here.

"No. Is that what I need to do?"

"You're for real, aren't you?"

"He won't be able to go on a mission if I'm pregnant. We'll have to get married. I'll be married, and I'm only 15."

"Sarah, how do you think you got pregnant?"

"I dunno. We lie next to each other sometimes while we kiss. We must have gotten too close 'cause I've missed my period."

Deckland starts laughing.

"This isn't funny, I'm serious. What am I going to do?"

Tears spring from Deckland's eyes. He clutches his chest and lies on the floor, still laughing.

The bell rings, and we slide down a little lower as students pass so that they can't see through the window and know we are still there. Deckland stops laughing and wipes tears from his eyes. "Meet me behind the band room for lunch, and I'll teach you about sex. I promise, if all you've done is kiss, and you kept your clothes on the entire time, you are certainly *not* pregnant."

"Are you sure?"

"Yes, I'm sure, little sis. See you at lunch."

I rush to put my flute away. I skip cleaning it because I can't be late for English Language Arts class. Ms. Caldwell is a stickler on attendance.

The minutes tick by slowly. I glance up at the clock more than once. Ms. Caldwell raps the front of my desk with her yardstick. "Sarah, back to work."

"Yes ma'am." I put my head down and read the first line of the paragraph for the millionth time. This is useless. I can't focus on the words right in front of my face. I count to 100 then turn the page without reading. I keep doing this during the rest of the class.

I can't concentrate during third hour either, so I count and turn pages again. Deckland sits behind me in fourth-hour Spanish. I'll find him before class. There's no way I can wait for his explanation until lunch. I look anxiously up at the clock; only three minutes left of third hour. I tap my toe on the carpeted floor. Two minutes. I shift uncomfortably in my seat. One minute. I slide forward in my chair, anticipating the bell indicating the end of third hour. I bolt out of my seat as soon as the intercom clicks on before the first chime of the bell.

Spanish is in the old building above the library. I run all the way there and take the stairs two at a time. I wait for Deckland at the top of the steps, right leg bouncing, worried that I missed him, somehow.

Finally, his head bobs among the last stragglers.

"I can't wait 'til lunch, come on." I grab his arm and tug him down the stairs after me.

"I guess I can miss Spanish today," he says. "Stop pulling me. I'm gonna fall."

I release his arm, and we hurry side by side across campus, past the intermediate school, and make our way to the Fine Arts building. We glance around to make sure no one is looking before we slip behind the building above the football field.

"Alright, Sarah, what do you know about having sex?"

"Well, Mom said sex is when a boy puts his sperm inside the girl's stomach."

"Yeah, and how does that sperm get inside a girl's stomach? It's not by magic… well, it's magical but not magic." His cheeks redden slightly.

"I don't know. Mom said it happens when you sleep together. I stopped sleeping next to Joey on our camping trips, just in case."

Deckland swallows hard and bites his lower lip. He's trying not to laugh.

"You think your brother can get you pregnant just from sleeping next to you?"

"Well, yeah. Why?" I hate feeling stupid. I know it's not intentional, but Deckland's reaction makes me feel foolish.

"Look, Sarah, I love your mother, but she isn't doing you any favors by hiding the details."

He's said this about my Mom before on different topics.

He picks up a large rock and, squatting in front of the path worn between the band room and the football field, he draws a vertical oval with pointy ends on the dry ground. Then he draws a line down the middle of it. "Pretend this is your pussy from a guy's view if you are laying on your back and he's looking right at it."

Near the top of the center line, he draws a smaller triangle thingy with a dot under it. "This pointy thing is called your clit. It's like a girl's tiny penis. It feels really good when guys touch you there, rub it, kiss it, suck on it… you get what I'm saying?"

I nod. I've always thought it was a tiny penis since that's where my pee comes from.

"This tiny dot underneath your clit is where you pee from."

"Wait, don't I pee out of my… tiny penis thing… my…."

"Clit," Deckland finishes my sentence. "And no, you don't, but lots of people think you do. Anyway, this little dot right under it is where your pee comes from."

"Okay…" not certain where he is going with his dust drawing.

Deckland draws a circle below the pee dot.

"When your legs are closed this looks more like a line, but when you spread your legs out to the side, it opens into a hole. It's warm and wet. Never let anyone put their dick in you unless you're wet down there or it will hurt like hell and bleed."

"How do you know all of this?" I ask, still not sure what to think.

"I read it, and I just know stuff." Deckland's face is crimson. I can tell he's uncomfortable, but I'm relieved that he keeps talking. "Anyway, the hole opens up really big. It's the same hole babies come out of, so it can stretch a lot."

That must be where Dr. Kline put his fingers in me to be able to reach inside my belly.

"That's the hole where the dick goes… that hole is your actual vagina. When you touch Johnny on his dick, it gets big, right?"

Heat rises to my cheeks, and I know I'm blushing. I can't believe I'm admitting to this out loud. I have to remind myself it's just Deckland. "Yeah, like really big."

"Lucky bastard." Deckland ignores me glaring at him. "Once a penis is hard, a guy will put it into that hole. Once they've done that, you're not a virgin anymore. Do you get it?"

He watches me closely.

My mind is racing, trying to take it all in. "Is that the only way you can lose your virginity?"

"Yeah."

Dr. Kline only put his fingers in me. "What if someone puts their fingers inside, does that matter?" A metallic taste fills my mouth from my chewing on the inside of my lip.

"It won't get you pregnant, and you'd still be a virgin."

Too stunned to respond, I place my palms on the reddish earth in front of me and stare at the scratches Deckland made in the dirt, letting this new information sink in.

I am still a virgin.

AUTHOR'S NOTE

It's difficult to understand why my father struggled so much with my sexual development. Around this time in my life, I recognized that it didn't matter what I did, how I covered my body, or how I interacted with boys, I was going to be in trouble for having a female body. Since I knew punishment or criticism was coming, no matter how I handled any situation, I lashed out and stopped caring about the consequences of my behavior. Looking back, I realize that all I cared about was being loved and unconditionally accepted by someone and being numb to the rest of the world.

A family counseling professional who worked with my parents and me explained that my father views women as either dangerous or simpleminded. That same professional theorized that Dad was subconsciously punishing me for the mistakes of his mother. I became the family scapegoat before I could talk due to my hypersexualized behavior, which started within my first year of life. As I became older, and naturally more independent, their attempts to maintain control of my life became more extreme and sometimes frantic. I feel they had a consistent fear that I would make them look bad if I wasn't an upstanding Mormon girl.

KIDNAPPED

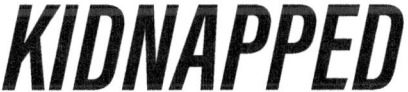

APRIL 1996

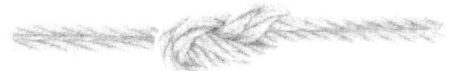

15 YEARS OLD

Johnny and I make a pact, promising not to go too far. I'm not entirely sure what that means, so I decide to just let Johnny take the lead. Gratefully, marching band season is over so there's less opportunity to make out on the bus, which is the only prayer we have of even remotely keeping that promise so we can be worthy to marry in the temple. When we do get to be alone, it's in the back of the beat-up red van Johnny drives. We park by the Taylor Rodeo Grounds where no one will bother us; it's more private and more intense, and before we know it, we've been making out for more than an hour.

"Crap, Sarah." Johnny scrambles to get into the front seat. "I was supposed to be home before now."

"Why don't you drop me off at my Dad's school?" I pull my shirt down over my belly and run my fingers through my tangled hair. "It's closer to your house." If Johnny gets grounded from using the family van for coming home late, he'll have to ride his bus home, and we won't have time alone together at all.

"Are you sure your Dad will still be there?"

"Yeah, he's always there late, grading papers." I'm not positive he'll be there, but I can walk to Zoe's house and call home from there. If they think I've been with Zoe, I won't be in trouble.

We kiss one last time, long and hard on the lips.

"You are incredible. I love you, Sarah." His crooked tooth grin and proclamation of love makes my heart flutter.

"I love you too, Johnny. Let's go." I push him back into the driver's seat.

Johnny presses hard on the gas and a few minutes later, we screech to a halt next to Taylor Intermediate School. I nearly hit my head on the dash as I shoot forward.

I risk one last quick kiss before jumping out. "See ya' tomorrow, outside the band room?"

Johnny has told me repeatedly he's not going anywhere, but I'm still terrified he will find something wrong and stop loving me. The closer we are physically, the more confident I am that he really does love me. He's so serious about going on a mission and marrying in the temple, I know he wouldn't risk being so close if it wasn't love.

"You better believe it, baby," he says with a laugh.

I barely close the passenger door before Johnny speeds away. I check to make sure that my clothes look okay. The only thing that gives me away is my messed-up hair, but I can blame that on the wind that plagues the Snowflake/Taylor communities.

I walk toward the entrance of the school along the sidewalk closest to my Dad's classroom. A whiff of Johnny's woody cologne from my shirt makes me smile. I love the way he smells. He held me so close at the last youth dance that I came home smelling more like him than my own scent, even though the chaperones reminded us multiple times that the Book of Mormon had to fit in the space between our bodies. They hovered over us until we separated to their satisfaction.

"That depends on what direction you put the book between us," Johnny had whispered, pulling me close again as soon as the chaperone moved on. I'd hidden my unwashed blouse from that night in my pillow-case so I could smell his cologne as I fall asleep each night.

"Sarah?" I hear my Dad's frantic voice and look up. Dad's entire face is pursed, his shoulders forward, and he moves swiftly toward me.

"What's the matter, Dad?" I ask; my heart skips a beat.

"Mom called and said that you didn't come home from school and that you don't have cheer practice for the rest of the school year."

My mind goes blank. I'm rooted to the sidewalk staring up at him, suddenly terrified of getting caught.

He stares intently at me, waiting expectantly for my response.

I can't tell him I've been with Johnny.

"We thought you were kidnapped."

"Kidnapped?"

"Did someone hurt you?"

I nod before realizing what that nod means. "I was with Zo…"

"Who was it?" His voice is shrill and unfamiliar. His eyes look around, frantically.

Dread overwhelms me. I don't know how to back out of this one.

Dad pulls my arm gently. "We are calling the police now."

My feet are heavy, and it feels like I'm walking through mud.

"It's okay, Sarah, you're with me now," Dad says, his tone softer, his eyebrows pinched together, his face still red.

Dad sits me down in a chair in the front office and leaves to go make calls. I can't sit still, my body is full of nervous energy, and I keep wanting to run away or go find Dad, tell him it isn't true, but I don't know where he is and I can't tell him where I really was. I wait for a long time, still trying to figure out my options when Dad comes back with two police officers.

Dad is speaking rapidly.

He keeps trying to give them his story, but the officer with the pen and the little notebook keeps interrupting him and asking questions… finally they let him just talk.

"Her mother called me. She hadn't noticed Sarah was missing right away because she normally has cheer practice after school, but the season ended last week…"

The taller officer interrupts. "May I talk to your daughter?"

Dad leans against the wall.

"I need to speak to her alone," the officer says.

"I'm going to kill whoever did this to my daughter."

"I understand," the officer's voice is matter of fact and not very comforting.

Dad keeps clenching and unclenching his fists, and he's grinding his teeth.

I relax a little when Dad leaves, muttering to himself.

"Sarah, I'm Officer Schmidt. Can you tell me what happened today after school?" The shorter officer leans casually on the high desk in the front office. I glance at him, then at the tall one, whose name tag says "Jones" on it. I drop my gaze to my lap, at my fidgeting fingers. I try to get the trembling to stop.

"I went someplace close to the rodeo grounds." My voice trembles, still not sure what to say. I'm pretty sure both these officers will know I'm lying if I say I'd been kidnapped.

"Who were you with?"

I shrug.

"Did you know the person you were with?"

I close my eyes, tears escape and run down the sides of my face. "No," I lie.

Dad told them I had been kidnapped. "They put a bag over my head," I said.

Both officers stand up straighter. Schmidt takes his notepad out of his breast pocket. Jones scribbles on his.

"What type of bag?" Jones asks. He looks at me over his glasses resting low on his wide nose.

I hadn't thought that far ahead. I scan my brain for a bag that I could breathe through. "The kind we use at church activities for potato races."

"Could you see through it?" Schmidt's voice is demanding now.

"No, it was solid black."

Schmidt raises an eyebrow. They know I'm lying, and I have barely even started. I start coughing.

"Do you need a drink?" Schmidt asks.

I need to pee, but I'm so nervous I'd probably trip. I decide to just tell my story and get it over with.

"They put the bag over my head…"

If they keep asking questions, I'm going to screw it all up. My stomach twists so hard my heart feels pinched tight.

"Who's 'they'?" Jones interrupts.

"The two boys. They were overweight. I could tell 'cause they lifted me into the back of their van. One boy drove crazy, and the other sat in the back next to me to make sure I didn't take the bag off and then…"

"Did you see their shoes?" Schmidt asks.

"No, I had a bag over my head."

"Like the burlap bags used for potato races?" he pushes.

There's something wrong with that answer. "Yes, like the itchy ones we race in," I confirm.

"And you couldn't see anything at all?" Schmidt stares directly at me.

Heat rises in my cheeks. I stare back at him, trying not to blink or break eye contact. "No, nothing."

Jones shoots Schmidt a warning look. "What happened next?"

"Well, they told me they would hurt me if I tried to fight them. They drove around for a long time, maybe an hour and then they parked by the rodeo grounds and carried me over to a tree, set me down, told me to turn around and stare at the tree or they would hit me. And then they drove off."

"How did you know where you were?"

Every question that Schmidt asks makes the lump in my throat grow a little larger. It's getting harder to swallow the spit accumulating in my mouth.

"I took the bag off my head, and I was at the rodeo grounds."

"Did anybody hurt you?" Jones asks.

I've decided I like him better. He has a kind smile, and he is obviously listening to me.

"No."

Schmidt won't just listen and leave it alone. He keeps asking me the same stupid questions over and over, like he has a problem with hearing or something. "Look," I snap. "No one hurt me. I'm home safe, just a stupid joke, no one should get into too much trouble for that, right? Boys play stupid jokes on people all the time."

They ignore my outburst and ask, "When they lifted you out of the van, did the bag slip? Did you see any clothing or shoes, the color of the van maybe? Take your time and think," Jones says.

I don't know if it's better to make up more details or not. "I didn't see the van."

"Then how do you know it was a van?" Schmidt demands.

"Hey, Schmidt, can you go get Sarah something to drink from the vending machine. I'm sure she's really thirsty after all that has happened today." Jones hands Schmidt a dollar from his wallet.

"Sure," Schmidt huffs. He stomps out of the office.

My heart slows as soon as the door snaps closed behind him.

"I think he's having a really bad day today," Jones says. "He's usually a nice guy, but he's kinda being a jerk."

I nod.

Jones grabs a chair and sets it backward in front of me. He swings his leg over the seat and straddles the chair, resting his elbows on the back of it.

"Can you start from the beginning again? Tell me what happened. Start from where you were before the bag was put over your head."

"I was near the band room, saying goodbye to my friends. Then two boys came up behind me and put the bag over my head. One grabbed my feet and the other put his arms under my shoulders. They lifted me into the van and closed the door. I know it was a van because I could hear the door slide, just like my parents' van."

Jones motions his pen at me to keep going.

"So, then we drove around a lot. One of the boys said if I cooperated, I wouldn't get hurt. They told stupid jokes 'til we stopped. They pulled me out of the van and sat me next to a bush and told me to face the other way. Then they drove off. I waited for a few minutes, then took the bag off and recognized where I was. So, then I started to walk to Dad's school hoping he would still be here." I can't see what Jones is writing, I can't tell if he believes me; I just need this to be over with.

"That sounds terrifying, Sarah."

Tears of relief wash over me. I pull tissues from a box on the end table to hide my face in.

"Part of my job is to ask you some questions. I know it can be frustrating when someone questions you, especially after you just told me the entire story, but this is how we make sure that you remembered everything right and I understood it all. Is that okay?"

So maybe I am not in as much trouble as I thought. The ache in my chest begins to subside.

"Where is the bag now?"

"I left it by the bush."

"Did they leave you by a tree or a bush?"

"Oh, a bush. I meant a bush the first time but said tree."

Jones smiles. "Sometimes my wife does that, too. That's why I was checking."

I smile back.

"Can you tell me if you saw anything, any flashes of color, could you see the floor of the van if you looked down under the burlap bag?"

He really wants me to have seen something, so I give him this little bit. "I saw my lap, and the seat I was sitting in."

"What color was the seat?"

"Light gray." My forehead crinkles, and my stomach drops. That's the color of the seats in my family van.

"Was it leather?" His voice is gentle, but his questions make me shift uncomfortably in my seat anyway.

"No, it was normal car fabric."

"Did you see anything else?" Jones writes on his notepad.

Schmidt knocks on the door and cracks it open. "Jones, do you need me?"

I jolt out of my chair and shake my head. If Schmidt comes back in here, he'll ruin everything.

"Nope, I'm almost done." He reaches for the root beer that Schmidt brought and hands it to me. "Please talk to Mr. and Mrs. Lee," he says to Schmidt.

The door clicks closed again. I sit back into my seat and force my shoulders to relax. I don't think I can take much more of this interview.

"Is my Mom here?"

"Would you like to see her?" Jones folds the notebook closed and slips it into his breast pocket.

"No, not yet," I say.

Mom has been paying way more attention to me since Dad's last freak out. She's actually a really good listener when she's not distracted, but I don't want to tell this story ever again.

"You seem to be handling all of this really well," Jones assures me.

"They were just stupid boys being stupid. I'm not afraid of stupid boys. Ha! You should meet my brother Joey. He's *really* stupid." I roll my eyes in pretend exasperation, hopeful the interview is over.

Jones smiles. "Yeah, my little brother was kinda dumb, too." We both laugh a little. I'm beginning to relax. My hands have stopped trembling.

"Do you mind if we all take a trip out to the rodeo grounds to look around?"

My eyes widen as I stare at him. He wants to go there. "It's really windy. I bet the bag blew away already."

"It wouldn't surprise me." He smiles and stands to leave.

We walk out.

Jones joins Schmidt who is talking to Dad. Dad's face isn't as red, and he appears more relaxed. Schmidt laughs at something he says, and they keep talking.

Mom looks ragged. "Did they hurt you?"

"I'm fine. I have to go to the bathroom."

I wait for Mom's nod indicating I'm allowed to go, then rush to the bathroom around the corner and lock the stall. I sit on the toilet, and let my tears come. Why hadn't I just told him that I'd been at Zoe's and forgot to call them. Now I've lied to the police. If they catch me, I'm going to be in so much trouble.

It only takes me a couple minutes before I pull myself off the toilet and wash my hands. I reach for the bathroom door, my hands still wet. I pull it open then freeze.

"You know that girl is lying, Jones. You know it." Schmidt's accusing voice churns my stomach.

"She's covering for something that she thinks is worse," Jones concurs. "I want her to feel safe enough to tell me."

How could Jones know that?

"Nah, Lees exaggerate, like father, like daughter. I've heard about him before. Mr. Lee is *never* wrong." Schmidt's sarcasm is unmistakable.

"There's a reason for the story, though. Something is going on, something so bad that she'd rather lie about being kidnapped than to tell the truth."

I can feel the tears well up again, threatening to spill onto my cheeks. I'm relieved to be understood. Maybe they won't tell my parents and things can just go back to normal.

The boy's bathroom door creaks as it opens.

"What exactly are we looking for Jones? You know just as well as I do, we ain't gonna find a thing out there."

Bile rises into my mouth. I spin around and gag into the sink. They know I'm lying, so why play along? I can't trust adults, they're too unpredictable. I blink at my reflection staring back at me. I've lied to the police, and they know it. I'm going to end up in juvie for sure.

I crack the girls' bathroom door open just enough to make sure the hallway is clear. I hold the door as it closes quietly behind me and hurry back to my Mom.

"Hey, kiddo, we are loading up." The lines around her eyes are deeper than normal. "Come with me and the kids. We are going to follow the police officers to the rodeo grounds."

I just need to lead them to a spot far from where Johnny and I were parked and pray the wind continues its crazed howling.

AUTHOR'S NOTE

How in God's name I got away with that cockamamie story is beyond me. As far as I knew, my parents never questioned my story. The police, on the other hand, did their due diligence to close the investigation, knowing that I was lying.

In lieu of the idea that I was hiding the truth, my story fell in line with my father's preconceived notions that I was in a world constantly under threat of being victimized by teenage boys. For some reason, my story relieved me of the burden of accountability. For the first time, I wasn't being blamed for the poor actions of someone else taking advantage of me. It also relieved both of my parents of the responsibility of having a daughter who wasn't living up to the Mormon standard's of chastity and virtue.

MOVING

SPRING 1996

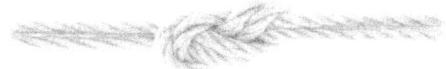

15 YEARS OLD

At the Taylor Rodeo Grounds, I don't "remember" anything useful. I also can't "find" the bush or tree that I'd been dumped off at, and of course there isn't a burlap potato sack in sight. Jones and Schmidt take a picture of the bottom of my shoes and say they will look for my footprints again in the morning when the light is better. They reassure Mom and Dad that they will call with any updates, and I silently hope I never see or hear from them again.

I feel a little guilty for lying to the police, but anything is better than getting caught making out with Johnny.

Mom keeps her promise, and we pick dinner up from the McDonald's drive-through on the way home. Mom and Dad don't ask me anything else about the "kidnapping," and I welcome the solitude of an early bedtime shortly after I finish my Big Mac.

When I arrive at school the next morning, Johnny is in his van parked across the street from the band room. My words spill out in a rush before he can kiss me.

"Wait, Sarah. What? Why didn't you tell the cops the truth?" Johnny asks as he leans back into the driver's seat.

"My Dad would completely freak. Not just for letting him think I was kidnapped, not just for embarrassing him, but if he found out where I really was, he'd ruin both our lives."

He knows what I am talking about. None of my friends like Dad much now that they know what he is like outside of his classroom. His teasing me in front of them is more mean than funny, which makes everyone uncomfortable. And he's always doing or saying something to be the center of attention around my friends, which is just plain weird. No one wants to hang out at my house because the rules are too strict, and the only boy Mom welcomes into our home is Deckland.

"The police are going to come here and ask you some questions because I told them I was with my friends before everyone left. I'm so sorry, Johnny. I ruin everything." My forehead crinkles, pleading silently that Johnny won't be furious with me. I can't stop my tears.

Johnny's mouth drops open. "You're beautiful when you cry, you know that?" My sobs come in gasping breaths.

"Stop, this is serious." He climbs out of his van and puts his arms around me. I continue to sob into his chest as he caresses my head. Once I've calmed down, I tell him about the police interrogation, leaving out the conversation I overheard between Jones and Schmidt.

"I understand if you want to break up with me, Johnny. I was trying to protect us. I didn't want you to get into trouble."

"I can't believe you lied to the police. That's kinda hot, like in the movies. What exactly did you tell them that I need to know about?" His brows come together in concentration. As long as things are okay with Johnny, I can get through this mess I've created.

"That I said goodbye to my friends who were parked here by the band room, and then I started to walk home."

"So that's Zoe, right? When I talk to the police, I'll need to say the same thing you did."

"I think Deckland was here. I'm not sure. We didn't leave for the rodeo grounds 'til all of them had left already. Remember?"

"Okay. So, I hugged you goodbye and drove away. Last I saw you, you were walking home. That's easy enough. Don't worry, princess. You can't get rid of me that easy."

I hug him fiercely, savoring his amazing smell. Last night, I had washed my clothes as soon as we got home from McDonald's, including the shirt hidden in my pillowcase that smelled like Johnny, just in case the police came by later and wanted my clothes or something for evidence. I didn't want them to connect the dots that I had been with him.

When Johnny and I walk into band, Mrs. Patterson is in her office on the phone and the entire room is in chaos. Half the class has their instruments out, the other half is standing around talking and ignoring the morning bell.

I sit in my place at the head of the flute section and put my flute together, hands shaking. Jones said he'd be by sometime later today to talk to my friends. I really, really don't want him to. I don't want my friends to know about yesterday, but there's nothing I can do to stop it.

At lunch, I get bombarded with questions. I ignore all of them and push through the crowd away from the cafeteria to the safety of the Fine Arts hallway.

"Why are the cops asking about you, Sarah?" Zoe corners me first.

"Some boys prank 'kidnapped' me," I roll my eyes and make air quotes. "Dad kinda freaked out and called the police."

"Who was it?" Cassidy asks.

I hadn't seen her come from behind me. "I don't know. I think they must have been from Show Low or something. I didn't recognize them at all." I try to sound nonchalant. I might be able to fool Cassidy, but Zoe is much better at reading me.

"You gave the cops a good description though, right?" Zoe asks.

Geez, she wasn't making this easy for me.

"No, I didn't see them."

"Then why do you think they were from Show Low?" Cassidy asks. Even if I come up with a good reason, they'll keep asking questions.

I sigh loudly, "I really don't want to talk about it." Cassidy and Zoe are so intense; I can't even look at them. I just want to move on. "They didn't hurt me, I'm okay. Dad is mad enough for everyone. Can we just talk about something else?" I beg.

Fooling Mom and Dad had been easy. My friends, not so much.

Johnny joins us and grabs my hand. "I passed with flying colors." He winks at me.

"You need to be more serious about this, Johnny," Zoe scolds.

"You're right, Zoe. Sarah, I'm glad you are okay and safe. So, what are we talking about?"

Cassidy and Zoe roll their eyes at him.

"We are discussing our summer plans." Maybe the change of subject will clue everyone into the fact that I'm done answering questions. "I'm still going to New York for a month to visit Grandma and Grandpa T at Otter Lake."

"I'm going to miss you. I'll probably just watch movies all summer." Johnny says, reaching for my hand.

I take his hand in mine and give him a little squeeze. "Don't worry, I'll call you long distance every day. Grandma and Grandpa T won't mind."

Johnny is such a part of my every day now, I don't know how I'm going to make it through summer vacation without seeing him regularly.

The semester is almost over. After two weeks with no leads, Jones calls Dad and tells him they're unlikely to solve this. Dad gets mad every time he sees more than one overweight boy hanging out together, thinking they might have been the ones who kidnapped me. I reassure him the voices are different and hope it all just goes away soon.

At home, Mom and Dad cope by pretending like nothing happened. We are back to our regular routine, but I'm constantly on edge.

Mormons are supposed to rest on Sundays, so Mom and Dad have us do our big chores on Saturday. Lees do not sleep in past 6:00 a.m., ever, not even on the weekends. Mom assigns the cleaning chores first thing Saturday morning, then she barks at us when we get distracted. All chores are to be done before lunch, and then we are expected to disappear until dinnertime so that the house stays clean.

This week I have the kitchen. I've been hyperfocused on finishing my chores early so that I can escape to my friend Jamie's house. School keeps us both so busy, we barely have time to hang out anymore, and this is my first free Saturday in months. I'm mopping the kitchen floor when the phone rings. I tiptoe around the wet spots and reach for the handset.

"Hello?"

"Hey, princess," Johnny's voice is a welcome surprise. "Can I see you today?"

"I'm supposed to go to Jamie's house. I can go for a walk once we check in with her mom. Meet me in a half hour in front of the intermediate school. I gotta go. Mom is coming." I hang up the phone and finish mopping.

Jamie and I don't get a lot of time to hang out anymore. Not since middle school because we have different elective classes. Jamie doesn't care that we are going to meet Johnny by the swings. She's cool like that.

"It's going to be weird not seeing you every day this summer," Jamie says. "Are you worried about missing Johnny?"

"Of course I am! I keep telling myself that I wouldn't get to see him much anyway if I stayed home. You know my parents won't let me hang out with any boy other than Deckland."

"That's so dumb." Jamie also has heard some of my Dad's rants about boys.

"Hopefully I'll be too busy to think about it much. My Grandpa lets me drive the speedboat, plus I'll be knee boarding, hiking…"

I see Johnny's red van parked in the staff lot just below the playground. He's up on a swing, his back to us, holding what looks like a disposable camera.

We break into a jog and run the rest of the way. He looks up as I get closer, but instead of his usual grin, his face is blotchy.

I slow to a walk.

He stands up and takes the last couple of steps toward me, closing the gap. I open my arms to him and he steps in for a hug, burying his head in my hair.

"I'm going to miss you so much," he says, barely above a whisper.

"I'll only be gone a month, and I'm not leaving 'til after the end of the school year."

He shakes his head in my neck. "My dad got a job in Portland, Oregon. We are going to be moving this summer. Actually, my mom and dad are moving at the end of this month. Jessica and I are going to stay with friends 'til the end of the school year, then join my parents there."

It's rare for people to move away from Snowflake. It's like some Mormon haven or something.

"You can't move away," I whimper.

We are both crying now. Jamie takes a few steps toward the slide in an attempt to give us some privacy.

"Here," Johnny says, handing me the disposable camera. "I brought this so that Jamie can take our picture. That way we'll have something to remind us about each other."

"I'm not going to forget you," I retort as I extend the camera to Jamie. Despite her distance, she has heard our entire conversation.

Jamie fills the entire camera roll with pictures of us crying, kissing, hugging, and crying some more.

Johnny and I mourn his upcoming move during lunch period, holding hands while I snuggle into his shoulder, breathing in the woody smell of him. My leg bounces constantly; the jumping frogs are back.

And then, seemingly so sudden, his moving day is upon us. Mom agrees to drive me to the hardware store near Johnny's house so that we can say our final goodbyes. Mom knows I like him.

"Now, Sarah, just because he's leaving doesn't mean you need to kiss him goodbye."

Whatever. She was too oblivious to know we were already kissing pros. If she did, she probably wouldn't be taking me to say goodbye.

"Sarah, are you listening to me? Promise me you won't kiss him goodbye."

"Mom, seriously. Stop."

"I'll give you fifteen minutes, then I'm going to come get you." The van bounces as her back tires roll over the curb. "Promise me, no kissing." She parks on the side of the building.

"Fine, I promise." I push the passenger side door open and leap from the van.

Johnny is waiting near the front entrance of the hardware store, his arms open wide, welcoming me. "Hey, beautiful."

The moment his arms wrap around my lower back, I release the sob I've been holding in all morning for fear that Mom wouldn't bring me. I feel him squeeze. His lips brush the top of my head.

"I love you, Sarah Lee. Wait for me, please wait for me." He tries to pull me away from him, but I refuse to loosen my grip. If I hold on, he can't leave me. I hear his soft chuckle.

"Look at me," he coaxes.

I release my grip and look up into his face. His eyes are bloodshot, his cheeks puffy. My heart fills with compassion seeing his hurt.

He lowers his head, leaning in for a kiss. I pull away.

"I promised my Mom I wouldn't kiss you today."

He cocks his head to the side. "Really?"

I am feeling foolish and yet determined that withholding the kiss is somehow extra romantic.

I remember Mom's 15-minute time limit, and I'm not about to go over it. I don't want her to walk around the corner and ruin our last moment together.

"I need to go. Mom didn't give me much time to say goodbye. I love you, Johnny. Please write to me." I hand him a wrinkled piece of paper with the address to the cabin on Otter Lake and our P.O. Box in Snowflake.

"I promise, I will write you."

I pull him in for one more crushing hug. He kisses my forehead.

"Promise me, Sarah, promise me you'll wait," his eyes pleading.

"I'll wait." I'm 15. He's 18 months older, which means I'll be 19 when he returns from his mission after graduation. I can wait five years. "I promise, Johnny, I'll still be here when you come back for me."

I release him and walk away without making eye contact. My chin quivers, and I swallow hard. I turn the corner and see Mom reading a book. I climb into the van, overwhelmed by a heavy emptiness.

"You okay?" Mom asks.

"No, I'm really not."

Mom seems to understand. I'm surprised when she backs out of the parking spot without saying another word. I twist in my seat hoping to see Johnny one last time and glimpse the back of his head for only a second before he disappears behind the building.

PART TWO

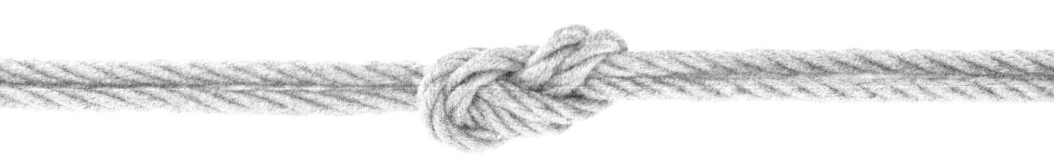

NORTH CAROLINA

SEPTEMBER 2009

28 YEARS OLD

"Sarah, where's the can opener?" Mason, my husband of 10 years, calls from the kitchen, the smell of pancakes heavy in the air.

Yet another new home. This isn't the first time I've moved our family of six across the country and unpacked alone, and it won't be the last. Such is life when the U.S. Army is your husband's mistress.

"Second drawer down next to the fridge," I yell back, not looking up from my textbook. "Did you find it?"

"Yep… Brigg, put that down. No! Don't hit your brother on the head with your plate. Just eat your food."

I chuckle at Mason's exasperated tone. Organized chaos is the norm in our house with four children under the age of eight. I stretch my neck from side to side and hear a loud pop, a nervous habit I'd developed to ease the tension that constantly lives in my neck.

The move to North Carolina had been a needed change for me. After five years in El Paso, my tribe of Army sisters had all moved on to new duty stations, and the loneliness left me with an ache I couldn't soothe. Besides, moving meant leaving behind the paranoia that I might run into my teenage love, Michael, or worse, his wife Megan. *Out of sight, out of mind.* Just what I needed to get back to avoiding the trauma of my youth.

That entire situation was so complicated I've chosen instead to immerse myself in learning how to raise my four young children differently than my parents had raised me. It has been easier to navigate the day-to-day nuances of marriage and family with my past emotions stuffed into the darkest abyss of my soul while focused on doing things right by my kids.

The move hadn't been without its own traumatic flare, though. Three months ago, Mason and I listed our home in El Paso in the rental market and were shocked when it rented within days. Rather than lose the renter, the kids and I moved out early and stayed with my parents in Queen Creek, Arizona, for a few weeks until we could close on the new house in North Carolina. Mason had just finished his bachelor's degree in Nursing and was assigned to go to Officer Basic Course, a 10-week training that was supposed to be like Basic all over again. Basic training, my ass. He had his cell phone the entire time and lived in a civilian hotel.

A few weeks into Mason's training, all hell broke loose—what a cliché, but so true. Brigg, our five-year-old son, had been different from all the other children we had fostered or cared for. His biological mother shared with me that bipolar runs in their family, but the Google search I did indicated significant trauma was always the catalyst for development of bipolar symptoms, with mood swings starting in the late teen years. *Don't trust Google* was my new mantra. Brigg spent his life screaming until his little brown face turned red, purposefully banging his head into everything, and barely sleeping. We had become used to extreme tantrums, poop murals on the bathroom walls, and erratic aggression. I struggled daily to keep everyone safe. Even at his young age, his tall frame was becoming increasingly more difficult for me to restrain. Living with my parents was the stressor that finally tipped Brigg's challenging behaviors into life-threatening territory.

Two weeks into our stay with my parents, Brigg had almost smothered Hayden, our three-year-old son, with a pillow while screaming, "You have to die, die, die." My father picked him up off Hayden and literally tossed him across the room. Gratefully, Hayden seemed to think it was all a game. The following morning, I caught Brigg strangling Kaydee, our 14-month-old, with yarn. I called Phoenix Children's Hospital and was told to bring Brigg to the Emergency Room.

Brigg turned five during his 10-day admission on the pediatric psych ward. I never knew a place like that even existed for children so young. It was reassuring to see that I wasn't the only parent with a child as challenging as Brigg.

Phoenix Children's was reluctant to release Brigg as he still wasn't completely stable, but if they didn't let us go, we would be homeless. With Mason in training and me in Arizona, there was no one available to sign the papers and take ownership of our new home in North Carolina. The seller wasn't willing to postpone closing, since their move was dependent on ours.

The psychiatrist finally agreed to release Brigg once his case worker had scheduled a follow-up appointment with a pediatric outpatient psychiatrist in Fayetteville. His diagnosis: "bipolar with psychosis."

A quick jolt pulls me back to the current moment. Squeals of delight carry above the kitchen clatter around Mason preparing breakfast, making it hard for me to focus on my homework. I lean back against the headboard, my pillow supporting my lower back. Mason's pillow is in my lap, keeping the laptop screen at a comfortable distance as I read yet another peer-reviewed article.

Developmental psychology is easy-reading material, as in easy to understand, but my God, it's triggering me left and right as I connect the dots from my own dysfunctional and abusive upbringing to my struggles in adulthood. I read a few paragraphs, then cry, then read a bit more, then cry a bit more; I always have a Kleenex box close by. My paper on developmental trauma becomes more of a burden to write with every passing day. The flashbacks and nightmares are crippling. So far, all I've learned is how much I am screwing up my kids because I haven't dealt with my own trauma. The familiar darkness of self-imposed mommy-shaming sits like a frozen piece of coal in the pit of my stomach.

I need Jim, my previous counselor, if I'm going to make it through this class.

Jim is another person I'm not sure I can survive without. He's the first counselor I ever saw more than once. He's taught me so much about myself the last three years, and I don't think I was as ready as he thought I was to transition out of counseling. It's not like I had a choice. When the Army says go, you go, and Jim wasn't willing to quit his job and move with me just because I wanted him too. Believe me, I asked… twice.

Kaydee's grunts from the neighboring bedroom indicate that my study hour is almost over.

I growl at myself for my lack of focus. "Mason, Kaydee is waking up. Do you need me, or can I keep hiding in here to finish my paper?"

I jump when his head appears through the door crack. His ability to move his lean body silently through the house is almost creepy.

"I'm good," he reassures me. "Where are the sippy cups?"

"In the same cabinet as the regular cups, just a shelf higher. Sheesh, it's like you weren't here when I unpacked or something," I tease.

"I know, right? How lazy am I to have sat around in a hotel, or in class, while you unpacked all by your lonesome?" His crooked grin always makes me laugh.

I grab the Kleenex box and chuck it at him playfully. He ducks, but the box doesn't even come close to hitting him.

He comes in and picks up the box. "Thanks, how did you know I needed to blow my nose?" He kisses my forehead as he places the box on the bed next to me.

I bat him away.

"The other girl in your life is calling you," I playfully scold as Kaydee's grunts evolve into warning whimpers.

"She's a beaut, just like her mama." He kisses me again, then walks out to retrieve Kaydee and eat breakfast with the three rambunctious boys already at the table.

With closed eyes, I take a deep breath. I hear Mason's moment-by-moment redirecting of the kids and reassure myself that he doesn't need my help. Mason has always been good with helping around the house and sharing the responsibility of our children, unlike many Mormon husbands. I'm grateful for his efforts. He really wants to do all he can to be a supportive husband. Despite all that, guilt nags at me for still feeling lonely.

I adjust to the laptop screen. I hate my glasses and refuse to wear them. I increase the text size and begin reading again.

Every word, facial expression, gesture, or action on the part of a parent gives the child some message about self-worth. It is sad that so many parents don't realize what messages they are sending. ~ Virginia Satir

Satir's words jump out at me. I pause to reflect on my words and gestures. What messages am I sending to my children?

My brain is overwhelmed after just another paragraph. Jim helped me recognize my "tells" to identify my "triggers." My mind races, I can't focus, I feel light-headed, I get flushed—hell, I even pass out. Neuro-cardiogenic syncope is what the cardiologist called the fainting spells that I have when the overwhelm consumes me. The neurologist called it a vaso-vagal episode. I call it humiliating.

Mom always said my fainting spells are "attention-seeking and fake." When I shared her opinion with Jim, he reassured me that fainting is a common trauma response.

"Are you pretending to pass out, Sarah?" he asked me gently.

"No, of course not. If I was, I suck at it, 'cause I had to get stitches from my head splitting open the last time," I explained.

No amount of physical evidence could convince my parents that I wasn't faking an illness. Jim taught me that the amygdala, or alarm system of the brain, causes a physiological shift in heart rate, respiratory rate, and blood pressure. Instead of my blood pressure increasing when triggered, it drops significantly, and I hit the floor. Learning more about the long-term impact childhood trauma has felt validating and formidable.

"The effects of early and severe trauma are extremely widespread, devastating, and difficult to treat. Because of the importance of safety and bonding in the early construction of the brain, childhood trauma compromises core neural networks. It stands to reason that the most devastating types of trauma are those that occur at the hands of caretakers… abuse by parents not only traumatizes children, but it also deprives them of healing interactions that would mitigate the effects of trauma." [7]

Another reason I had decided to pursue a degree in behavioral health was to find answers for Brigg. I wasn't expecting it to be this hard on me.

---

7   Louis Cozolino. *The Neuroscience of Psychotherapy: Healing the Social Brain.* (New York: W.W. Norton & Company, 2002), 329.

My parents weren't overtly physically abusive, but I showed all the signs of someone who had been emotionally battered, manipulated, and neglected. Hell, at 28 years old, I constantly questioned my own reality and went into most interactions expecting my position to be belittled and discounted.

A small chip on the laptop casing scrapes against the palm of my hand as I close it with a soft click. I set the laptop on my nightstand, shove Mason's pillow back into its place, and slide deeper under the covers, frustrated at needing yet another break. My breathing slows, letting memories of early childhood flood in, and like a book-on-tape, my mind begins to narrate the past.

AUTHOR'S NOTE

Post-Traumatic Stress Disorder (PTSD) can be a total mind fuck. The alarm system in the brain—the amygdala—hijacks logical reasoning and sends false signals of pending doom in otherwise safe environments. Sometimes the takeover is manageable, and other times it can be so intense the experiencer loses time and the ability to function.[8]

I was diagnosed with complex PTSD (c-PTSD) in 2013, just as I was finishing my master's degree. Honestly, I was shocked, which seems so odd because I had studied trauma intensely for several years and was working with teenage foster children at the time. Where PTSD is more commonly a result of a single traumatic event, c-PTSD is developed usually due to chronic childhood abuse and neglect, domestic violence, imprisonment, or repeated/systematic abuse/neglect. A person is more likely to develop c-PTSD when there does not appear to be an escape.[9]

---

8   "How PTSD Affects the Brain," *Uniformed Services University of the Health Sciences, Human Performance Resource Center.* May 30, 2017. Accessed Jan. 16, 2023. https://www.brainline.org/article/how-ptsd-affects-brain.

9   Shirley Davis, "Complex Post-Traumatic Stress Disorder (CPTSD) and Adverse Childhood Experiences," CPTSDFoundation.org, Nov. 18, 2018. https://cptsdfoundation.org/2018/11/15/complex-post-traumatic-stress-disorder-cptsd-and-adverse-childhood-experiences/.

Academically, I understood the effect of trauma, yet I was blind to seeing it in my own life because what I had experienced wasn't "that bad compared to the foster children I was working with." Sure, my parents never tried to kill me, they never starved me, and I was only hit a couple of times, etc., etc., etc. Trauma is trauma, whether it's a collection of micro-traumas throughout your life or the "big T" traumas, like combat. It changes the way our brain works, thus changing the way we experience reality. For me, the emotional flashbacks were all-consuming, probably because I was severely emotionally neglected from the moment I was born.

As you continue to read this book, you may find that my story triggers your own emotional flashbacks, just like studying human development and psychology triggered mine. After all, you don't have to have a formal diagnosis to experience the hard shit life throws at us.

NEW KID

SUMMER BAND CAMP 1996

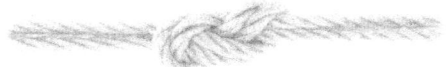

15 YEARS OLD

I miss Johnny so much that my body actually aches. A constant heaviness in the pit of my stomach took away from the beauty of the lake and the deep green of New York. I feel slow, tired, empty, and so sad. It took over two weeks for me to stop crying myself to sleep at night.

Mom and Dad can see that something is wrong, and of course they know I'm depressed about Johnny's moving to Oregon. Dad responds by teasing me all the time with his childish kissy noises. Mom scoffs at the idea that I thought I would marry Johnny. Shortly after Johnny had left, Mom leaned over the dinner table before Dad arrived and said, "I heard that Johnny watches R-rated movies."

My eyes widen as I take in her raised eyebrow, indicating how terrible that made him. I know what she is trying to tell me… Johnny isn't marriage material.

I don't care what kind of movies he watches, I think to myself. I just want to be with him. He loves me and accepts me and he defends me. Plus, he has a lot of what Mom wants on the "husband" list. Mom's expectations are impossible for anyone to live up to.

Mom loves matchmaking. A little red-haired boy in her Cub Scout troop was the first of many potentials on her list. I was in first grade!

"He's so polite, and he cleans up after himself. He comes from a strong Mormon family. I think he'd be the perfect husband for you." He was polite… when adults were watching. When they weren't watching, he pushed me down on his trampoline.

A few days after I get back from New York, the letter containing information for band camp comes in the mail. Knowing Johnny won't be there dumps me into an even deeper depression. I don't want to go if Johnny isn't there. It's bad enough at home, but everything at school, especially in band, will remind me of him. Mom refuses to let me quit. She doesn't understand love. I don't think she really loves my Dad. I mean, I know she loves him, but she doesn't love-love him. At least, not from what I can tell.

On our first day of camp, I scan the crowd. Most of the faces are familiar, including many of the rising freshmen from middle school, but there's one tall boy with thin, blond, wispy hair, standing alone with his shoulders hunched. For a second, I think I recognize him, but I can't place it. My gaze lingers on him a little too long, and I feel a twinge of guilt when my heart skips a beat.

"Did you meet the new kid yet?" Zoe comes up behind me, clarinet in hand, her reed poking out the side of her mouth like a flat cigar. "He seems a bit weird." She points at the skinny blond-hair guy I'd just been staring at.

"No, I haven't. I just got here. Have you seen Deckland?"

"Deckland got a job at McDonald's. He won't be here for another hour. Let's go talk to the new kid."

I don't share Zoe's enthusiasm for meeting new people, but he's been standing alone since I first spotted him, so I follow her.

"Welcome to Snowflake High," she extends her hand, but he doesn't take it. He looks me up and down slowly, his trombone resting on his bony shoulder.

"Hi, I'm Sarah Lee."

He stares at me, his mouth slightly open, saying nothing. I notice how striking his blue eyes are, but when he doesn't break his gaze, I have to look away.

"I'm Zoe."

She pulls her offered hand back, but he doesn't seem to notice.

"Or not." Zoe leans in a little closer.

I escape his blatant staring by pretending to be distracted by a group of freshmen who are laughing, pointing at something out of view.

"Ummmm, helllllooooo," Zoe waves her hand in front of his face. Her tone seems to break him out of his trance.

He turns toward Zoe. "Oh, sorry. Hi, I'm Michael Iles."

"Good to meet you," Zoe says. "Where did you move from?"

"Phoenix."

"What year are you?"

Michael resumes his staring while Zoe's face is growing red with annoyance.

I shift my weight from foot to foot. I have no idea what Michael sees that is so interesting, but I wish he'd stop seeing it. I avoid eye contact.

"Senior."

"That must really suck to move to such a small school, especially right before your senior year," Zoe laments.

Michael finally stops looking at me and turns to her. "I'm not too excited about it, that's for sure."

Now that Michael has stopped staring, I can find my words again, and they're filled with disdain. "Why would anyone choose to move to Snowflake?"

I want to move to Portland to be with Johnny. I don't understand why anyone would want to move to this poor Mormon town in the White Mountains of Arizona.

"My parents wanted to get out of the valley. My grandma owns a cabin in Show Low, so my parents bought some land out east of Snowflake and we had our home built here." His explanation is even more grating than the creepy staring was.

"Well, another Mormon out east of town isn't unusual," I snap.

Michael's eyes widen and he stands up a little straighter. "I'm not a Mormon, thank God. Are you?"

I feel a rock of shame settle in my stomach. "Yes." I shift my weight again, searching for a reason to walk away.

"Doesn't sound like you are too excited about that," Michael says with a soft smile.

I want to slap the smile right off his face.

The new band teacher claps and waves his hands to get everyone's attention. Mrs. Patterson told us that she was leaving at the end of the school year. I don't remember if she moved away or just got another position, but no one was sad to see her go. She never really seemed to like teaching us.

Mrs. Patterson's replacement is a short, thin man with a lump in his cheek and an obvious tic that I'm guessing is Tourette's. I read about Tourette's Syndrome in one of Grandma T's *Reader's Digests* over the summer, and his twitching looks just like what I imagine Tourette's would look like.

"My name is Mr. Douglas. This is my first teaching job out of college. Don't think I'm going to let you get away with stuff since I'm new. We will start today by teaching you how to march in formation with cadence from the drum section."

There are chalk marks sprayed on the asphalt road in front of the Fine Arts building. "I don't care where you are in the formation, we'll march you in sections later. Just find an open x and stand on it."

In the shuffle to locate an open x, I sidestep far away from Michael. Some of the upperclassmen get into a small wrestling match over their x. Zoe and I look at each other and roll our eyes.

"Boys," I mouth at her.

Mr. Douglas points at each of the wrestlers, one by one, demanding names. I watch Michael balance his trombone on one shoulder while he uses the tail of his T-shirt to wipe sweat off his forehead. Mr. Douglas finishes scolding the disrupters and returns to the front of our formation, his head twitching a bit more than normal.

"I will give you eight counts before you step forward with your right foot, marching to the beat. We will stop after twenty-four beats," Mr. Douglas instructs. "Give me a beat," he says to the percussion section.

The snare drum hesitates. Our beat usually comes from Deckland, who is a natural metronome. They've never had to keep our time without Deckland there to lead the section.

When the beat finally starts, I count to eight and start marching forward. At 24 steps I stop, and the freshman behind me slams into my back.

"Oops, sorry, Sarah." We giggle at her mistake, and she moves back into place. I looked around. She wasn't the only one who kept marching past the 24th beat.

"Look around you," Mr. Douglas calls again. "Are you directly behind the person in front of you? I cannot hear you!"

My eyes rest on Michael. He's staring at me. My heart skips in my chest and I look away, shifting uncomfortably on my mark.

Some of us holler "yes," and others "no."

Some smart ass from the trumpet section yells, "Hell no, I'm in chaos."

Mr. Douglas ignores the joke and continues. "What's our goal?" Mr. Douglas challenges.

We look at each other confused, not sure what to say. From the trumpet section comes the shrill, "Eliminate chaos."

"Good enough for me," Mr. Douglas confirms. "Back to the beginning, let's go!"

We repeat this exercise over and over for several hours. We are hot, sweaty, and frustrated by the time Deckland arrives, still in his McDonald's uniform, and takes over the marching cadence. His ability to keep time helps our formation maintain its shape. By lunch we can march in formation up and down the street in front of the Fine Arts building without our instruments.

"After lunch, we will repeat this exercise with our instruments to the tune of C-major scale. You have thirty minutes," Mr. Douglas's voice cracks.

"That was pathetic," Zoe says as she comes up behind me.

"No kidding. It's like most of us have never marched before." I wipe the perspiration from my forehead on the bottom of my T-shirt. "How long is he going to march us like this! It's July in Arizona!"

"One thing's for sure," Michael adds, "none of us are ready to join the military."

I chuckle, and he grins at me. I kick at a pebble and pretend to ignore him again. He's not handsome, not in the way Johnny is, and yet, I feel like I've known him for years. I chew on my bottom lip, fighting the urge to chatter.

"Who are you?" Deckland asks.

"This is Michael," Zoe introduces. "Michael, this is Deckland. Michael moved here from Phoenix this summer; he's a senior like us."

"Welcome to Snowflake." Deckland extends his hand, and Michael takes it.

Everyone catches up on summer events while eating, but I'm lost in thought. I wonder what Johnny's doing right now, what it would be like if he was here, what he'd think of Mr. Douglas, and what smart-ass comments he would be making to lighten the mood.

Michael is less fervid toward me with Deckland there, but his irritating stare occasionally distracts me from my daydreams.

With a few minutes left in lunchtime, Zoe and I gather around the piano with some other students to tune our instruments. As a sophomore, I'll be playing the loaner piccolo for marching band. It feels like French kissing a bumble bee, and my fingers aren't used to the tiny instrument. I prefer my flute.

"Outside!" Mr. Douglas booms.

Zoe and I jump.

Mr. Douglas takes a few minutes organizing us by section. "Auditions for chair placement will occur at the end of the week."

I take my place in the first-chair slot both because it is familiar and because I am confident that I will keep my spot. No one protests.

Mr. Douglas works us into absolute exhaustion right up until the 4 p.m. dismissal.

Zoe and I say goodbye to Deckland and head for her car.

Michael intercepts us along the way, practically skipping. "I'll see you tomorrow," he says to me, his tone light.

"Ummmmm, okay," I answer. I shut the car door and avoid eye contact.

"The new kid has a major crush on you," Zoe warns. "There is something off about how he just stares at you."

"Yeah," I agree. "He'll be disappointed. I'm not into being stared at constantly, and I'm waiting for Johnny, anyway."

"Good choice," Zoe says.

Too tired and dehydrated to say much, we drive to my house in silence. Zoe waits for me to open the front door before she backs out of my driveway.

When Zoe and I arrive at the band room the next morning, most of the students are already outside standing on the freshly re-sprayed chalk marks. I don't see Michael anywhere and am instantly annoyed with myself for looking.

"Three minutes," Mr. Douglas says into the megaphone, his face already twitching worse than yesterday.

Zoe pops her reed into her mouth as she assembles her clarinet. I click the two pieces of the piccolo into place and head for the door without tuning.

"Good morning, Sarah Lee," Michael says as he falls in place beside me. My throat goes dry. I don't know why he keeps seeking me out, and I don't really want him to stop either.

"Good morning. You don't have to call me by my last name. Sarah will do."

"But I love your name. It has a beautiful ring to it." His blue eyes sparkle; he looks floaty and high.

"Uh, cool beans, I guess. Just don't sing the jingle from the commercials or I'll have to jab my piccolo into your stomach," I warn. His entire body bounces with his deep laughter.

"I don't think I would mind that type of abuse from you at all," Michael winks.

I roll my eyes and stifle a smile before taking my place on the chalk x in the upper left corner of the front row. A girl I don't recognize, about my height with curly brown hair and freckles, takes the x just to my right. She smiles and extends a hand, but as soon as she tells me I can call her Kat, Mr. Douglas gets started.

Once again, we take our places. Deckland kicks off the drum line and gives us his eight-beat starting count. We march up the block, playing the half-steps to the chromatic scale. When we end, only a few freshmen are out of position. They correct themselves quickly. On and on goes the drill, same as yesterday; only today, Mr. Douglas stops us occasionally to teach the freshman how to stand in parade rest or march in place while we continue playing.

We break for lunch in our usual spot, and all I can think about is the fact that Michael has barely taken his eyes off me all morning. I know because I keep double-checking. I haven't been encouraging his attention, and I've been careful to make my glances toward him seem casual. I stretch my neck, and out of the corner of my eye, I see he's making a beeline straight for me.

HE'S WEIRD

LATE AUGUST 1996

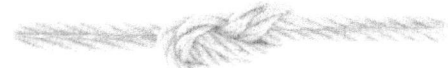

15 YEARS OLD

I'd made a promise to marry Johnny, and I know that adultery is a sin. I love Johnny and want to marry him after his mission, so there has to be something wrong with me because just being around Michael makes me feel nervous and a little bit excited. It's not like I love Michael, but he occupies far more of my thoughts than I want anyone else to know about. I've even started to dream about holding his hand and going on romantic dates.

"I don't understand why he makes me so uncomfortable," I grumble to Zoe as we drive to school.

"Because he *is weird*," Zoe retorts, brushing the black curls that have escaped her ponytail away from her eyes in frustration.

"In what way?" I push.

"He has red flags all over the place," Zoe explains. "For one," she holds up her pointer finger near the rearview mirror without taking her eyes off the road, "he's had a bunch of two-day relationships in the month that he's been here. He asks a girl out, and then for some unknown reason he dumps her, or she dumps him almost immediately."

I feel my face flush hot and turn to the window so she won't see. Zoe doesn't know that I've talked to every girl Michael has shown an interest in and warned them about how dangerous he is. In some ways, my warnings are sincere. Something *is* up with Michael, and just because I don't under-stand it doesn't mean there's nothing wrong with him.

He's jumpy and "off." Just the way he stares at me, his blue eyes all lost and dreamy, is kind of creepy. He hasn't said anything about his feel-ings for me, but why would he? Everyone knows I'm devoted to Johnny. I've made sure to talk about it, especially in front of Michael. But even though he knows that, he's still obsessively focused on me and then asks other girls out.

He's disloyal. I feel like I have to do something to protect them, and I'm pretty sure he knows I'm the one who is ruining his other relationships. I don't even care if he knows. I hate the way he looks at me, but I love it, too. I must be losing my mind.

"Okay, so other than burning through like, four girls in two weeks, what's wrong with him?"

"Sarah, do you really need me to spell it out for you? He's creepy. C-R-E-E-P-Y. The way he gapes at you with his gaunt face is gross. He can't just talk to you... he's always touching you." In imitation of Michael, Zoe puts her hand on my knee and says, "Oh, Sarah, you're so funny!" I didn't tell her that I'd grown to kinda like it. "Once he has a girlfriend, he drowns her in at-tention. You should have heard the poem he shared in English last week. He compared love to the sounds of an orchestra warming up. It was over-the-top sappy romantic. He wouldn't know what real love was if it hit him square in the nose. Seriously, no woman could be what he expects them to be. He lives in the clouds, and he's clingy. He's like a leech that won't let go."

Michael had shared that poem with me before turning it in. It was beautiful. It's the first poem I've ever read that I didn't have to decode in order for it to make sense. He told me he's going to submit it to the high school's poetry contest, but after that he promised I can have the handwritten copy of it. He wasn't the best-looking boy, his face almost mousey, but the way he focused just on me when we talked was captivating and arousing.

"Have we actually *asked* him to go away?" I ask Zoe as she pulls into her spot outside the Fine Arts building.

"Well, no. Anyone can tell you aren't interested in his attention, though."

Honestly, I'm not so sure. Some days, when we are alone, I flirt with him, and the way he responds feels so good. But then I think of Johnny, and I feel so bad that I can't help but be angry at Michael, even though it's not his fault. I tried ignoring him. When he asked if he had done something wrong, I snapped at him and walked away. When he finally cornered me and asked what he did to upset me, I lied and told him I was about to start my period. He was so gentle and sweet about it, it's like nothing I do is wrong in Michael's eyes. When he shared that poem with me, I felt special… noticed.

I haven't felt valuable since Johnny left three months ago. Over the summer, I was Dad's helper when he rebuilt Grandma and Grandpa T's deck. Dad, Joey, and I spent hours on the lake, knee boarding, tubing, and driving the motorboat. It was the first time since before middle school that Dad had had a real conversation with me. He even thanked me for being the best helper while rebuilding Grandma and Grandpa's deck.

I'd hoped that meant he'd forgiven me for whatever it was that I did to make him stop loving me, but as soon as we got back to Snowflake, he went cold again. No hugs, no kind words, nothing. It was as if I'd stopped existing again.

Johnny's weekly letter is all I have to look forward to, and since school started for both of us, his letters aren't coming every week. I can't be mad about that either because I'm so busy with cheer and band that I haven't written him back for at least two letters. It was so easy this summer, but now every time I try to write to him, I don't know what to say, like I'd run out of new information.

"Look, Sarah, just keep ignoring him. Eventually he'll get the hint and go away," Zoe advises, drawing my attention back to Michael.

I decide to stop complaining to Zoe about this. She doesn't understand. It's not exactly that I like Michael in my life, or that I have any intention of being with him, but I feel good around him, and I am not giving that up.

AUTHOR'S NOTE

It's hard to put into words why Zoe and I identified Michael as "weird." He was always very polite, full of genuine compliments, and the epitome of a Jane Austin gentleman. He often came off as unreal, and an over-the-top romantic whose "love language" was physical touch. Looking back, I think he was pushed away by so many because he wasn't Mormon, and he came on too strong and held on too tight.

That combination of traits, while off-putting to many of our peers, meant he filled my need to be noticed. Despite his romanticizing everyday occurrences and touchiness, he filled the emotional deficit I was experiencing from being pushed away from my father. I desperately needed a male to notice and love me. I needed his physical touch and praise to feel valued. That need has been a pattern at different points in my life, and when I was experiencing an emotional deficit, the intensity with which Michael gave me attention filled the void.

TREASURE HUNT

SEPTEMBER 1996

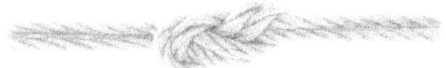

15 YEARS OLD

I roll my eyes at Michael, who sits in the driver seat with a sheepish grin on his face. I look down at the dozen red roses nestled in green tissue paper draped across the passenger seat. "That's not a cliché or anything," I taunt.

"Right…" Kat agrees from the back seat. Deckland's girlfriend is along for the ride to the Sweet Corn Festival Run in Taylor since she lives down the street from Michael.

Our friend group is meeting at the Taylor Rodeo Grounds to cheer Cassidy on as she crosses the finish line. Michael and Cassidy have been dating for less than a week, too soon for him to know she abhors roses.

"Do you mind holding these?" He lifts the roses from the seat and holds them out to me, "I don't want them to get crushed in the back."

"Gee, thanks asshole," Kat chides, rolling her brown eyes.

I can't answer. I can't even look at him. No one has ever paid attention to me the way he does to Cassidy. He just sits there holding Cassidy's stupid bouquet out to me while I take my time settling in. I fumble with my seat belt. Once the belt is pulled securely in place, he lays the flowers in my lap.

"I figure running thirteen miles warrants something special."

Kat groans loudly, and I glance back at her. She sticks her forefinger in her mouth and mimics retching. I smile at her over my shoulder.

I don't even know exactly what it is I'm feeling, never mind why. I was the one who pushed Michael to join the cross-country team to get closer to Cassidy, but now that they're actually a couple, my chest twists itself into a knot just from thinking about them. Seeing how he immediately started doting on her annoys me. He barely knows her. Gratefully, Cassidy doesn't appreciate his overtures either and told him to back off several times in front of us at lunch.

"Are you okay?" Michael glances at me as he pulls into the Taylor Rodeo Grounds and shifts into park. "You haven't said a single word since you got in the car."

"Fine," I force a smile. "I'm sure Cassidy will love the roses."

I glance down at the delicate petals looking for bruises or brown spots. I don't see any. With a heavy sigh, I climb out of the car and hesitantly hand the flowers back to Michael. We gather at the finish line and wait for the runners to come into view.

Cassidy finishes the race, first in her class. She smells like feet and is completely soaked in sweat. Wisps of wet hair are glued to her bright-red smiling face.

I look down at my feet when Michael hands her the roses, then embraces her thin frame in a silver space blanket to protect her from post-race chills.

"Sorry," Cassidy takes a step back, "I'm all gross."

"You're beautiful," Michael protests.

I cringe a little, watching Michael fawn all over Cassidy, telling myself that I'm only bothered by it because it makes me miss Johnny; Johnny always called me beautiful. It's been more than two weeks since his last letter. I can't call him because it's long distance and will cost too much.

"You must be thirsty, starving?" Michael keeps one attentive hand on Cassidy's elbow, smiling at her like she's a prize he doesn't want to let go of.

I can't help but think that if Johnny were here, we'd be snuggling on the rotting wooden bleachers. I don't know how I'm supposed to get through the next four years on sporadic letters, especially while everyone around me pairs off.

"I'm pretty thirsty," she admits. "I think they have drinks in the racers' area."

Cassidy and I walk together so she can cool down while Michael trots away in search of something for her to drink.

"Seems like things are going well for you two." I raise one eyebrow to tease her; secretly, I don't see their relationship lasting very long.

"Yeah," Cassidy laughs. "The roses are a bit much, but he's sweet."

I want to be happy for her, but she doesn't seem that into Michael. Jealousy churns my stomach.

"I didn't even know you two really knew each other, but here he is bringing you roses and wearing your sweat."

"Gross, Sarah." She digs in her duffle bag and wipes her face with a towel. "We didn't know each other until he joined the cross-country team. I don't know why he joined; he sucks at running."

He joined because I'd suggested it, pushing him toward Cassidy, even. Seeing them together, though, I was starting to regret it.

"He smokes like a pack of cigarettes a day. It's probably hard to be in good shape when you smoke that much."

"Very true," she says as Michael comes up behind her with a room temperature Gatorade.

"Your order, Milady," he says with a small bow, holding the drink out to her.

I ignore the sting of jealousy. In six months, I'll be 16 and will be "allowed" to date. I keep thinking that it wouldn't be so bad if Johnny and I could stay promised to each other and just date other people socially, not seriously, but I can't suggest that to Johnny without the risk of losing him.

A week later, I slide into the front seat of Michael's 1986 Buick Century and shove my book bag down at my feet. "What, no flowers?"

"Flowers?" Michael's brow furrows.

"Isn't there a cross-country meet today?" I know Cassidy broke up with him yesterday. She called me last night and told me all about it, but I want him to tell me.

"Cassidy broke up with me. I quit the team since I'm not a runner."

"Maybe you should stop smoking," I snap at him.

Any amount of guilt that I *might* feel for what I said to Cassidy is overshadowed by knowing that it wasn't going to go anywhere anyway.

"Someone's saucy today." He's right. I don't know where my anger is coming from.

"I guess you should be a little more choosy about who you give flowers to next time."

"Really? Like who?" Michael's tone is harsh. "Should I have given them to you?"

I feel my pulse quicken. No one's ever given me flowers before. "Yeah, maybe you should."

"Why would I give you flowers when you're so devoted to Johnny? You never stop talking about him."

Heat rushes to my face. In my most recent letter to Johnny, I had hinted at how it might be nice if we could still do normal high school things, like homecoming, with other people who understood and respected our relationship with each other. I'd had a hard time focusing since I'd mailed it. I kept having nightmares of Johnny tearing up my letter and calling me a slut for even thinking about it.

"We are kinda on hold for now." I force my voice into a softer tone, giving in to the fact that I need someone to look at me the way Michael does.

"What?" His jaw muscles relax, and I breathe a little easier.

"We're trying to be realistic. I might want to actually go out on a date with someone when I'm old enough, you know?" As the words leave my lips, I know they are wise. I'm way too young to promise myself to someone several states away, and I won't even see him for at least five years.

He pulls into the lot and parks by the Fine Arts building.

"When is your birthday?" He winks at me.

"You can sit with me." I move over in the seat, making a show of extending a charitable welcome to Michael on the band bus. Most people around us are paired off, as usual.

Michael plays along and slides into the seat. Between the hum of the engine and the commotion of students, the bus is so loud that we can sink down into our seats and talk for hours without anyone overhearing.

Now that I've told Michael that things are less certain with Johnny, there are no other girls to envy. At home, Michael is that nonmember kid who smokes. At school, Michael is that weird kid we include and tolerate. Alone, Michael is a well of acceptance and love. The closeness we have is just for us, and that's enough.

"Hey, what's the deal with Jenny Fellows?" Michael sinks lower in the seat and wraps a loose thread from my blanket around his finger. "I keep hearing rumors, and each one is a little more extreme than the last. Is she really pregnant?" Jenny and I were in Young Women's together. She seemed nice. I felt awful for her, not just because she was pregnant, but because of how she would be treated now.

"My Mom said she tried to keep the pregnancy a secret, but once she started to show, well, you've lived in this tiny Mormon town long enough to get the rumor mill." My parents were talking about how sad the entire situation was at dinner on Sunday, and how they expected us to never be so foolish, like they always say.

"It really sucks that no one is celebrating the beautiful life that's about to come into this world," Michael's voice incredulous. I study his face. I've never heard any boy talk about women or children the way he does.

"No one here thinks like that, Michael. My Dad told us about one family that sent their daughter to live with her grandmother so no one would know she was pregnant. She didn't want to, but they made her put her baby up for adoption through LDS social services. That's the church's adoption agency. My Dad said it was her fault for sleeping with half the football team. I guess she didn't know who the father was."

"If any girl disappeared for months like that, most people would think she was pregnant or institutionalized."

"You don't have to disappear in Snowflake for everyone to know your business," I say matter-of-factly. "Between the rumor mill and church doctrine, we are all experts on everyone else's lives. No one in this town gets to go through anything quietly. Especially if they are Mormon."

Michael shakes his head in disbelief.

"What's institutionalized?" I ask, swiping a potato chip from the open bag in his lap.

"You know. Put in a mental hospital."

He isn't wrong… that is exactly what people did say.

"I think Jenny is keeping the baby. Dad said she's telling everyone Kyle Johnston is the father." It makes sense to me since Kyle is her boyfriend, but Dad had said it like he thought she was lying.

"Is he the father?"

"Probably. They've been going out for a while. I don't think Jenny would lie about something like that, and Kyle's dad looked pissed at church on Sunday. He's in our bishopric. According to my Dad, the Johnstons' reputation is ruined forever. He says he wouldn't be surprised if Jenny is lying in order to be attached to a strong Mormon family like the Johnstons."

Michael yanks the thread off the blanket. "Your family is intriguing. What does your Mom say?"

"Nothing really. Mom is really quiet… unless she's yelling at us about not doing our chores right. She yelled more when I was little. She mostly just listens to Dad's rants because it's pointless to disagree with him." It feels so natural telling Michael about my family.

Michael scratches his chin, his eyes cross in consternation. "But if Jenny knew the Johnston family's reputation would be ruined by a pregnancy, why would Jenny want to be attached to them to be viewed as a 'strong Mormon family'?"

"I dunno. My Dad says a lot of things that don't make sense like that. I just try to lay low when he gets like that. Once he gets going, he'll start lecturing us. My Dad thinks that anytime a boy has premarital sex it's because the girl seduced him."

"So, your Dad believes it's the girl's job to control the guy's sexual impulses?"

"More than that. He also says once you are married, if the woman gets the man worked up, she has to follow through with sex. I'm not even allowed to say no if a boy asks me to dance. He says boys are terrified of girls, and if they work up the courage to ask, the girl shouldn't embarrass him by saying no."

"That's insane."

Dad's position on that idea has always bugged me; I'm relieved to hear that Michael thinks it's dumb, too.

"If Kyle is the father, I hope he claims it."

I imagine Jenny trying to raise a baby alone in a community that thinks she's a slut. "Lots of boys around here lie and say the baby isn't theirs, and most people believe him," I say. The whole thing is terrifying to me. I'm expected to follow a boy's lead, but I'm also responsible for making sure things don't go too far, and if I fail, it's my fault, and mine alone.

Michael shakes his head. "I'd never do that."

"Never have sex?" I tease.

"No, silly. I'd never just bail on the mother of my child like that." His blue eyes stare right into mine. "Seriously, *never*." His face is earnest. His gaze pierces my soul, and I believe him.

I'm not surprised that Michael feels so strongly. He'd told me that his mom got pregnant when she was my age. I don't know much about his biological father, just that his stepfather loved Michael as if he was born to him. He'd said so, even after his mom and stepdad divorced, that he considered Michael his child. I wonder what it would be like to have a child with Michael. A blond-hair, blue-eye angel that would be loved by her father no matter what.

"I just don't understand why your parents are so weird about all of this… falling in love, having sex, and babies. I mean, sure Jenny and Kyle weren't married, but it happens. Why not love them and embrace new life?"

"I don't get it really, either." I hate the way Mom just sits there and listens to my Dad go on and on and doesn't say anything even when he's so mean about women. "It's hard disagreeing with Dad. It's his way or no way. Dad trashes anyone who disagrees with his opinion. Besides, Mom *never* talks about sex. Deckland was the one who explained the birds and the bees to me." I chuckle at the memory of Deckland drawing female anatomy in the dirt.

"That's awkward," Michael laughs.

"Nah, Deckland is like my big brother. He did a good job making sure I didn't say anything stupid or embarrassing in front of our friends."

"He's a good guy. I have a lot of respect for that man. Seriously, though, sex is natural and normal and beautiful when two people in love come together by choice." I wonder if he knows this from personal experience or if he's basing it off of something he read in a book. I search his face for signs of a hidden agenda but don't see any.

For most of marching season, we spend most of the bus rides like this, practically alone, in the dark, under my blanket. We talk about our families, our hopes and dreams, about serious things that matter to us. He really listens to me and values my ideas. Despite his making very little effort to conceal his infatuation with me, he's never even tried to push anything physical. We haven't even kissed.

"Don't you think sex is a little gross?" I challenge.

"Not when it's consensual and with someone you are devoted to." He sighs. "It just seems like people in this town get their panties in a twist over things that are a normal part of life. Teens have sex, sometimes they get pregnant. It happens. I think new life should always be celebrated and cherished, and no one should ever be *forced* to place their baby for adoption."

I love that Michael and I can just talk. This isn't a conversation I could ever have with anyone at church or home. Even when Zoe and I talk about church or my parents, I know she's on my side, but she doesn't put nearly as much effort as Michael does into just understanding. I wonder if Jenny and Kyle love each other or if she'd had sex with him to keep him close. How ironic would that be, because Sunday was her last day in Young Women's, even though she wasn't 18 yet. Once you're pregnant, you have to go to Relief Society, the class for adult women, even if you aren't an adult. Mom said it's so the other girls aren't encouraged to get pregnant too. Jenny had seemed so sad, and I was sad for her, but I knew better than to try to be her friend with all the adults around.

I squint as the bus passes under a streetlamp. I look out the window and recognize the familiar rock formations of Payson. We still have over an hour before we get home. I turn back to Michael; he stares at me, making eye contact longer than is comfortable. He tilts his head to the side; his blond hair needs a trim and almost covers one of his piercing blue eyes that seem to plead with me. The same look that used to creep me out makes me feel appreciated and special. I'm afraid if I don't take the next step, he might not always look at me that way.

I smile back at him. There's nothing I can't tell him. I've told him things I never told Johnny or even Zoe. When I tell Michael things that have caused me pain or make me feel ugly, he just listens. He shares stories about his past that make him feel the same way. I've never felt like anyone has understood me the way he does.

I pull the blanket up to my neck. "Want to go on a treasure hunt?"

Michael leans in closer, a sly smile on his face. "What kind of treasure hunt?"

I look up at him in the low light, then down to the blanket. He pulls up one corner and slides in next to me. We pull the blanket over our heads. I click my "reading" flashlight on. He looks into my eyes then leans his face in, closer to mine. I smile and close the distance between us. Our lips meet, and I close my eyes. His nasal exhalation warms my upper lip. I press more firmly into him. Ignoring and being ignored in all the chatter and commotion around us, Michael continues to kiss me. I click the flashlight button off, and the light disappears. I take his hand in mine and place it on my stomach under my shirt. He is slow and takes his time, noticing and responding to my body's reactions to his touch in the dark.

THE POEM

DECEMBER 1996

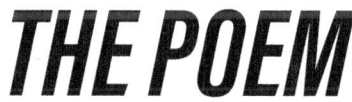

15 YEARS OLD

My relationship with Michael grows powerful, so fast. It's not just the physical stuff, either, although we do make out every chance we get, but it's emotional things, too. We talk about everything, our pasts, our futures, our families now, what we wish was different, and what kind of parents we want to be. We read each other's writing assignments and offer critiques, and we write just for each other almost daily. It's deeper than anything I experienced with Johnny. I never have to choose my words carefully with Michael, never worry about how what I say will come across, never have to be anything other than what I am in that moment in order to be loved, completely.

"My best friend, Sawyer, is coming for the weekend. I really want you to meet him. Can you come hang out with us?" Michael asks as I put my flute away after rehearsal.

"Sure, wanna pick me up after Friday night's football game?"

"We can do that. I have to take my brothers home before we do anything, though, or mom will be pissed."

Michael struggles with his mom the same way I struggle with my Dad.

"I can't be out too late either," I add. I won't bother asking for permission since the answer will be no.

Friday morning, I tell Mom it's my turn to help reorganize the cheer supply closet, so I'll be home later than normal.

After the game, Sawyer, Michael, and I sit in the front seat of Sawyer's pickup. Luke and Brian climb into the bed of the truck. They don't seem very happy about the arrangement since it's freezing outside, but Michael doesn't give them a choice. Sawyer and I chat for a few minutes before Michael starts kissing me. Sawyer steals glances at us from the driver's seat, and I see him from the corner of my eye trying not to smile.

Sawyer parks the car in Michael's driveway. I straighten my cheerleading warm-ups and fumble out of the truck behind Michael. Luke and Brian grumble about how cold they are, and once again, Michael ignores them. I take in the grandeur of his house in the low light, the columns on the front porch, and between them, a swing. All the lights are off on the second floor, but I can see a woman through a window on the first floor. I'm excited to get to know Michael's mom. He always talks about women with a ton of respect, and I figure she must be pretty amazing. I've only said hello to her once before. I redo my ponytail and straighten my uniform again. I want to make a good impression. I hear the horses whinny a hello to the boys. Michael opens the front door for me to go in.

His mother looks up from the dining room table and smiles as we walk in. Her thin blond hair and blue eyes catch me off guard. It's like looking at a female version of Michael with soft wrinkles on her forehead. I've seen her before, but she always had makeup on and her hair done. Meeting her in her natural state accentuates the similarities she shares with her firstborn.

"Hello, Mrs. Iles," I greet her.

She lowers the playing cards in her hands and glances at her husband seated next to her. Her expression changes from warm and welcoming to livid in an instant.

"That is *not* my name." Her voice is controlled, but her thin face is pinched.

"Oh right, sorry, Mrs. Vincent."

"What is *she* doing here?" she asks, looking at Michael.

"He made us ride in the back of the truck all the way home," Luke mutters.

"Take. Her. Home. Right. Now."

"I'm sorry," I stammer, cold shame filling my chest. I don't know what I did wrong. Sawyer grabs my shoulder and tries to spin me around. I don't move, so he grabs my wrist and pulls me back into the cold night air.

"Shit," Sawyer says, kicking a rock.

"What did I do wrong? Where is Michael?" I look back over my shoulder.

"You didn't do anything. She's just in one of her moods. Get in the truck, Sarah. You'll be warmer there." Sawyer climbs into the front seat and starts the engine, cranking the heater up. "I'm gonna go rescue Michael. Whatever you do, don't come back inside the house."

He swears again and slams the truck door behind him. I chew on my bottom lip, feeling confused and afraid that I've gotten Michael into trouble somehow. About five minutes later, Sawyer returns with Michael, who is shaking.

"Are you okay?" I ask as he slides into the truck next to me.

"Let's get the fuck out of here," he says to Sawyer.

"Hell yes, that was fucking insane."

Sawyer guns the engine. The tires squeal and the truck bed swerves behind us. We ride in silence most of the way home. Michael holds my hand and stares out his passenger window.

I reach for his hand. "Are you in trouble because of me?"

"No, I'm in trouble because she's my mom."

"Don't worry too much about it, Sarah. Michael and I will go for a long ride; she'll cool off before we go back."

Sawyer pulls up to the side of my house.

"It's not your fault." Michael cups my face in his hands and kisses me.

"Are you sure? I don't want her to hate me forever."

"I'm sure. No one could hate you. This isn't the first time mom has freaked out over nothing; it won't be the last. It's just how she is."

I get out of the truck and walk around to the front of my house. Sawyer waits to drive away until I wave at them from my bedroom window. I rest my chin on my hand and gaze at the stars in the night sky, running the scene from Michael's house over in my head, trying to figure out how I can make this right. A few minutes later, Dad knocks on my door.

"Sarah, may I come in and talk to you?"

My shoulders stiffen. "Yes." I push away from the window, the curtains brush against the back of my head. I sit crisscross on my bed and brace myself. "Come in."

"How was the game tonight? It must have gone long since you got home so late."

"Zoe and I lost track of time talking to Cassidy, and then I had to help coach with the supply closet. Sorry."

"Thanks for telling me. I saw a truck parked on the side of the street a minute ago. Did you see it?" He walks over to the window and draws back one side of the closed curtain to look out. "I want to make sure you are closing your curtains all the way so that no one can see in."

"I didn't see the truck. Were the curtains closed enough just now?" I ask.

He lets the drape fall back. "Yes, make sure you keep them that way, especially at night."

Dad glances around before he walks out of my room. I stand and close the door behind him, lifting up on the knob to make sure the latch caught. I listen for his retreating footsteps then collapse on the bed. I'm so pissed at myself for calling Michael's mom by the wrong name. Now she's going to hate me like so many other grown-ups do.

I glance at the notebook sitting open against Michael's knees. There are more lines crossed out than intact.

"I'm thinking about submitting a poem for publishing. Would you be willing to read it over?"

"Of course."

He flips a few pages before handing me the notebook. I fold the left side behind the right and begin reading.

The Legs of a Child

He comes to his knees, at first he's slow
Quickly his confidence begins to grow.
He's on his feet, wobbly and unsure,
And looking around a bit insecure.
The world is so big to so small a guy
But hope shines forth so bright in his eye
And at last, he ventures that first little step-
And quickly is toppled and run short of breath.
He tries it again, more cautious this time,
And Mommy is there to help in the climb.
One little step, wobbly, unsure,
But no longer is he so insecure.

He runs forth free, so carefree and wild,
I'd love to travel the world on the legs of a child.[10]

Can a man really be so insightful toward children? Can a man see these fragile details and want to nurture them? I want my husband to see my children like this.

"Michael, this is beautiful," I gush. "Wow, you're so talented."

---

10   Michael Iles, "The Legs of a Child." Snowflake, AZ, December 1996.

"You really think so?" His face lights up as he accepts the notebook back.

"It's so, I don't know, *real*." I love the way he observes children. I wish my parents had a softer view of me.

He leans over and kisses me. I push back from him and place my hand on his hollow cheek. "You'll be an amazing dad." He touches his forehead to mine.

"You can have the poem if you would like, Sarah." He tears it out of his notebook and hands it to me.

I stare at him in wonder.

TWENTY DOLLARS AND A NEON

MARCH 1997

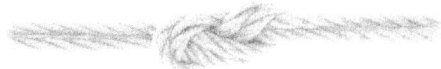

16 YEARS OLD

Dear Johnny, I *miss you so much. Nothing here is the same without you. I miss your movie quotes and laughing at your dumb jokes.*

I chew the end of my BIC pen, the noise of crunching plastic helps me focus. I haven't written a response to Johnny's last two letters. Since the "treasure hunt" on the bus with Michael, anything I try to write feels gross and wrong. I do miss him, and I love him, and if he hadn't moved to stupid Oregon, I wouldn't be in this mess.

He'd probably want to break up with me if he knew what I'd been up to. I've gone too far with Michael, and I can't take any of it back. I don't even want to take any of it back. I don't feel lonely with Michael in my life, like I've finally found something I didn't know I'd been missing. If I lose Michael now…

> *Hey, guess what? I'm not quitting my job at Ed's anymore. I don't know how I'm going to keep up with band, and cheer, and homework. Dad says I have to get my license when I turn 16 and pay for the insurance. He got so mad when I said I was fine just walking that he screamed in my face, said that I should want to help Mom drive the little kids around. If I have to work, I might as well save up for a Dodge Neon. Grandpa T said they're an excellent starter car, but Dad said I can't have one, even if I buy it. I wish you were here so you could make me laugh about this like you used to.*

I feel that familiar knot in my stomach. If Johnny came to visit that would be a disaster. Maybe not… no one really knows about Michael except Michael.

> *Will you pray for me that I can keep up with my schoolwork and band and cheer… and working at Ed's. "I swear" I'm praying for you, too.*

> *Sarah*

I crumple the paper and carefully hide it in my waste basket under tampon wrappers and tissues. I stare at the blank notebook. I really don't know how I'm supposed to keep up with everything at school and work at Ed's, too. Mom wasn't very happy about Dad's decision, but once he started yelling in my face again, she backed off, as usual.

At first, it didn't look like Mom and Dad were going to let me get my driver's license. Dad said that the car insurance would skyrocket with a teen driver on the policy, and I didn't need a license yet since everything is within walking distance.

I tried to explain that I *was* being responsible by waiting to get my license until I could afford to pay for my insurance like he said I had to. That just made him madder. Mom tried to stick up for me, but it didn't go very far. I think she's afraid of him.

"If you weren't so selfish and immature, you'd be happy to do your part and work to pay for YOUR insurance so that you can help your mother when she needs it," he screamed, his spit hitting my face.

"When am I going to have time to drive the little kids around? I'm never home during the week, and I work at Ed's most Saturdays."

His hand whipped across my face.

My mother had gasped, but she didn't utter a word of protest.

The rest of what he said is a blur.

Sleep was impossible. I had stared at the ceiling counting the popcorn blobs until the rising sun filled my room with light. I roll out of bed, fighting my brain's push to think. I need Michael before I can let my guard down.

I pace the parking lot, waiting for Michael to arrive before first hour. As soon as he pulls into the parking lot, I grab his hand, leading him behind the band room where I lay my head on him and sob.

Michael gathers me in his arms and holds me.

"I love you, my princess." He caresses the back of my head with his fingers. He rocks my body back and forth in unison with his. I tell him my story in hysterical bursts.

"Good God, Sarah. What is he thinking?"

"I don't know, I don't know what I did wrong. He was my best friend when I was little, and all of a sudden, he just stopped loving me."

"Don't worry, baby. Shhhhh. Don't worry. I'll get a job and pay for your insurance. Don't even give it a second thought. I'll always take care of you. It'll be okay."

He pulls away from me and looks in my eyes. He wipes the tears from my cheek and kisses my nose. "You're safe with me." He gently leads me by the hand to a shady spot against the cement wall. When the bell rings for first hour, I turn to head back to the band room, and he says, "Not yet." He sits down, leans against the building, and invites me to sit next to him. Instead, I curl into his lap. He rocks me back and forth and tells me that when we have kids, they'll feel safe, they'll know they're respected. We won't scream and hit, we'll reason and talk, have harmony in our home, and work together to solve our problems. I relax and listen, content to be soothed.

"Sarah, I will give you anything. All you have to do is ask. You know that, right?"

I pull away from him and smile. "All I want is twenty dollars for my trip to Flagstaff on Friday and a Dodge Neon."

He laughs, "Twenty dollars and a Neon it is, Milady."

The next morning, Michael holds his trombone over the trash can. He presses the lever on the spit valve and blows into the mouthpiece. Built up condensation and saliva trickle into the trash can.

"That is soooooo gross," I manage to squeak out before being hit with an involuntary gag.

"I thought you liked my spit."

I shudder again. "Not like that."

"Wanna go for a walk with me after you check in with Mr. Compton for theater?"

"Absolutely."

The theater director, Mr. Compton, dutifully takes attendance at the start of class but then disappears to work with all the students who are actually interested in theater. If the rest of us want to build sets for the upcoming production, cool. If we'd rather take an extra hour before lunch, no one notices or cares. Everyone he likes gets an A, the rest of us get a B. Since I have seminary the hour after lunch, I have almost three hours of free time in the middle of my day if I decide to skip class.

Michael meets me just outside the auditorium entrance shortly after the start of fourth period.

"Can we walk to my house? I forgot to grab the blue panties that go under my bloomers for cheer."

"Will either of your parents be home for lunch?"

"No, they are both at work, and they never lock the door." As soon as Charlie started full-day school, Mom quit her babysitting gig and started working as a teacher's aide.

As soon as we are off campus, Michael reaches for my hand and pulls me closer to his side. I rest my head on his shoulder for a few steps; he kisses my hair gently.

We never actually talked about keeping our relationship a secret, we just did. I would have too much to explain, and I think Michael likes being the treasure I keep to myself.

"Are you excited for your cheer competition this weekend?"

I shrug. "We've practiced for weeks. We know the routine so well, I don't even have to think about it anymore."

"I brought you something," he says with a smile. He lets go of my hand, and we stop walking. He digs into his front pocket and presents me with a $20 bill. "I will always give you what you want." His voice is intently sincere.

"Wow, I was just teasing you when I asked for twenty dollars."

"I know. I'll get you the Neon someday, too."

"Thank you, Michael, you didn't have to." He kisses my forehead and tugs my hand to lead me the rest of the way to my house.

The van and Dad's blue truck aren't in the driveway, but I call out, "Hello!" anyway just to be sure we're alone before I invite Michael in.

He follows me to my bedroom and sits on my bed while I dig in my closet cubby searching for my blue underwear.

"I like your doggie bedspread." He plays with one of the yarn ties.

"Thanks, my Mom made it for me years ago. It's starting to get a little thin, but I love it."

"Did you paint your room? It looks good."

"I helped Mom do it. It's called feather duster painting. It went really fast. Mom picked three different shades of blue to match my bedspread."

"Blue is my favorite color."

"Really? It's my favorite color, too. Aha! Found them!" I proclaim, triumphantly holding my panties high in the air like a trophy.

Michael laughs at me, "That's cute."

I shrug. "Do you want to make some lunch?"

"No, I'm good. Thanks, though."

I sit on the bed next to him. "Soooo, what do you want to do for the next two hours?"

He raises his eyebrows at me. I smirk at him, then lean in for a kiss. He raises his leg and rolls on top of me, gently pushing me back onto the bed.

Elder Rogers, one of the 19-year-old missionaries who looks fresh off the farm, leans earnestly off the edge of our couch toward Michael. "What we'd like to share with you, today, Brother Iles, is The Lord's Plan of Salvation. What do you know about The Lord's Plan of Salvation?"

Michael glances at me on the opposite couch, looking a bit confused.

"The what, now?"

He is so lost I choke back a giggle.

"Brother Lee, can you help Michael?" Elder Rogers looks to my Dad, who after months of trashing Michael, has his best church-face on for his "hosting a troubled kid" role, even though he thought Michael was un-trustworthy with young women and a disgusting smoker.

I fidgeted nervously in the background. Before Michael had arrived, Dad had a conversation with the missionaries about Michael. It was more like a warning that they were wasting their time on him. I wasn't expecting Dad to write off a potential Mormon baptism where he could be the "Savior" of some lost boy's life, and realized as I listened to him lecture the missionaries that virtually all of what Dad said to the elders was from overhearing my phone conversations with Zoe at the beginning of the school year.

Guilt churned my gut; if Michael ever could have had a chance with Dad, which was the whole purpose of Michael's meeting with the missionaries, I'd ruined that before they even met. They listened and nodded while my father told them not to get their hopes up. Elder Larson wasn't convinced that Michael was "too far gone" to be saved and led us in a prayer that Michael's heart would be softened. Then he reminded us that even the hardest heart could be touched by Christ's message.

When Michael had arrived, I invited him into our home as though he hadn't been here several times before when my family was not, enjoying forbidden pleasure. He smiled as he came through the door, reached past me, saying "Hello, Sir," to offer a handshake to my father, who just moments before had referred to him as "worthless."

Dad cleared his throat before responding to Elder Roger's request. "Well, Heavenly Father's plan for us starts with faith and repentance," my Dad speaks directly at Michael. "And when we have sufficient of both, we are baptized by total immersion and receive the Gift of the Holy Spirit to guide us in our lives."

"That's similar to what I believe as well," Michael answers politely.

"Our hope is to take what you already know to be true and add to it." Brother Rogers pulls out a picture and asks, "Do you know where you were before you came to earth?"

This might be the first time I've really considered what all of this sounds like to an outsider, or how the elders, who are teenage boys themselves, speak with absolute authority. I'm worried that if Michael thinks this is ridiculous, he'll think I am ridiculous and break up with me.

I'll be 16 in two weeks, which means I'll be old enough to officially go on dates. There is no way my Dad will let me go on a date with Michael. He loathes Michael. Michael had suggested that maybe the missionary discussions would help my Dad see him differently.

I stare at Michael who is trying so hard to be enough for my parents.

This guy, who doesn't have any desire to be a Mormon, is going all in just to make my father like him so he can date me. I'm doubtful it will work to change my Dad's mind, but I think Michael is amazing for trying. No one has ever put this much effort into loving me. The deepening frown on my father's face confirms that it won't be enough.

AUTHOR'S NOTE

My father hated Michael, in some part because I had talked badly about him to Zoe in front of Mom, who probably gave Dad the rundown on this overly dramatic, clingy kid. I never went back and corrected the misrepresentation of his character to my parents. I didn't think it would have mattered. I never did with my friends either. Fortunately, after a few months, we accepted him into our friend group, and their opinions of Michael were based on their own interactions with him, not rumor and judgment.

My own incriminating words about Michael and his smoking made my parents nervous, but the fact that he wasn't Mormon made him un-qualified for me in their eyes. I was allowed to be friends with non-Mor-mons, but not "in love" with one.

I was incredibly young to be looking for a husband at only 15, but that was common in Mormonism, and especially so in Snowflake. Many of my Mormon girlfriends were married within weeks of graduating from high school. The pressure to be married young and have babies right away was very intense. At home and at church, I was constantly being taught to look for marriage qualities in young men, whom I wasn't allowed to date *seriously* until I turned 18 and graduated, according to their rules.

Whirlwind romances, on the other hand, were normal and encouraged in my culture as a way to prevent sex prior to marriage, which would threat-en one's worthiness to marry in the temple. Without a temple marriage, a family would be ripped apart in the afterlife, thus threatening the eternal nature of the family.

Michael and I had talked about marriage and kids and a future together, but his not being Mormon, among his other "faults," meant that he was not "worthy" to take me to the temple—would never be worthy in my parents' eyes—and was therefore perceived as a direct threat to my eternal condition.

BODILY FLUIDS

APRIL 1997

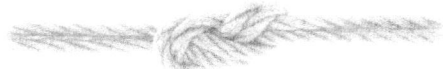

16 YEARS OLD

When I step out of the shower, I hear Michael's voice calling me from my living room.

"I'm in my bathroom," I call back to him, shocked that he's here in the middle of the school day when I came home alone.

"Are you okay? I heard some asshole in the hall talking about how you had bled through your pants down to your ankles."

I wrap a towel around my wet body and pull my mostly dry hair out of the scrunchie high on my head. I open the door, "More like, bled through to my knees, but yeah. I'm bleeding pretty good. Can you grab the 409 off the dryer and bring it to me? I need to get the blood out of my clothes before it stains."

"409? Really? Do you have hydrogen peroxide?"

"Yes, in the hall closet."

"Give me your clothes. I'll get the blood out."

"It doesn't gross you out?" I'm not sure I feel comfortable with this level of care from my secret boyfriend. Even my Mom gets exasperated at having to clean up the blood stains.

"Not at all. It's a part of you. It's beautiful."

"Ummm, you might be the first person who thinks period blood is beautiful."

I feel a warm drip run down the inner side of my leg. "Damn it."

Michael follows my eyes.

Heat rises to my cheeks.

"Sarah, it's just part of being a woman. Here, give me your clothes and get cleaned up."

I squint at him, trying to decipher his motivation before sliding my soiled clothing across the floor with my foot.

Michel leans down and picks them up. He kisses my cheek and heads for the laundry room. "You look amazing in that towel by the way," he calls back to me over his shoulder. I roll my eyes at his compliment.

I fish a clean pair of stained underwear from my hidden stash under the sink and hold it between my front teeth while I grab a pad and tampon and hurriedly try to clean up. Michael is in the kitchen with a large bottle of hydrogen peroxide in his hand.

"Michael, what are you doing?"

"Removing the blood. Watch." He pours a small amount of peroxide onto the blood left on the crotch of my jeans. White bubbles appear. "How are you feeling?"

"Fine, it wasn't a ton of blood, just caught me off guard. It used to be way worse than this before I started taking birth control pills. My period started two weeks earlier than I expected. I'm bleeding pretty heavily, but not enough to feel shitty yet."

"Wait, you're on birth control?"

"Not anymore. I stopped taking it at the beginning of the school year. I was hoping whatever's wrong with me would have fixed itself by now. Obviously, it hasn't, but it's a lot better than it was last year."

"So, why don't you start taking it again?" He winks at me, and I shove him playfully.

"Dad doesn't like it. He says taking birth control is like giving me permission to have sex." I roll my eyes. "I'd rather bleed to death than argue with him."

"That's still a lot of blood." Michael looks concerned as he rinses the peroxide away.

"How would you know?"

"I have an older sister, and her periods never cause her this much trouble."

"You do?" As much time as we spent talking about our families, I can't believe he had a sister and never mentioned her before.

"Well, a stepsister."

"I didn't know that."

He smiles at me. "Do you want me to make you lunch after I start your laundry and then maybe we can go to your bedroom so you can get some rest? I'll hold you and make sure you wake up on time."

"You're going to do my laundry?"

"Is that okay?"

"Yes, it's just… my Dad never helps my Mom like this."

"He has no idea what he's missing out on," Michael says, planting a kiss on my forehead.

Michael always follows my lead on our midday school-ditching dates. He's gentle in his care of me and never pressures me to go farther than I'm comfortable, but I know what is expected of me next. It's the woman's responsibility to make the man happy when he's providing for her, otherwise she's taking advantage of him.

I obsess for days: I don't want him to feel like I'm taking advantage of him. Once my period stops, I write him a note. *I'm ready for more… let's pick a day.* I'm not sure I am ready to go all the way, but I am sure that I don't want him to leave me.

It's only been a week since Michael agreed to take the discussions with the Mormon elders, and we've already had three. I didn't tell my parents that he'd agreed to be baptized so we could have a relationship; hell, they didn't even know we were dating. The missionaries have been playing off each other for more than an hour, with Michael saying very little.

At the end of each lesson, missionaries are supposed to get the interrogated to make a commitment. I'm just waiting for them to get to that point.

"Brother Iles, will you commit to reading a little bit of the Book of Mormon each day?"

"I can do that," Michael says.

I'm sure he is just trying to get through this discussion, but I remind myself that he asked for this torture. My Dad still won't like him, but maybe he won't forbid us from going to prom or even just to the movies together.

"Great!" Elder Larson grins so that all of his perfect white teeth show. "And will you pray to know that it's true?"

Michael gives a thin smile.

My Dad invites Elder Crocker to offer a prayer, and just like that, Michael is dismissed from our home.

Michael shakes my hand on the way out the door. It feels weird to be so formal when we are so familiar with each other.

"Thanks for coming. See you in school tomorrow," I tell him.

"Twenty dollars and a Neon," he winks.

The next morning, before band, Zoe approaches me, her face pinched, her tone angry. "Is Michael *really* taking the missionary discussions in *your* home? You know he's only asking because he wants to be with you."

"He wants my Dad to like him."

"Look, Sarah, Michael is weird, but he's growing on me, kinda like a fungus, but I like him. Don't make him be a Mormon just so that he can be accepted by your Dad. It's not fair."

"I know that, Zoe."

"Sooo, are you like, a thing now?"

"I don't know what we are." I'm not lying, not entirely. This feels way more committed than anything I had with Johnny. Still, I can't lift my eyes to meet Zoe's. "He and I talk a lot. He really listens, and he understands how hard things are for me at home. Besides, Johnny has stopped writing to me, so I think it's okay to move on." I don't tell her that Johnny stopped writing to me because I stopped responding to him after Michael's "treasure hunt" on the bus last fall or because of how much Michael has filled a void in my soul that I didn't know I had.

Dad doesn't think that Michael's efforts to learn the gospel are sincere. He's right, they aren't, but I'm pretty sure he'd say that even if they were. Once Dad makes his mind up about somebody, there is no changing it. Not even after Michael apologized for all the "things" he had done wrong. Dad said Michael's apology wasn't sincere either, which makes sense, since Michael didn't actually *do* anything wrong.

Right after my birthday, Michael invited me on a date. He even set it up as a double date to make sure he was following all the rules. At first, my parents had said I could go, especially since Deckland would be our double. At the last minute, Dad changed his mind, saying he's had a prompting that I wouldn't be safe. I didn't believe it, but then Michael wrecked his car.

Michael said he wasn't speeding, just that he took a turn too fast on a gravel road and lost control of the wheel. Deckland, his date, and Michael walked away without a scratch, but the car was totaled. My Dad is convinced that if I had been in the car with them, I would have died.

Between my "near-death experience" and the missionary discussions, Dad seemed to feel it was his place to teach Michael "valuable life lessons." At the Jazz Band fundraising concert, Dad kept interrupting Michael's and my dancing by purposefully dancing into us. Then he told Michael it was inappropriate for him to ask the same girl to dance over and over again.

He said it was a man's responsibility to make sure all the girls got a chance to dance.

I wasn't surprised when Michael told me what Dad said. I'm familiar with Dad's double standards about men and women, but I was surprised when Michael told me it was creepy advice.

"It's like training someone to have an affair. If you are looking for someone to date, then yes ask more than one girl. But if you have found someone to date, you dance with them," Michael's voice had been firm and almost angry, which was a side of him I hadn't seen before.

He had a good point too. I had never thought about it in that way. When Michael acquiesced to Dad's suggestion and danced with Kat, I tried to ignore them, but I couldn't get rid of the lump in my throat, even though I knew they were just friends. Besides, Johnny never danced with other girls at any of the church dances when he was my boyfriend, and no one ever told me it was wrong. Johnny may have made sure he was always the first one to ask me though, because he knew I wasn't allowed to tell a boy no. Dad said it was my responsibility to make sure the boys' feelings weren't hurt.

The next day during lunch, Michael told me that Dad had lectured him on sex when Michael had formally apologized for all the things he didn't do.

"Oh my God, Michael, I am so sorry." I put my sandwich down, trying to swallow my bite. There's no way I'll be able to eat now.

"It's not your fault." His attempt to reassure me isn't working. I'm horrified. I feel like I should have known my Dad would do something awful.

"It feels like my fault. What did he say?"

"He said that after a woman has sex, she either hates it or can't get enough of it, so it's important to wait until after you are married, just in case."

I inhale my spit. "Wait, what?" I stammer between coughs.

"What I learned from your father is if I have sex with you, you will either hate it and *never* want to do it again, or you'll turn into a nympho-maniac… unless you are married first." I'm grossed out and embarrassed thinking about Dad talking to Michael about sex. It feels icky… inappropriate even.

"Threatening someone with a nympho for a girlfriend? That's not much of a deterrent," Deckland points out.

I snort, and Dr. Pepper comes out my nose. Michael pounds me on my back while Deckland, Zoe, and Kat laugh at me.

I'd heard Dad say that before. Women either hated sex altogether, or they were promiscuous.

"So, what exactly did you apologize for?" Kat asks, her freckled nose scrunched up, drawing her thin eyebrows closer together.

"I apologized for my behaviors that led to his feelings of mistrust." Michael pops another fry into his mouth. "I didn't specify anything since none of us actually know what those behaviors were." I swallow hard; I'm responsible for at least some of what Dad is thinking. "As soon as I got my words out," Michael continued, "his lecture on sex began. It was… awkward."

I shift uncomfortably next to him before stealing one of his fries. I chew on it slowly, feeling the gritty salt dissolve on my tongue. Michael smiles then reaches his arm over my head and pulls me in for a short hug. I smile back at him, and he kisses my cheek.

"Do me a favor," Michael whispers in my ear. "Once we have sex, like it so much that you'll be insatiable."

I shove him playfully. "Tomorrow, okay."

With his pen Michael writes, *Yes, my love. Tomorrow,* on the palm of my hand.

On the walk to my house the next day, Michael and I don't talk as much as we usually do. Part of me is excited, part is nervous, and all of me is wondering if it's too late to back out; I still don't know if I'm ready. If it is too late, I wouldn't even know what to say.

When we walk in my door, I yell out, "Hello!" as usual, half expecting that my parents know and are waiting, but the house is silent.

We head to my bedroom. I can't relax, don't know where to put my arms, what to touch, or how to lay down. Michael stops kissing me to pull my shirt over my head and remove his clothes. He stands naked in front of me. I let my eyes linger on his thin, muscular body.

I startle right off of the bed at a loud bang from somewhere in the house.

"Get in the closet," I hiss at him. My shirt gets caught on my ponytail when I yank it back over my head.

He stands up and scowls at me, an edge of irritation in his voice. "Are you serious? Just go see what it is."

"No, get in the closet."

I shove Michael's shirt at him. He steps backward a few feet, then reluctantly lets me shove him to the floor and slide my hanging clothes up to his face.

I ignore his half-laugh, half-grunt as I slide the closet door closed.

No one answers when I call out. The front door is still locked, no cars are in the driveway. No one in any of the bathrooms or bedrooms, and I don't see anything obvious that has fallen over.

"You heard it, too, right?" I ask, as I extend a hand to Michael.

He pulls against me to stand and steps out of the closet.

"Sounded like the cat knocked something over?"

"I didn't see him or anything out of place."

As if to prove me wrong, Maestro, the cat, slinks into my room and rubs his arched body against Michael's leg.

I scoop the cat up. I set him in the library next to his food bowl, then return to my bedroom and close the door behind me, lifting up on the knob and listening to ensure that it latched before I lock it.

I shrug Michael's hand off my shoulder; my heartbeat hasn't returned to normal. He tries to pull me back on the bed with him.

"Just give me a second."

I try to calm the panic I'm sure is irrational but won't go away. I lay back and Michael takes that as a sign I'm ready to pick up where we left off.

With an eye on the door, I feel Michael peel my pants and underwear away from my skin. I lift my feet as he tugs them the rest of the way off before tossing them to the floor, and I tug the blanket up to cover me. I feel the warmth of him seep into me as I watch the door, listening for sounds in the house. I moan softly when his mouth explores between my thighs. He gently pulls my hips into his face.

A moment later he says, "Hey, I think I lost you there for a minute. Do you still want to do this?" I don't even know, I'm so afraid we are going to get caught.

"Yeah, I'm here," I tell him, even though I'm incredibly distracted. "I'm just worried someone is going to walk in on us."

"If someone walks in right now, we are fucked, anyway." I look at him, sharply. I know he's right, but it doesn't help me relax. Instead, I'm annoyed that our most intimate moment is somehow the moment he's the least in tune with me.

I turn from the door, back to him, sinking under the covers a little deeper.

He whispers, "Are you sure you are ready?" I don't know, it's happening so fast; his voice is raspy, face flushed.

I can feel his erection pressing into my leg.

I just can't tell him to stop now, we're too far gone. Besides, the way he is kissing and caressing me feels amazing. I do want this. I nod at him.

He kisses my lower abdomen, then my belly button, then just below my breasts, my chest, my lips. He presses his hips into me, and I rub against him. He leans down and whispers, "Will you marry me?"

My heart skips a beat, and I hear my own voice whisper, "Yes." I have to anyway, now that we are doing this.

The wet tip of his penis enters me. Suddenly, I smell sterile metal and hear the sound of the speculum clacking. A flash of Dr. Kline's face enters my mind. I cry out in pain. Michael pulls away from me.

A hot stickiness spreads across my stomach.

I look down and realize what has happened. "Get it in me. Get it in me!" I cry, frantic to stop the spurt of penis fluid.

I squirm, but I can't get away from it. Liquid from him is *on* me, instead of *in* me. He presses himself back into me, thrusting gently, but his flaccid penis slips out. He uses his hand to guide himself back in, but it is no use. The moment has passed.

This is *not* beautiful.

AUTHOR'S NOTE

Teenagers. Looking back, I understand the normal progression of teenage relationships. It's important to note what led to me having sex before I was ready. I can't identify the exact moment or incident when I received the message that a man wouldn't stay with a woman unless she met his sexual needs. I can say it's something I learned young and didn't unravel until after my professional training. I feel the combination of my religious culture and my father's illogical ideas regarding sex and relationships were contributing factors.

From an early age, I was indoctrinated with the idea that men couldn't help themselves, that if they weren't sexually satisfied, they would leave. I also learned that my body was the cause of male sexual arousal and that it was my job to cover my body to keep the men in line. This was communicated as early as my baptism, when I was eight, and I was shamed for wearing bright-color panties with statements like "do you want to give men the wrong idea?" or "men will look at you."

The idea that girls weren't allowed to say no to a boy's request to dance is still alive and well in Mormon culture. I was listening to a Mormonism Live episode where moderator Maven expressed that she received the same message as a young single adult, which encompasses men and women ages 18–35 (see Mormonism Live Podcast Episode 087).

My father espoused the idea that if a boy or man built up enough courage to ask, a woman was not allowed to dash his confidence by saying no. I found it extremely confusing to be told that refusing a boy's request was antisocial, but at the same time, I was responsible for making sure things didn't go too far. Boys, on the other hand, were told to control their impulses (which I understand to mean avoiding pornography and masturbation) and that by doing so they will be less likely to experience deviant desires or be sexually and physically abusive later in life. I agree with Bill Reel and Radio Free Mormon (RFM) that the Mormon Church grooms compliance, especially in their women, and that this culture of compliance within the patriarchal system is a breeding ground for all types of abuse.[11]

---

11   Bill Reel, host, "Mormonism LIVE: 087: Mormonism Grooms Compliance" Radio Free Mormon (podcast), Aug. 4, 2022, accessed Jan. 16, 2023, https://radiofreemormon.org/2022/08/mormonism-live-087-mormonism-grooms-compliance/.

TRAPPED

APRIL 1997

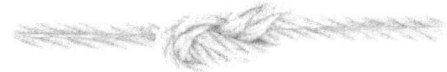

16 YEARS OLD

I can't stand the thought of pulling my clothes on over this sticky mess, but I don't want Michael watching me clean his goo off me with wet wipes. "Can you give me a few minutes to get dressed?"

He nods then stands slowly, his skinny legs still wobbly. "Take all the time you need, sweetheart." He kisses my forehead and walks out of my room.

As soon as I'm alone, I flip the sheets back and grab the Kleenex. I wipe my skin, trying to avoid letting salty cum touch my fingers. It smells. I feel… gross. I'm nauseous, and I need to hurry up or Michael might come back in here. I clean up as best as I can, flip the comforter over my bed and grab my cheer uniform. Cheer photos are this afternoon. I try not to think about what just happened.

Michael is standing at the counter, eating a sandwich over the sink. He looks like a stranger to me. His mouse-like face lights up when our eyes connect. Everything is moving too fast. I'm trying to understand what the hell all of this means, and I don't know how to. We forgot to use a condom, and even though he mostly came on my stomach, there is a chance I might be pregnant. I can feel hysteria rising. I wasn't ready, and I can't take any of it back.

Tension crawls up my spine. Michael smiles at me. I break into uncontrollable sobs, gulping for air, desperate to slow my mind and fix this mess. I want to bolt, to run away from him, from my parents, from Snowflake. I want to start anew somewhere else and pretend like none of this ever happened.

Michael drops the rest of his sandwich into the sink and reaches for me. He guides me to the couch. We both sit down, then I lay my head on his lap. He smooths my hair and speaks in soft tones that I can't discern over my own crying. I feel the need to explain to him why I'm crying, but my thoughts are shifting so quickly I can't find my words. He holds me on the couch and I close my eyes, feigning sleep to avoid conversation, my head still in his lap.

"Sarah, Sarah." I feel Michael gently shaking my shoulder. "We need to go back to school before your Mom gets home."

I look at the time and stand slowly. The school day is over in a half hour. I grab my uniform for cheer pictures. I try to fix my hair in the mirror, it's flat where I lay on Michael, but I don't care; I feel empty… numb… dirty.

"We need to go the long way, or Mom might drive past us on her way home from work." My voice is flat. He smiles at me again. I avoid eye contact, and we walk back to school, hand in hand, listening to each other breathe.

I change into my uniform in the locker room and wait for my individual photos with the rest of the squad. The photographer keeps telling me to smile and says stupid crap like, "Your team is winning," and "Show me your spirit!"

The after smell of sex is threatening to overrun my brain. I can't believe we forgot to use the damn condom, and I'm right in the middle of my cycle. How could I have been so stupid? I glare at the photographer in frustration. He keeps interrupting my thoughts with posing instructions. I won't be allowed on the team next year if I'm pregnant. Today is a bad day for me to have team pictures. One more thing I didn't think through before having sex.

Eventually the photographer gives up on me and just takes shots of me in the usual cheerleader poses with no "spirit" in my facial expressions. After the photo shoot, Coach comments that I'm not my usual enthusiastic self and asks me if I'm feeling okay. I tell her I think I might have the flu, and she releases me from practice. I walk home in a daze. I just wish I could hit the reset button and start this day over.

"Sarah, do you want a snack?" Mom asks when I walk in the door. She doesn't even notice I'm home two hours earlier than normal. I wish I could talk to her, but she wouldn't understand. She'd probably just yell at me or drag me into the bishop's office to repent.

"No, I need a shower." I breeze by her and rush to my room, scanning for any evidence she might have seen that Michael was in here. I grab my period sweatpants and an old T-shirt and lock myself in the bathroom. The shower heats up while I yank my uniform off, stumbling and hitting my knee on the toilet.

I grunt as my foot catches in my skirt and bloomers.

I wonder if anyone could see it on me, but the mirror is too foggy for me to inspect myself. I scrub my stomach until it's pink and my skin squeaks. I scrub between my legs, even though he mostly missed. I shampoo my hair and shave my legs, just to be sure I've gotten all the sex off me. I rub my skin raw, and when the water runs cold, I stand there a little longer, shivering and covered in goosebumps. Is this how I'm supposed to feel? It only hurt a little, and Michael was basically prancing all the way back to the high school. I just feel—confused. I thought sex was supposed to be romantic and beautiful and fulfilling. I feel… violated.

I swipe a towel through the condensation on the mirror and lean in; sad eyes stare back at me. I wonder how long I have before everyone in town finds out. Jenny kept her pregnancy a secret from everyone, even her parents, until she couldn't hide her belly anymore. Will I be shunned like she was? At least Kyle had been Mormon and willing to marry her right away.

I get dressed then head to my room so I can strip my bed and throw my sheets and clothes in the wash. My bedroom smells musty, and I retch. Hopefully Mom didn't come in here and smell this. I leave my door open, hoping the smell will dissipate.

Mom comes up behind me. "Sarah, it's not Saturday, why are you doing laundry?" Mom takes one look at me in my period sweatpants and her annoyance softens, "Oh, never mind. Do you want me to put them in for you?"

"No," I practically yell at her. "I can do it."

She raises her eyebrows in a half-questioning, half-threatening manner. I sigh heavily.

"Sorry, Mom, thank you for offering, but I've got it."

As usual she doesn't inquire as to what is bothering me and returns to her kitchen chores. As long as I don't yell at her again, things will be okay. I need to get myself under control.

234

While the sheets are in the wash, I dump the crusted tissue from my wastebasket into a plastic grocery bag, tie it, and stuff it upside down into another plastic bag and tie that one, too, and take it to the outside can.

With my wet hair pulled back and comfy sweats on, I sink onto my navy-blue bean bag chair. I hit play on my boom box, and Bon Jovi's voice fills my bedroom. My room still smells like Michael. I open my window to let the fresh air in.

I hum along to track eight on my *Crossroads* album. I know every word to every song; *Bed of Roses* is my favorite. The tension in my shoulders fades a little, and my stomach growls. I haven't eaten since breakfast, but I am not leaving my bedroom. I don't want to face anyone in my house. I need food, but more than that, I need some time to think.

Even after a restless night, I don't skip school the next day. Michael and I don't even discuss what we did, like some unspoken agreement. He seems to be able to read my need for space, which is good, but still grates my nerves. I *need* to talk about what happened to someone other than Michael, but who?

I make my way to theater class. After Mr. Compton takes attendance, I stick around and help paint a backdrop to look like a brick building, trying but failing to act normal. I think about all of my friends and contemplate the reasons they can't be trusted with this information.

At lunch, Michael finds me sitting with Zoe and Deckland in our usual spot. I sneak glances at him. He looks well-rested, which irritates me because I was up half the night, replaying the day before and wishing I'd done everything differently or maybe not at all. Sometime around 2 a.m., I'd gotten out of bed and written Michael a letter.

My stomach has been in knots all morning, worried that Michael will brag that he had sex with Sarah Lee, or act so weird people will figure out what we did. Instead, he seems happier than normal, almost giddy. I can't stop worrying about being pregnant. Even though he'd proposed and has told me multiple times he would never leave the mother of his child, I can't believe him. It's easy to break promises you've made about things before it really matters. Now that he got sex from me, does he still want to be with me? Tons of boys wouldn't.

"Hey, nice of you two to finally join us," Kat says curtly as she sits down. "It's been days since we've seen either of you. Where do you go when you aren't here with us?"

I'm so used to having to go home midday to change my clothes, I don't even have to think through the lie. "I'm having issues with my period again. I've been skipping theater after Mr. Compton finishes taking roll so I can go home and take a nap. Michael swings by during lunch to wake me up so I'm not late for seminary."

Kat snorts, "That is *very* generous of you, Michael."

Zoe's thick, dark curls catch on the brick wall as she slides to the floor next to Kat.

"I wouldn't want Sarah to miss out on her spiritual nourishment," Michael teases.

"Speaking of spiritual nourishment, how are the discussions with the missionaries going, Michael?" Zoe asks.

I'm grateful that Zoe is focused on Michael and not me. It's easy to act like nothing's wrong with Kat, but Zoe knows me too well.

"Well, Zoe, I can't say the Book of Mormon is true, and you can't get baptized unless you do… I'd say they are on hold until I'm ready to do something drastic like marry a Mormon girl."

She smiles and pretends to wipe her nose to hide her scoff.

"Wait, so Mr. Compton just lets you leave class?" Kat's mouth hangs open. "I need to take Theater," she cajoles.

"It also helps if you have Sarah's bizarre body," Zoe raises an eyebrow at me. "If she says she needs to go home, everyone just lets her. No one wants her passing out or bleeding to death in their classroom."

"Oh, that's awesome—never mind, you can keep it." Kat shakes her head.

"It's why no one has called my house to tell my Mom I've been absent again. They just assume I'm cleaning myself up."

"You need to start taking the birth control pill again, Sarah. I don't want you to get as bad as you were at the beginning of freshman year," Zoe says.

"I know. I really do need to." She's right. If I'm not pregnant, Michael will expect me to keep having sex. I guess Dad was right, taking the pill does make having sex a lot less stressful.

Michael slides a note into my lap. I slip it under the brown lunch sack perched across my legs. I hope I can open and read it in glances between bites of my sandwich. The letter I'd given him this morning had taken forever to write. I just want to know that if I am pregnant, he won't bail on me like so many guys do, and if I'm not pregnant, we'll take some precautions next time... if there is a next time.

I thought this next step would make us closer, but I don't feel any closer. I still love Michael, but I'm not sure I want this anymore. It feels like everything is going so fast, and now that I've had sex with him, it's not like anyone else would ever want me. My stomach feels uneasy.

Deckland and Kat start talking about prom. I put my sandwich down, unable to eat and zone out. Michael is always talking about our life together and our future family like it's already a done deal, and now that I said yes to his proposal, he probably thinks that it's a done deal for me, too.

I open his note discretely in my lap, trying not to make noise crinkling the paper.

My Dearest Sarah, Of course I'll marry you if you're pregnant, I'll marry you if you're not. In my mind, we are already married. In Matthew, Jesus says, "Therefore what God has joined together, let not man separate." We are now joined in the eyes of God, my love. In Everything, I am yours, Always, Michael

I shift into a more comfortable position and lean away from Michael. I'm not sure how this relationship is going to work. I've never heard that sex meant we were married in the eyes of God. Maybe that's why my parents and church leaders teach us to wait. I thought sex prior to marriage made me used and unworthy, like a chewed-up piece of gum that no one else will want. Do I belong to Michael now? My stomach twists more. Dad will hate Michael for asking me to marry him. If I'm pregnant, Dad will absolutely lose his mind.

It doesn't seem to matter how I look at this. No matter what happens, Michael is my only option.

AUTHOR'S NOTE

It seems silly that I thought I might be pregnant since Michael missed the target. And yet that's what I thought. Just the idea that his penis had gone inside me, even for a moment, and that fluid was present was enough to make me concerned.

Arizona does not require that schools offer Sexual Education, and in schools where a program is offered, it is required both that the curriculum stress abstinence and teach that abstinence is the only 100% effective way to prevent pregnancy.[12] To my knowledge, Sex Education was not taught in my high school, but if it was, parents may easily opt out of participation for their child. Deckland's lesson was the primary reference I had for how a girl got pregnant. Combine that with the fear of becoming pregnant that had plagued me since middle school, and I was a bit quick to assume a baby would follow most forms of sexual contact.

12   "Arizona State Profile" SIECUS.org. Oct. 26, 2022, accessed Jan. 15, 2023. https://siecus.org/state_profile/arizona-state-profile-22/

DISCOVERY

MID-APRIL 1997

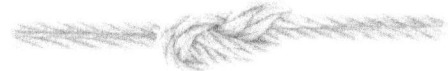

16 YEARS OLD

Michael and I sit at the top of the Fine Arts hallway with Deckland, Zoe, and Kat, going through papers in our backpacks. We're getting close to the end of the school year, and I don't need most of what's in mine. It's been a week since Michael and I had sex, and we haven't ditched school since then.

I shift closer to Michael so I'll have more room on the other side to organize books and school supplies. I unzip the front pocket of my backpack and dump it upside down on Michael.

"What are these?" he asks, setting down his checklist for graduation, his lap littered with notes and love letters dating back to the fall.

I wink. "I don't know, but you can have them if you want."

He grabs one, opens it, and smiles. I'm not ready to have sex again, at least not until I know if I'm pregnant. Gratefully Michael doesn't push me or bring it up, and things have gone back to normal other than more intense kissing the few moments we have alone before and after school.

"How many of these are there?" He organizes them like miniature files. "Someone must be infatuated with you."

The door at the top of the hallway opens, and my parents burst through. My father looks sick. Mom hovers behind him, face pinched. Somebody must have died.

"What's wrong?" I slide away from Michael.

"Get your flute and come with me right now," Dad demands. For a moment, when his eyes rest on Michael, Dad looks feral.

I lean over to retrieve my books.

"Leave them," Dad snaps.

I stand up and look to Zoe, who shrugs. I point at the books, and she nods. I follow my parents out the door toward the main building of the high school, confused, but too afraid to ask more questions. They are walking so fast I jog to keep up.

"We're going to your locker and then we're going home," Dad growls at me over his shoulder.

"What's wrong?"

"We'll talk about it when we get home," Mom huffs, her short legs matching the pace of mine.

Dad holds open the door to the sophomore hallway, and I walk tentatively past him to my locker. Mom follows behind me then hands me paper bags from Ed's that she's been carrying under her arm.

"Clean it out," Dad instructs, his voice gruff.

"Why?" I ask. "School's not over for another six weeks. I still need my locker."

"I said. *Clean. It. Out.*"

I put my remaining textbooks and personal belongings into two of the paper sacks. Finally, I slide my flute into my open and empty backpack.

"Is that everything?"

I look at Dad's red face, trying to figure out how best to respond.

"Well, yeah. My cheer uniform and the school's piccolo are at the house, but I have all my stuff. Zoe will get the textbooks I left on the floor in the Fine Arts building."

"Don't worry about that. Mom can bring your uniform and your piccolo back to the school tomorrow."

I turn to Mom who has remained silent, as usual. She has dark circles under her puffy eyes.

"What's going on?" I mouth silently.

"Obey your father, Sarah." Her voice is flat, and she won't make eye contact.

"Don't forget the lock," Dad adds.

I grab it and close my empty locker, following them to the parked van outside the front office. Neither of them says anything on the short drive home. I'm terrified to know where all of this is going. I set my belongings down in the entryway to the house, and Dad tells me to sit on the couch. Once again, I obey.

He turns to me. "Are you still a virgin?"

It feels like I've been punched in the stomach. "Of course I am, why?" My voice is too loud.

"Michael's mother called. Said she found a note you wrote to him. So, I'm going to ask you again. *Did. You. Have. Sex. With Michael?*"

I look to my mother. Her eyes are so sad, it hurts me to see. She wipes a tear away and breaks eye contact with me. I look back to my father. His knuckles are turning white from clenching the arms of his recliner. I look down at my feet.

"Yes," I whisper.

Dad lets out a wail that fills the air and makes me cringe.

Mom buries her face in her hands.

"Why would you do that?"

I shrink into the couch. "Because I love him."

"He's not worthy of your love, Sarah." Spittle flies from Dad's mouth.

"What else have you lied about?" Mom asks.

We've been sneaking away from school for weeks to make out when no one is home; I'm suddenly panicked they may have found out about this, too.

"What do you mean?"

Dad huffs, his hands open wide and swinging wildly. "I'm only going to ask you this once, Sarah."

I freeze in anticipation.

"Were you kidnapped last year?"

I feel cold and numb. Johnny is safe in Oregon now, so what does it matter? "No."

Dad jumps out of his recliner and kicks it. "Tell me the truth. Where were you that day?"

"I was with Johnny."

"What were you doing with Johnny?" His voice is filled with disgust.

"Kissing."

He kicks his recliner again, and it slides backward. He jumps toward me. Towering over me, he screams, "What have you done?"

I flinch, sure he's going to slap me again. I feel trapped between the couch cushions and Dad's face.

"David, stop!" Mom's voice is shrill. She stands up from her spot on the love seat but doesn't move to stop him.

"Get me the phone! I'm going to have that worthless piece of crap arrested for statutory rape."

I leap from the couch and grab at Dad's shoulder to stop him. "He didn't rape me!"

"He's eighteen, you're sixteen. That's statutory rape, Sarah." He pushes me off of him.

I stumble back into the couch and begin to cry.

Mom hands him the receiver. He dials a number.

"I need to report a rape," he yells into the phone. He pauses to listen. "No, he's a student at Snowflake High. Are you serious?" Dad gives his name and phone number before hanging up.

"They have a special person who deals with this 'type of situation,'" he mocks. "I have to wait for him to call me back," he tells my Mom. "Unbelievable."

He deflates onto the couch, his body still for the first time since we arrived home. I try to quiet my sobbing while my mind races. He reaches out one arm to me, the way he does to Charlie and Ev when they're hurt. I crawl into his lap, shoulders hunched, sniffling and gulping for air between shudders. He strokes my hair, pulls my head to his shoulder and lets me melt into him. I want so desperately for him to love me the way he used to, before sixth grade.

The phone rings. Mom reaches for it, but Dad shoves me off of his lap and lunges to grab it first.

"A student at Snowflake High School… Michael Iles… He raped my daughter… No… What do you mean by age of consent?"

I can't make anything out of one side of the conversation.

"I'm telling you, he raped my daughter… No, you may NOT talk to her… What good are you? You can't even keep our children safe!" He bellows into the phone, then hangs up.

I release the breath I didn't realize I was holding.

"What did they say?" Mom asks.

Dad looks at me then back to her. "I'll call them back later."

His disgust is written in his furrowed brow and sneer.

"Sarah," Mom asks quietly.

"Yeah?"

"When was your last period?" My heart sinks.

"Two weeks ago," I admit.

Dad groans, and Mom inhales sharply.

"You'll put the baby up for adoption," Dad says.

"No, I won't, if there even is a baby." I practically scream at him, my worst nightmare being realized. This is one fight I refuse to lose. If I am pregnant, I *will* keep my baby.

"Of course there's a baby. Your mother gets pregnant when I walk by her." His face has turned purple, and a vein pulsates near his temple.

"I will not give my baby away! I won't. Michael and I will get married, and we'll raise the baby together." I'm hysterical.

"No, you won't." I watch his fists clenching and unclenching. "You're sixteen. You don't have a choice in the matter. The baby will be placed for adoption. I will not be grandfather to that bastard child."

"D-D-David," Mom says in a shaky voice. "Why don't you take a break."

Dad stands up and kicks the couch I am sitting on. He leans right into my face.

"You're a promiscuous little bitch, aren't you?"

He abruptly spins on his heels and walks down the hallway toward his bedroom, punching a hole in the wall and swearing some more. My Dad doesn't use language like that, not even to talk about people he hates.

Mom remains glued in her seat.

I need to make her understand, but she's lost, staring off into space.

"I'm sorry. I didn't mean for it to happen, but I love him," I plead.

Mom very quietly says, "You must, to have given yourself to him in that way."

I curl up into a ball and sob.

Dad returns to the living room only a couple minutes later. His face is its normal color again, the anger gone, a look of determination about him.

"I have something to tell you." His voice is flat and direct.

He looks at Mom, then back to me.

Mom cocks her head and moves forward in her seat.

"After my mission, when I was at BYU…"

Mom gasps. "No, Dave, don't," she begs.

"Yes, Emma. She needs to know."

Mom folds her arms and looks away, fiery anger in her eyes, her mouth clamped shut.

"When I was at BYU, I used to let my dates ride behind me on my motorcycle. My girlfriend, Lucy, would pull her body snug against mine and reach her hands below my waist. At first, I loved it."

I'm incredulous as he details the events that led to intercourse with the girlfriend whom he hates so much that we aren't even allowed to say her name in our house. He tells me she is the reason he and Mom struggle with intimacy. All this time he talks about how evil people are for having sex before marriage. And here he is telling me that's exactly what he did. I stop listening to the details of his story.

"Sarah, did you hear what I said?" His voice brings me back to the living room.

"Did Mom know?" I look at her. "Did you know about this?"

Mom bites her bottom lip and nods. "I did," she whispers.

"I've paid a steep price for what Lucy did. It's ruined our marriage, Sarah. Ruined it."

I gape back and forth between them. I can feel my Mom's hurt when she cringes. "How did it ruin your marriage?" I ask.

"I hurt your Mom when…" He falls silent when Mom stands up and glares at him. He hesitates and says, "I will keep you away from Michael at all costs. Emma, call the school to confirm that she will be unenrolled today."

"No!" I scream. "I'll fail."

"Not if I withdraw you today. Your grades will stand as they are as of this moment."

"But what about my concert? My flute solo?"

"None of that matters. You want to act like a woman. You're going to take responsibility for what you have done to this family." He starts yelling again. "Your mother will follow you everywhere you go."

"No, Dave. I have work." She sounds determined, but he isn't really listening to her.

"Then Sarah will go to work with you. Do not argue with me on this, Emma. The stake president said this is what he would do if his child did something like this."

"When did he say that?" Mom challenges.

He ignores her and turns back to me. "Mom will take you to your job at Ed's and sit in the parking lot to make sure Michael doesn't come in or you go out. Then she'll bring you home. She will take you to seminary and wait in the parking lot until class is over. You will go nowhere alone. And you will NEVER go back to that school. Not as long as an Iles boy goes to the same school. The decision is made." He stares me down, daring me to protest, but I know better.

"If your mother is not with you, you will not leave this house. Now go wash the filth off of you."

I think back to the pink Gillette beckoning me to slice into my wrists and end this nightmare. A shiver runs down my spine. My head is throbbing. It started after Mom told me to get out of the shower and hasn't stopped. My limbs won't stop shaking either. I pick at my dinner. The table is silent.

"Sarah, you have an appointment at the police department first thing in the morning," Dad proclaims triumphantly.

I drop my fork onto my plate. "What? Why?" There's no way I'm going to tell them anything that would help get Michael in trouble. Dad ignores my question entirely and keeps talking; his expression is smug.

"Your Mom is to go with you. You are going to admit to ditching school and lying to the police."

I pick up my fork and continue to slide my uneaten food around on the white Correll plate. The little kids all look scared and aren't even pretending to eat.

"You'll be lucky if they don't arrest you for lying to them," Dad sneers.

Arrested? My head spins.

"And the next day you will see the bishop in the evening to confess your sins as long as you're not in Juvenile Hall." He bangs his fist on the table for added emphasis.

I just sit there, motionless. The phone rings.

"Emma, answer the phone," Dad snaps.

Mom stands obediently and walks over to the phone.

"Hello… Oh, hi Zoe… I'm sorry, Sarah can't take calls right now… It's going to be awhile before you can talk to her again, sweetheart… Thanks for checking in… No, she doesn't need a ride for the rest of the school year. We love you too, sweetheart." Mom hangs up the phone.

Panic fills my chest and rises into my throat. How long is "awhile?"

"I'm not even allowed to talk to Zoe?" I interrupt the silence.

"No one is going to know that you slept with that filth!"

"Dave, not in front of the kids."

Joey, Evelyn, and Charlie sit staring at us, wide eyed.

"Sarah," Mom's face is pinched. "Take a bite of your food."

Another shiver runs down my spine.

"TAKE A BITE!" Dad screams, pounding his fist on the table.

Charlie starts to cry.

The mashed potatoes taste like chalk in my mouth. I force myself to swallow and repeat the process until my plate is clean. "May I be excused?" I don't recognize the sound of my own voice.

"Just go to your room," Mom says.

I stand and put my dishes in the sink.

"Don't even think about sneaking out," Dad warns. "I will be up every hour to check on you to make sure you are still in your bed."

I nod and head to the bathroom where I throw up my dinner. I go to bed without changing into my pajamas and pull the covers over my head. I'm a prisoner in my own home. Dad will never let me see Michael again.

I really did miss my chance with that pink razor.

AUTHOR'S NOTE

I've shared with my clients the scene of seeking comfort from my father and abuser many times over the years. It's a common trauma response. My world was collapsing, I needed comfort, and I had a deep desire to feel like my Dad still loved me. Any behavior on his part that gave me hope that he did was welcomed by me. It took many more years for me to recognize that any gesture of love or kindness always came at an emotional price and eventual re-traumatization. Such is the cycle of abuse. The scene here depicts what is known as "rapid cycling," meaning the stages of the abuse cycle, occurred in a less than 24-hour period.[13] (Rapid cycling is also a term used in reference to multiple, severe mood changes in less than a 24-hour period often seen in bipolar disorder.)

Statistically speaking, some research suggests it takes an average of seven attempts for a victim of domestic violence to leave their abuser.[14] This statistic goes out the window for minor children who are being abused, as they depend on their parents for basic survival. Even if I had been able to get away that day, I would not have had anywhere to go, or any way to get there. Death truly did feel like my only way out, and I chose to live for a baby that did not exist. I am grateful every day that pink Gillette stayed on the bathtub ledge.

---

13   American Psychiatric Association. 2022. Diagnostic and statistical manual of mental disorders. 5th ed. Text rev. https://doi.org/10.1176/appi.books.9780890425787.

14   Family Violence Prevention Fund, "Domestic Violence Statistics," DomesticAbuseShelter.org. Accessed Jan. 15, 2023. https://domesticabuseshelter.org/domestic-violence/.

TRUTH INCRIMINATES

APRIL 1997

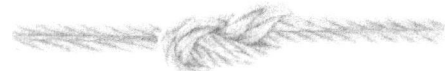

16 YEARS OLD

What do you wear to get arrested? Should I bring a change of clothes or personal hygiene supplies? I hear Mom rush the little kids out the door to meet the school bus. It's time for me to come out of my room.

"What am I supposed to wear to the police station?"

"Normal school clothes should be fine."

"Do I need to pack a bag?"

Mom stops wiping the table and looks at me. "You are not going to school after the police interview. I have to support your Dad. He's the priesthood holder and head of this home."

"A suitcase?"

"Stop that. What on earth are you planning on bringing?"

"Never mind." I return to my room and change my shirt. I pull my hair into a high ponytail and head back to the living room to wait for Mom.

"Let's go," she snaps. I wish she would slow down, but Mom doesn't know how to go slow. I need more time. I stand slowly and drag my feet out to the van.

We drive the few miles in silence. The police station is in an old, musty-smelling building. Mom checks in with the receptionist, and soon we are ushered into a small office crowded with cardboard boxes filled with papers. The smell of coffee makes me cringe. Even if I wasn't Mormon, I don't think I'd drink coffee because it smells so bad.

I look up and see the kind face of Officer Jones smiling down at me. "Good morning, Mrs. Lee, Sarah. Do you remember me?"

I nod.

"Your Dad said you had something to tell me."

He drops a notebook on the desk, positions his chair before he sits in it, and keeps smiling. I look to Mom and back to Officer Jones. I'm not sure what I expected was going to happen, but I figured one of them would start the conversation.

"Umm."

He waits patiently and quietly; Mom is no help. She just stares at me, expecting me to talk.

"Well, I never got kidnapped." I close my eyes and wait for him to put down his coffee cup and put handcuffs on me.

"Can you tell me what happened that day?"

I open my eyes. He's stirring sugar into his mug nonchalantly.

"I was making out with my boyfriend near the rodeo grounds." I glance at Mom. I know she already knows, but I don't want to say it in front of her.

She's sitting with her purse in her lap, ankles crossed, body rigid.

"We lost track of time. He dropped me off at Dad's school so that he could get home faster."

Officer Jones jots a few notes on his pad, then peers over at me. "Why did you say you had been kidnapped?" I think back to that day and the fact that both Jones and Schmidt had known I wasn't being truthful.

"Dad kind of freaked out and asked if I had been kidnapped. I just nodded my head. Then you showed up." I pause and look up at him. He smiles encouragingly. I sigh, dropping my elbows to my sides. "I didn't know how to get out of it." As the truth comes out of me, I feel lighter somehow, like a knot in my neck has released and I can move more freely.

"Lying to the police is a crime, did you know that?" He looks at me above the rims of his glasses and takes a slow sip of his coffee.

"I didn't mean to lie. I was scared, and once I started, I didn't know how to stop and just tell you it was just a misunderstanding. I'm sorry." My heart pounds in my chest as I wait for him to stand up and cuff me.

Officer Jones writes something on the large pad of paper on his desk in front of him. I shift nervously in my seat, wishing he would just get this over with. Finally, I summon the courage to confront the inevitable.

"How long will I be in jail?" My voice cracks.

Jones startles in his seat. He shoots Mom a questioning look, then scowls at her. "Sarah, what makes you think you're going to jail?" His question is slow and tentative.

Mom adjusts in her seat, crosses her legs, then taps her foot rapidly in the air.

"Ummmm, isn't that where criminals go?"

"It is. Are you a criminal?"

"Well, I've been ditching class, and Dad says that's illegal."

Officer Jones takes a small sip of his coffee, then leans back in his chair, still holding his mug. "We don't put people in jail for ditching class or for being afraid of their fathers." He watches me for a long time, takes another drink and leans forward again. He sets his mug down and picks up some papers, tapping them on the desk to straighten them out.

"If I didn't know where my daughter was, I'd probably think she had been kidnapped, too. Scared fathers say some really weird things. I appreciate the courage it took for you to come talk to me."

"Am I going to have probation, or go to jail, or do community service?" My body shakes with relief.

"No, I think we are good. I assume you learned your lesson about not lying to police?"

A single tear tumbles onto my cheek as I nod in agreement. I want to go home and go back to bed.

"Good, we don't want to waste time or resources. Plus, I don't want you to miss any more school. Isn't the year almost over?"

"Yes, but I'm not allowed to go back to school."

Officer Jones raises his eyebrow at me and glances at Mom with his jaw set.

My Mom jumps to her feet. "Well, thank you, Officer. I'm sure my husband will be in touch." She is almost out of the room when she says, "Let's go, Sarah."

I stand still, examining his face. Usually his look is kind, or completely unreadable. His lips are pursed. His eyes squint toward Mom, full of fiery... hate, no... loathing.

Mom grabs my arm and yanks me out of the tiny office.

Her pace is fast, and I stumble behind her. I pull my arm free and peer down at the tiny fingernail marks left on my pale skin.

"Mom, when are you going to return my cheer uniform and piccolo?"

"Hmmmmm? Oh, tomorrow morning before I go to work." Her words are non-committal, as if she's not even aware that she's said them.

"What am I going to do while you are at work?" My tone measured. Saying the wrong thing here would be disastrous, especially since I'd heard Dad tell Mom she was to tell him everything that occurred this morning.

She shrugs and sighs with defeat. "Stay at home, I guess."

"Do I have to go to seminary?"

She whips her head around and glowers at me. "Oh, yes," she says through clenched teeth.

I'm taken aback by her sudden awareness. I feel guilty for asking so many questions. I know she hates it, but I hate not knowing what comes next. This is new territory for both of us. I can tell she's overwhelmed, but still she obeys Dad, like one of his minions. I almost feel bad for her.

I wish she would just take us all away and hide from Dad, but he's a "good man" and we all have to make "sacrifices" in relationships. Like me, she's being forced into this even though she doesn't agree with him. At least, I don't think she does. In that way, we are both at Dad's mercy.

I promise myself, there in the parking lot, to *never* allow anyone to abuse my future child. Not ever!

"I can't miss more work today, so I guess you can skip seminary since I can't trust you to be there on your own," Mom says breaking into my thoughts. "We'll start our new schedule tomorrow. I'm going to take you home." She heaves another deep sigh. "I guess I will have to call you every thirty minutes. If you don't answer, I will call your Dad and come straight home."

"Okay," I say, feeling resigned. At least she won't be staying home with me. I stare out the passenger window. I'm not used to being on Main Street on a weekday morning. Most of the parking lots are pretty empty.

Mom drops me off a few minutes later and tells me to clean my room as she dashes off to work later than expected. I sit on the couch and stare at nothing, waiting for her calls. They do come every 30 minutes as promised.

After the fourth check-in, the doorbell rings. There is loud pounding on my door.

Zoe is on my doorstep, frantic. "What in the hell is going on?" she demands.

"My parent's found out I had sex with Michael and now I'm not allowed to see him, ever again. I'm not even allowed back in school as long as he's there."

As soon as the words are out of my mouth, I burst into tears.

"Dad says if I'm pregnant I have to put the baby up for adoption. They won't even let me have a choice. They made me go to the police."

"Are you serious, the police?"

I wipe roughly at my face, embarrassed that I am crying but glad to be able to tell someone what I'm going through.

Zoe's eyes are wide in shock. "God, your Dad is so fucked up. Are you alone here?"

"Yes."

"Well, that's dumb. Michael's gonna figure that out and come see you."

I shake my head. "I'm only alone today, tomorrow is when the new routine starts. I don't even know what it is." I wipe my eyes, grateful Zoe is here to think for me.

"Oh, come on, Sarah, they can't watch you 100% of the time."

"Dad says Mom has to follow me everywhere, even to Ed's and seminary. She has to sit outside in the parking lot in case Michael tries to come visit me."

"That's insane!"

Zoe's fury is comforting in a way.

"I don't know what to do. Dad is so mad."

"Oh, I know. He called my mom and Kat's parents and yelled at them, saying we're bad friends because we didn't stop you from sleeping with Michael. Neither of us even knew you two were going out. I bet he called Cassidy's dad, too."

"Are you serious? Why would he do that? This doesn't make any sense. He doesn't want anyone to know, yet he made me go to the police, he's pulling me out of school *and* calling all of you. The entire town is going to be gossiping about me before Sunday." I pace my living room frantically.

"Yep. If he wanted to keep this quiet, he royally fucked up. He's the one who started the gossip chain." Her wild curls frame her red face.

"Shit, what is everyone saying at school?" My heart pounds so hard I can see my shirt vibrate above my breasts.

"That you're pregnant. Are you?"

"It's too soon to tell. We won't know for at least a week or two." Her eyes lower to my stomach then back up to my face.

"Now would be a really good time for your period to do its thing and show up early," she growls.

The phone rings, and I shush her.

"Hi, Mom. Yes, I'm alone. Okay." I hang up.

"This is nuts, Sarah. What can I do?"

I grab paper and write Michael a note.

Don't come to my house. It's not safe. Mom is going to take me to seminary and sit outside and watch. Same for my shifts at Ed's. Dad is trying to get you arrested. I'm sorry. I love you.

I hand the note to Zoe. "Give this to Michael. It's not safe if he tries to come visit me right now."

Zoe hugs me. "I'll find ways to come check on you, even they can't keep you locked away forever."

I hang onto those words.

Mom starts cooking dinner as soon as she arrives home from work. I hide in my bedroom to avoid talking to my siblings. They know better than to ask what happened, but I have no patience for their concern. The entire house seems to be on edge. Despite being nestled under my covers, I hear Dad's voice roar over Joey and Evelyn's bickering.

"What do you mean they did nothing?"

I crawl deeper into the bed and pull my pillow over my ears, trying to block the fact that my own father wants me to go to jail. He really does hate me.

"I'm calling his supervisor," he bellows over the now terrified cries of Charlie and Evelyn.

My Dad is my captor. I'm a prisoner in my own home.

The smell of morning pancakes is nauseating. Dad sits at the head of the table as usual, with a smug look on his face.

"Sarah, I spoke with the supervisor of Officer Jones late last night. You have been assigned probation for skipping school."

I remain silent.

Mom continues to flip the pancakes, which sizzle on the electric griddle.

"You will join Mom in her classroom as a kindergarten teacher's aide for the remainder of the school year, at which time, your probation will be over. Mom can take her lunch between the morning and afternoon sessions so that you can still attend seminary. Do you have any questions?"

"Officer Jones said it's not against the law to ditch school, so why do I have probation?" I feel betrayed... I thought Jones was a little bit on my side, at least I thought I could trust what he said. I wait for Charlie to finish drowning her pancakes before taking the sticky syrup bottle from her.

"I wouldn't argue with the police, Sarah. You're lucky they didn't arrest you for lying to them about being kidnapped. Be grateful they're going so easy on you." He leans forward in his chair, his tie tucked into the space on his shirt between buttons to keep it safe from our sugary meal.

I slump back in my chair, losing the energy to fight with him. He'd already told me two days ago that I had to go to work with Mom, which seems weird, but I'm too defeated to put much thought into it. "All right, sorry. I'm just confused."

"Sarah, you need to dress professionally for the classroom." Mom sets the platter of remaining pancakes at the head of the table in front of Dad and Joey. "Please put on one of your Sunday dresses when you are finished eating. We leave in about twenty minutes."

"What about my piccolo? If I don't turn it in, we'll get charged for it."

Mom releases a low growl. "Tomorrow. I can't be late for work again."

I like kids, so my probation during Mom's class doesn't seem too bad. Mom tells me how they had to call the principal and get special permission for me to go to work with her. I don't really care. If it's such a big deal, why not just let me go back to school? Dad has already ruined my reputation. Not attending high school so that I can babysit at an elementary school doesn't seem like a good way to punish me for not going to my classes.

Mom pulls into a parking spot in the staff area for Highland Primary. I climb out of the van and straighten my dress. Just before we enter the building, Mom stops me.

"You have a meeting with the bishop tonight to confess your sins."

They've pulled me out of school and won't let me talk to my friends. I'm not about to go be humiliated in the bishop's office and listen to him lecture me about the evils of sexual sin.

"Mom, no!"

"You have to."

I spend the remainder of the morning emotionally numb, and sit in the far corner table, cutting things out and coloring with kids, but not saying anything.

At lunch, she takes me to seminary. I don't know why she bothers. I can't focus, and I have no idea what the lesson is on. We head back to Mom's school immediately after. I am assigned recess duty. The other teachers gather in small groups and chat while I wander around the playground thinking about Michael and wondering if he's in trouble with the police, too.

After school, we go home, saying nothing. Mom boils hotdogs for the kids. Dad stomps in and says nothing to me or anyone else. We eat in silence, except for Mom giving Joey babysitting instructions for the evening. The threat of having to confess to Nephi's dad that I had sex looms over me. Nephi is in my third-hour English class, and we've gone to Sunday School together since my family moved back to Snowflake after Dad finished his graduate degree. He and his parents have always been kind to me, but still it's weird. Supposedly, Bishop has the power to judge me as if he were God. I ignore the slimy hot dog and pretend to sip my milk.

Forty minutes later, Mom, Dad, and I walk into the empty church house that feels eerie without other people there to warm up the building. Bishop Blyth greets us formally and then his gaze turns to me. He invites me into his large, cold office, alone.

He sits on a rolling chair behind a big executive desk. Pictures of the prophet adorn the wall behind him. President Hinkley is a tiny man. His wrinkled-up eyes seem to jump out of the picture and stare into my brain.

"Sarah, let's open this meeting with a prayer, would that be okay?"

I stare at his thick brown hair and nod. No one is really allowed to say no to a prayer.

"Would you please offer it?"

I clench my jaw and glare at him for a moment before looking at an adjacent wall.

"That's okay, I can say it this time," he concedes.

He bows his head and folds his arms across his chest in the way I've been taught to pray my entire life. I stare at him with his eyes closed, fighting the impulse to run. The only thing keeping me in my chair is knowing my parents are on the other side of the closed door.

He finishes his supplication by asking for the Spirit to be with me so I can be sufficiently humbled and open to receive my Savior's love once again.

My blood boils. Why is it that the Savior won't allow me to feel his love unless I confess my sins to my bishop? Why would he stop loving me in the first place?

Bishop must feel the Spirit because he opens his eyes and jumps right in. "Sarah, the Savior has manifested to me how much he loves you. What did you want to tell me tonight?"

"I didn't want to. They're making me." I gesture with my head toward the door.

"Your parents?"

I nod.

"Why do you think they wanted you to come talk to me?"

I stare at him. He already knows. I heard Mom telling him about it on the phone when she set up the appointment. I wonder if his son Nephi knows now too, not that it matters since Zoe said the entire school is buzzing about my being pregnant.

I sigh. There is no getting out of this. I might as well get it over with so I can go home back to my prison. "Because I'm not a virgin anymore."

He doesn't even look shocked, or mad, which is a huge relief.

He starts quoting scriptures and telling me how much Jesus loves me. He tells me about the woman from the Bible who was dragged into the city center, pulled away from her lover in the middle of sex. I'm only half listening. I look at the bishop and think of Jenny Fellows from church and how she has to go to Relief Society now that she's pregnant. At least I won't be the only teenager in Relief Society.

"What do you think, Sarah?"

"About what?" I startle and my face flushes.

"Do you understand what I'm asking of you?"

"Can you ask me again? I think I tuned out there for a second." I inwardly scold myself. Ever since Mom and Dad showed up at the school, I've been extra jumpy, and I can't seem to focus on anything for very long.

"Of course. Our Savior loves us, he loves you. I love you, and your parents love you." He cocks his head to the side, his face soft.

I huff. "No, they don't. Well, maybe Mom does, but Dad hasn't loved me since before middle school."

The bishop sits upright. "What makes you say that?" I rise from my chair and knock the small picture of Jesus on the corner of his desk to the floor.

"He never hugs me. He used to, until I started to grow boobs. He's always picking on me about my looks, teasing me about my frizzy hair and my acne. Nothing I do is ever good enough, and he only gives me compliments if I'm the best at something." I pause to catch my breath then add, "Oh yeah, he yells at me all the time, and he's slapped me. He told me it's my fault Joey looks at porn, and he goes on and on about how my behavior is tempting boys, and how I'm going to mess them up because I'm a girl and boys can't help themselves." I realize I've been screaming at him and look at the heavy wooden door, expecting my Dad to burst through it and "correct" me.

Bishop's face appears sad. He just looks at me, deep in thought. I slump back in my chair.

"My wife used to feel that way. It's not true, you know." His voice is almost a whisper. "Boys are responsible for staying morally clean, too."

I roll my eyes. "I'm not sure anyone else agrees with you, even if you are the bishop."

He furrows his brow. "Would you like to speak with my wife? She experienced something hard like this when she was younger."

Yeah right, I doubt her dad wanted her to go to jail, I want to scream at him, but don't. He's just trying to be nice. It's not his fault my Dad is a bully and that my Mom won't stand up to him. "No, but thanks. Can I go now?"

"In a minute. I have just a few more things we need to cover."

I shrug, feeling defeated. Once again, I'm at the mercy of "my priesthood holder."

"Sarah, the Lord requires us to be worthy in order to partake of his sacrament. These restrictions are meant to help you on your path to repentance. I ask that you not take the sacrament until I tell you otherwise. You may not pray in church, and you will attend Relief Society with your mother until your probation period is up. I'd like to meet with you every Wednesday night for the time being. Do you understand what I'm asking of you?"

Bishop Blyth is a kind man, but I don't care. The Savior gave no punishment to the grown-up woman pulled from her lover's bed, and all He did was say, "Don't do it again." But I have to stay away from all of my friends, not be allowed to go to school, go to work with my Mom on probation, and have her follow me everywhere? Jesus is an asshole if you ask me.

I walk out of his office, past my parents, and out the double doors. I start walking home and then realize that will only get me into more trouble. So, I turn back and lean against the van as the sun sets behind the large trees planted by the Mormon Pioneers when they built the Main Street Chapel. It takes almost an hour before my parents join me. By that time, I'd counted every green shingle on the roof of the church building.

"Sarah, Bishop would like for you to talk to a counselor from LDS Family Services to help you understand the repentance process a little better." Mom seems calm and reassured that speaking to another man whom I don't know will fix this whole mess.

She has no idea how wrong she is, even if I am not pregnant.

AUTHOR'S NOTE

The Mormon Church teaches that serious transgressions, such as premarital or extramarital sex, must be confessed to the bishop, who receives revelation from God that will guide the penitent individual through the repentance process so that they can receive forgiveness.[15] While the Mormon Church does not directly teach its members to drag sinners to confession, it is common for desperate parents or hurt spouses to manipulate, pressure, or even force these meetings.

In some cases, the bishop may respond by calling a disciplinary council (now called a Council of Love) made up of male leaders in the church who decide together what action, if any, should be taken. Possible outcomes of a disciplinary council include being disfellowshiped, where a church member is prohibited from holding callings, offering prayer at church, and partaking of the sacrament, or being excommunication, where a person is no longer considered a member of the church at all.

In theory, confession to a bishop and the variety of actions that may follow are meant to provide support in healing and change, and to help those who participate feel healthy, whole, and loved. In practice, it left me feeling traumatized, shamed, publicly humiliated, unloved, and unworthy; unfortunately, I have lost track of the number of my patients, friends, and acquaintances who were similarly failed.

---

15   "32. Repentance and Church Membership Councils." Church of Jesus Christ of Latter-Day Saints, August 24, 2022. https://www.churchofjesuschrist.org/study/manual/general-handbook/32-repentance-and-membership-councils?lang=eng.

FIRE

END OF APRIL 1997

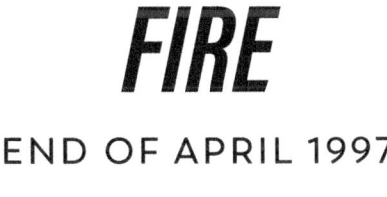

16 YEARS OLD

Being stuck in a kindergarten classroom with nothing to do sucks! After recess, Ms. Eleanor, the kindergarten teacher with whom Mom works asks me to read a story to the kids. One of them whines about being tired and begs me to let him lay down, so I say yes and then all the kids copy him. I'm not even halfway finished with the story before most of the kids are sound asleep, which I think is great. They are obviously tired and now we get some quiet time, but Ms. Eleanor tells me, "This is why you don't let them lay down."

On the playground the kids don't listen to me. They call me the "fake teacher." I tell Mom and she says I have to be firmer with them. I try, but they still ignore me. I'm not allowed to discipline them; I can't even tell them to sit out for a little while, so they have little respect for me and act like heathens.

Mom says I have poor classroom management skills. "How am I sup-posed to keep them from touching each other if I'm not allowed to make them take a break and sit by me for a minute?" My protests are ignored.

Mom keeps telling me things will get better once I talk to the coun-selor. I remind her that she still hasn't returned my piccolo. Amy is on the JV cheer line, and one Sunday at church, I give her my uniform to turn in for me, but the borrowed piccolo still sits on the shelf in the kitchen. I suggested that Zoe could come over and pick it up to turn it in for me, but I got yelled at and reminded of my sentence, which didn't appear to have an end in sight.

Mom is sick of following me around everywhere. She told Dad after the third day that she wouldn't wait for me while I work at Ed's anymore because she had better things to do. They decide that Mom would just drop me off and pick me up, instead of allowing me to walk the four blocks to and from work.

I make sure Zoe tells Michael, and he comes into the store the follow-ing Saturday, drops a note into my smock pocket, whispers, "I love you," and walks out. The heat of his breath on my neck feels familiar, and I want to grab him and wrap him in a long embrace.

Ten minutes later, his stepdad walks into the store looking furious. Michael is long gone so I pretend not to recognize him and ring up the next customer, hoping my shaking hands don't give me away.

As soon as I get a break, I lock myself in the bathroom and unfold the note.

Sarah, my love, being apart is killing me. I haven't been able to think about anything else since your parents came to get you. My heart aches just imagining what you're having to endure. I'm so sorry that I kept the note, I should have known that my mom would snoop through my keepsake box. I've got a plan. Have a bag packed, be ready to go at a moment's notice. I'm coming to get you. We will have the beautiful life, marriage, and family we've been dreaming of. I'll be a devoted husband. You'll never want for anything. I love you so much, Michael.

P.S. If you are pregnant, I will refuse to sign the adoption papers. No one will take our baby away from us.

My packed suitcase is in my closet, ready to go. I just need Michael to come for me.

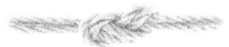

Monday morning, Mom remembers to stop by the band room on the way to work so that I can return my piccolo. I stare out the window at a tumbleweed, listening to the sound of gravel crunch under the van's tires in the parking lot across the street from the Fine Arts building.

"You have five minutes." Mom picks up the novel she has been reading and flips through the pages before finding her spot. "If it takes you longer than that, I'm coming in after you."

I hop out of the van with the tiny piccolo case and sprint across the street. In the band room, everyone starts calling my name and pointing.

"Hey look, it's Sarah!" Someone slaps me on the back.

"What did you do? Your parents are insane!" Soon, I'm surrounded by band members.

"Where's Michael?" I demand.

"I'll go get him," Layla calls, "he said he would be in the library."

Zoe asks, "Do I need to go stall your Mom?"

"No," I say, shoving the case into her hand. "Can you make sure Mr. Douglas gets this, so I don't get fined?"

"Of course. I'll stand watch for you."

I frantically look around the room for Michael. I need to see him. Even if it is just for a minute. I need to touch him and feel him. Deckland and Kat refuse to make eye contact with me.

I didn't blame them for being mad. Dad had called their parents and reamed them out. Thanks for ruining more of my friendships, Dad.

I look up at the clock, my time is up.

Michael bursts into the band room from the inside doors. I rush into his arms and hug him hard while he kisses the top of my head. A few kids catcall, but most just stare at us. I can hear him panting from running and feel his heart pounding against my breasts.

"I have to go, sorry." I kiss him quickly on the lips and run out the door towards the parking lot.

"I was just about to come in there after you. What took so long? Did you see Michael?"

"Mr. Douglas was on the phone. I finally gave up, and Zoe said she'd turn the instrument in for me."

The next day, Michael sneaks into seminary and drops a note in my lap. He slides into the seat behind me.

"Did my Mom see you?" My heart jumps into my throat. Seminary is the only time I have with people my own age, and I don't want his presence to ruin that for me.

"I'm wearing a hoodie."

"That doesn't make you invisible," I hiss.

Less than a minute later, the door opens and my Mom is standing there. "Let's go, Sarah," Mom calls out.

I can feel the redness creep up into my face as I walk by her through the door. In the empty parking lot I yell, "You didn't even give me a chance to leave on my own! How will you know you can trust me again, if you never even give me the chance?"

She looks genuinely sorrowful.

"You're right, I should've given you a chance." She pulls into our driveway instead of going to the elementary school. "You can have the rest of the day off."

Once I'm safely alone, I open Michael's note.

I love you, wait for me. I'll find a way, I promise.

I clutch the note. I need him to find a way. It's not just that this is the first time I've been alone in two weeks, it's that my parents treat me like I'm a criminal, and my Dad doesn't even try to hide his hatred and disgust. I change out of my Sunday "work" dress and head for the bathroom. My period has started. Not pregnant. I show my underwear to Mom when she gets home from work, and she falls to her knees.

"Thank you, Heavenly Father," she says over and over again.

I sit on the couch, watching her clasped hands and tear-streaked cheeks turned to the sky in gratitude. She looks crazy.

I thought she was reaching for the phone to call my Dad, but a moment later she says, "Hello, Maria, this is Emma, Sarah's mom. Yes, of course you know who I am. No, I wanted to let you know that Sarah's period started today."

I don't wait to hear the rest of Mom's conversation with Michael's mom. I go to my room, climb into bed, and stay there through dinner.

How much longer am I going to be a prisoner? I lay awake, staring into the dark. I think about Johnny. I wonder if it had been Johnny instead of Michael, would the punishment be so bad? I sit up with a start, remembering that my journal is filled with details about all the times Johnny and I made out.

I leap from my bed and dig in the bottom corner cubby of my closet, searching for my secret journal. I open it up and several pictures of Johnny and me kissing fall into my lap. I flip through the pages. If my parent's find this, they will call his parents in Portland and make things even worse for both of us. They already called them to tell them he and I had made out the day I said I was kidnapped. Who knows what else Dad said. I wonder if he told them about Michael too.

I shove the shoebox full of letters and love notes from Johnny and Michael back into the cubby and stuff my journals on top of it. I slide the pictures into my pillowcase and lay down on them. My parents come to say goodnight at eight. I listen, waiting for the familiar sounds that the house is quiet for the evening.

Once I am sure everyone is in bed, I roll over and flip my lamp on. I slowly flip through the pictures, sometimes smiling, sometimes laughing, sometimes crying as I burn each image into my memory forever. I creep out of bed and read my journals, reminiscing, taking the time to close my eyes and relive my favorite moments. I focus on the smells, Johnny's cologne, Michael's roses. And then I say goodbye.

I check the time on my alarm clock. It's 3:30 a.m. Dad is usually up between 4–4:30. I put the pictures and letters back in the shoe box, stack the journals on top, then I cover them with my clothes. I climb into bed and close my eyes only to wake a few hours later to the familiar smell of pancakes.

"Breakfast is ready!"

It's 6 a.m. I roll out of bed, ready to get my Saturday cleaning assignment. I stumble into the kitchen, still groggy from sleep. Evelyn is bright-eyed and talking Mom's ear off. She falls silent when Dad enters the kitchen.

"Dad?" I keep my voice timid. His face is unreadable. "I want to erase all my bad memories. Can you help me burn my journals and letters from Michael?"

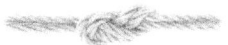

The smell of ash and smoke fills my nostrils. It's not hard to get a fire going in the high mountain Arizona desert. I throw everything into the flames, all at once, to ensure that my Dad won't get nosey and try to read any of it. Dad rakes at it to make sure it catches. I stay and watch until I am certain the words have been devoured. I gaze at the ink dripping off each photo image before it melts. I blink away tears as the photo of me kissing Johnny under the swing set curls in on itself and burns into wisps of ash. Finally, I walk away from it all, completely numb.

I finish my chores and take a quick shower to wash the smell of fire out of my hair. I have the afternoon shift at Ed's. The grocery store is quiet today. I am sitting on the floor, rotating and restocking small jars of baby food, when I look up and see Jamie next to me; we've barely talked since freshman year. It's ironic that she shows up here the same day the picture she took of me and Johnny melted away in my own mini book burning.

"Michael is dead, you fucking bitch!" My brain races through the confusion, trying to comprehend the words she's just said to me.

"Wh… wh… what?" The world is closing in on me.

"He's dead. He and I had sex last night and then he killed himself, and it's your fault."

I put my hand to my mouth. "What, how… what?" I don't understand. Michael can't be dead, he wouldn't kill himself, he's coming to rescue me.

"He drove his car off the Salt River Canyon. It's your fault, you fucking bitch, for breaking his heart like that. And he told me a secret. He said you weren't his first. He's had sex lots of times before you."

I need Michael to be alive, I need him to save me, to love me.

I try to stand, but I'm too dizzy. An older gentleman shopping nearby grabs me by the elbow and steadies me. "Take a breath, sweetheart, you need to breathe." I grab onto his shoulder. My body shakes uncontrollably.

"I hope you feel better, bitch, about what you have done!" she screeches. I can't support my own weight; my legs are wobbly.

"It's time for you to go home, young lady. You have delivered your message, now go." The man wraps his arm gently around my waist. I want to tell him I can't live if Michael is dead, but I can't speak.

Jamie startles and stares at him before scurrying away.

"Let's get you to the back so you can call your parents, okay?" The boxes are still on the floor. I'm not sure what I should be doing.

"The baby f… f… food."

"Just leave it. I know the manager. He won't mind."

The gentleman walks slowly, guiding me past the produce section and into the back. He sits me gently down on a chair in the lunch area, then flags my manager down. They talk in hushed tones. My manager must have called my Mom, because a few minutes later she walks into the breakroom and guides me back out into the van. I sob, speechless the four-block drive home.

I stumble out of the van and vomit in the grass. "He's dead," I sputter over and over between sobs. "I can't believe he's dead."

Mom pulls me into the kitchen, probably so that the neighbors won't witness my hysterics. I drop to my hands and knees as soon as she releases me. She fills a glass of water then crouches in front of me, offering me the cup.

"What exactly did Jamie say?" Mom seems genuinely concerned.

"Michael slept with someone last night and lots of people before me, but last night he drove himself off the Salt River Canyon."

Mom reaches over and rubs my back. "Breathe slower, Sarah. You're hyperventilating."

"Don't tell me to breathe, not right now." I feel a sharp pain. I can't focus. My body continues to quiver. "Sorry, I just... I can't."

Mom wipes a tear from her own cheek. I feel like I'm going to throw up. Mom picks up the phone and calls Mrs. Vincent.

"Hello Maria, this is Emma... Well, a girl came to Ed's today and told Sarah about Michael... That he was in a car accident last night... Oh, really... Well that's wonderful... She also told Sarah that Michael has slept around quite a bit... I completely understand, I would be upset too... Yes, the rumors are awful... I understand... I know the young lady's mother... I will absolutely be making a phone call to her... Yes, while she was working... Yes, in front of customers... Buh-bye."

Mom sets the phone receiver back in its cradle on the wall. "Michael is alive and doing just fine. He's at home doing chores." Mom sits on the floor next to me and lowers her voice. "Mrs. Vincent assured me that Michael has not been with other girls before or after you." She clears her throat and rubs my back for a few minutes before standing. "I'm going to call Jamie's mom now. That was an unacceptable and cruel joke to play on anyone."

I don't think I would be able to live if Michael dies.

CASTING OUT THE DEVIL

MAY 1997

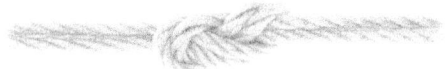

16 YEARS OLD

Mom drops the roast into the crock-pot and covers it with potatoes and onions. "Sarah, don't forget you have your first counseling appointment this afternoon with Brother Artus."

Ignoring her, I whine, "Do I have to go to work with you today? It's so boring." My probation has no official end date, and I wonder what I'll have to do over the summer to fulfill my obligation. I haven't talked to Officer Jones since I'd confessed, and he'd lied to me about not being in trouble.

"Yes," her voice is firm. "We need the extra adult hands for supervision during end of the school-year games."

I sigh, "Will you at least let Zoe get my yearbook and bring it to me? I've done everything you've asked. Can she come over and talk to me sometime soon? It's not like she and I are going to have sex."

Mom rolls her eyes. "Not tonight, Sarah, I just told you that you have counseling. She can probably come over tomorrow night or another night you aren't working or at counseling."

Tears of relief bubble out of me. I wipe at them quickly, hoping Mom doesn't see them. She walks over and puts her arms around me. I stiffen.

"I know the isolation has been hard on you. I'm sorry, this is just the way it has to be for now."

I know better than to ask her why. None of this makes sense to me. If I keep my mouth shut, maybe they'll ease up on all these new rules.

"Thanks for letting Zoe come," I say softly, trying to swallow my anger toward her, especially since she just offered to let me see a friend for the first time in weeks and I don't want her to change her mind. I can't stand her hugging me, though. I shouldn't have to be grateful that she might allow me one friend, and I know that if my Dad decides that I can't see Zoe, Mom will pretend like she doesn't have her own opinion and go along with whatever the head of the house thinks is best, especially since he holds the priesthood.

I go back to hide in my room until Joey, Evelyn, and Charlie leave for the bus stop and Mom is ready to leave for school. I miss journaling because it helps me think, but I stopped writing when I burned all my childhood memories since I don't trust my parents to honor my privacy anymore. I just sit and stare at the wall, trying not to cry so that my eyes won't be red when it's time to go to work with Mom.

The workday passes in a blur of snot-nose kids and supervised trips from the playground to the bathroom. Dad had said being a teacher is the best job for a woman to have so that she can have the same schedule as her children. The last five weeks in a kindergarten classroom have ensured I will never be a schoolteacher. I'm not a fan of babysitting almost 30 kids for seven hours a day.

Mom switches into wife mode as soon as we get home after a long day of work so that she can have dinner ready as soon as Dad walks in the door before my appointment with the Mormon therapist. I've never seen a therapist before, but I suspect it'll be a lot like my visit to the bishop.

Dad rushes in late, and Mom sets a plate on the table for him, instructing him to eat quickly. I try to get my food down, but it just came out of the crock-pot, and it's still too hot. Besides, any time Dad is in the same room as me, my stomach is in knots, and I feel sick. I cut the potatoes into small bites and push the food around my plate while Mom gives babysitting instructions to Joey.

We pull into the parking lot of the Beehive Clothing and Cannery 12 minutes later. It's a windy day, as usual in Snowflake. I squint at the sun, low in the sky, wondering how long this is going to take.

"Why are we at the cannery?"

"This is also where LDS Family Services is," Mom explains.

"So, you can buy temple clothes, garments, canned food, *and* see a counselor all in the same place? That's efficient." Mom shoots me a warning look, and I check my sarcasm.

The building smells like the back room of Ed's. Down a short hallway, there's a door marked *LDS Family Services.* The waiting room is cold and bland. There is a picture of Jesus in a red robe on the wall. A tall man with silver hair enters the room and introduces himself as Brother Artus.

Mom pulls some paperwork out of her purse and hands it to him. He flips through it quickly then looks up. "I'd like to meet with Sarah alone for the first bit. I'll invite both of you in after I get to know Sarah a little."

Dad leans forward and opens his mouth; I'm sure he's going to object and tell Brother Artus that I'm a liar, or something, but then he closes his mouth and stares at the floor.

"Sarah?" He extends an arm of welcome to follow him into his office.

I step inside, peering around the office. It's almost identical to the bishop's office, except the desk is pushed against one wall and there's a couch to the side of it instead of several fabric folding chairs.

"Where do I sit?" I ask tentatively.

"Most people sit on the couch." Brother Artus points toward a worn sofa. "But you can also sit in my chair if that makes you feel more comfortable." He motions to the executive rolling chair directly across from the couch. There is a small coffee table with a box of tissue on it between them. The desk is a mess of overturned papers and several books, including the Book of Mormon, the Bible, and Spencer W. Kimball's *The Miracle of Forgiveness*, which Dad had already forced me to read and write a book report on.

I sit on the couch thinking about how awful that book had made my heavenly future sound and how hard it had been to write a book report on a book with no plot. Brother Artus lowers himself into his chair and closely reviews the papers Mom had handed him.

"Your Mom dropped off a letter for me last week telling me about you, and I spoke with your bishop. It sounds like you've been through a lot recently. I'm interested in what you have to say about all of it. Would you be willing to share that with me?"

Irritation that I have to recite what happened when he already knows makes me grind my teeth. I roll my eyes and sigh heavily. "If Mom wrote you a letter, let's go with that version."

Brother Artus smiles gently at me, and the sides of his eyes crinkle. "It doesn't seem fair that I know so much about you when you've never even met me, does it?"

I huff and he continues, "Everything you and I talk about is confidential, that means I'm not allowed to share it with your bishop or your parents unless I think you are going to harm yourself or someone else. I also have to get help for you if I think someone is hurting you. Based on what I've read and heard, it sounds like you've had a really rough few weeks."

Something in me breaks. I scoff in derision, "Everybody in this shit town thinks they know, but they don't. They just gossip and make stuff up."

He chuckles at me, "Yes, I've learned not to believe the rumors. Usually they are mean and not very accurate."

I stare at Brother Artus for a few seconds, waiting for him to tell me I shouldn't say "shit" because it offends the Lord, but he doesn't.

"So, I can tell you whatever I want, and you can't tell my parents?" I challenge.

"Unless I think you are going to hurt yourself, like suicide, cutting your body, or dangerous drug use," he assures me.

"What if I lie?"

"Well, if you lie to me, I won't be able to help you much. I tend to believe my clients, so I won't know you are lying. I'm hoping to help you and your parents work through some of the things you are going through. I understand they've put some… parameters in place that probably have you feeling very isolated. It is my hope that the work we do here will help you be understood and gain your freedoms back."

"That's not likely to happen. Did they tell you Dad wants me to go to jail for ditching school, so now I have to go to work with my Mom for probation? The cops said they don't do that, but Dad convinced them to anyway." My tone is full of hate and disgust, but Brother Artus just nods encouragingly at me.

"That's interesting. Are you checking in with a probation officer once a week?"

"No, Dad says he's doing that for me, since I'll only lie to them to get out of it sooner." I chew on my inner cheek to keep myself from crying in front of this stranger. He's the first person who hasn't immediately come to Mom and Dad's defense since this entire mess started. Actually, Officer Jones hadn't either, but then I got probation, even though he said I wouldn't.

Brother Artus scratches something on the yellow legal pad of paper perched in his lap. "I think I'll check in on your probation then. If you really are on *legal* probation, the officer has to talk to you, not your parents, usually once a week, sometimes less, but almost always monthly."

I shrug. I'd rather talk to Officer Jones once a week, even though he lied to me, than to Dad.

"Your Mom and Dad need to feel like you're safe before they will trust you again, but you *need* your social group. I want you to hang out with your friends, and I want your parents to feel comfortable with your doing so."

I stare at him with squinted eyes, searching his face. I wonder if he's just saying that to get on my good side, since that's what I want too.

Brother Artus leans back in his chair. "It feels like you don't believe me."

"I don't," I say matter-of-factly. "Sorry." I shrug. I want to believe him, but so many adults have lied to me, I don't trust any of them.

"Don't be sorry. It's good that you don't trust me just because I say you can. Trust is something you earn. I have a paper I like to show teenagers who come to see me." He stands up and opens a drawer on his desk, which is full of files. He fingers through the tabs looking for the one he wants, then pulls a page out.

"Here you go," he says, handing me the paper with a few lines high-lighted in bright pink ink.

I look at the paper and read what looks like a law about counselors having to maintain confidentiality.

"If I tell your parents what we talk about without your permission, I could get into a lot of trouble and lose my license, which means I would lose my job as a counselor forever."

I hand the paper back to him, still skeptical.

"Okay, so… what do you want to know?"

"I want to know what you think I need to understand to help you heal your relationship with your parents and this boy… what's his name? Your Mom told me…"

"Michael."

"Yes, that's it."

"Nothing is *wrong* between Michael and me, except we aren't allowed to see or talk to each other, and I'm not allowed to go anywhere without my Mom following me. It's creepy." I think of how often I look over my shoulder now to see if Mom is following me like a stalker.

"I don't think I'd like it very much if I got followed all the time either," he concedes.

I'm not used to adults actually listening, never mind actually considering what I say. He seems very relaxed and calm, smiling in his chair. I sink into the couch, find a comfortable spot, and then I tell him everything.

I knew Brother Artus's promise was too good to be true. I shouldn't have told him anything. I take off my shoe and throw it at my closet door as hard as I can. It leaves a small black mark on the paint. I throw the other one just as hard, leaving a second mark. I lay backward onto my bed and stare at the ceiling through a blur of tears. My head pounds from crying; I'm exhausted.

I'd told him everything, answered all his questions, and not just about what happened but how I feel, and then he asks to speak with my parents alone. He told them they should put me back in school. He told them that keeping me isolated is a form of abuse and that it needs to stop. At first, I was so grateful to have an adult on my side, but that was the reason Dad discounted everything Brother Artus said.

"I AM NOT ABUSING MY DAUGHTER!" Dad screamed at Mom the whole way home.

"Maybe we have been too hard on her, Dave. What he said about brain development makes sense. She needs to be with her peer group."

"That man does not know what he is talking about. He should have his license revoked. When he said he would let his fifteen-year-old daughter go to prom if prom was three days prior to her sixteenth birthday, he lost all of my respect. And telling us to let her go to the yearbook signing dance? She lies, sneaks around, skips school to commit immoral acts IN MY HOUSE… she's been disfellowshipped from church, and we're supposed to reward that with a dance?"

"Dave, please, be reasonable."

"No. He's an idiot. What kind of professional would recommend that we allow our daughter to have a relationship with a rapist? As if it's okay, so long as we more closely supervise her interactions with said rapist. And we *are* providing more supervision. That's why you are following her, so she has *more* supervision."

"Dave, I can't keep following her everywhere." Mom's voice is soft, but firm.

The fighting doesn't end when we arrive home. The little kids scatter to their rooms, and Dad keeps at it.

"And I'll tell you what else, Emma, she is not going back to that therapist again!" I'm not surprised, considering all the rude names Dad had called Brother Artus since we left his office. Dad discredits anyone who questions his opinions, especially his parenting. He's a self-proclaimed expert on how to interact with children and youth. I stare at nothing, feeling heavy with loneliness.

Mom calls the younger kids to the living room for evening prayers.

Evelyn eyes Dad while she kneels next to me, folding her arms, and breaks the silence, "Dad, why are you being so mean to Sarah?"

Dad leaps toward her, his hand raised high in the air.

I jump in front of Evelyn, "DON'T YOU HIT MY SISTER!" I scream.

His hand comes down hard against my cheek instead.

I whip my head back to him, "Go ahead, hit me again."

He grabs my arm just below my shoulder and drags me through the library.

I try to wriggle free, and he strengthens his grip.

"Dave, stop!" Mom yells after him.

Charlie's hysterical cry drowns out Mom's yelling.

Dad yanks me into my bedroom and pulls my face to his, "Don't you EVER tell me what to do," he hisses, and then shoves me hard away from him.

I stumble backward and fall against the metal bedframe. I hear a loud crack, and pain sears through my back, just below my shoulder blades, knocking the wind out of me. I look up at Mom's pale face, but I can't speak yet to ask her to help me. She turns and walks away, and Dad slams the door behind her. I can hear him stomping back into the living room. "Go to bed," he yells at the little kids.

I'm trembling from the terror and pain. I roll to my hands and knees. Something warm drips down my side. I reach under my shirt. My fingers slip through blood.

I can't wear my bra without it opening the thin scab that has formed over the cut across my back. I show it to Mom after Dad leaves in the morning. She acts like it's not a big deal, but her voice is shaky, and she tells me that I can stay home from work for the day. I want to run away, but I don't know where to go, and I'm in too much pain.

I rinse my T-shirt and bedding with water, then pour hydrogen peroxide over the blood stains like Michael taught me. I'm so numb, I don't even cry when I think about him. I lay down on the couch, positioning myself precariously on my stomach to avoid reopening the wound and sleep off and on all day.

When Mom makes it home from work, she tells me that she invited Zoe over for dinner and that I'm allowed to call her again as often as I want to. When Zoe walks into the house, I want to collapse into her and release the tension I haven't been able to escape from in weeks. Instead, we stare at each other awkwardly, knowing we are being watched.

I don't tell Zoe anything. I don't tell her about Dad, about the bishop, or Brother Artus. So far, telling has only made things worse, and I don't want Dad to ban me from ever seeing her again.

She tells me Michael ditches most days and won't be able to graduate because he's missed too much school. She picked up my yearbook for me and brings it over.

I flip through its crisp pages mindfully. I want so much to hug her hard and talk like we always have. She seems sad and angry, and I'm not sure if she's mad at me or just mad in general. From now on, I'm going to have to fend for myself, since no one is safe when I open my big mouth.

"This Friday is the yearbook signing dance. I'll ask your Mom if you can go. I'll promise her to keep Michael away from you."

"I doubt they'll let me go." I sit crisscross on my bed, leaning forward to protect my back. Our eyes meet and she gives me a pitying look, so I drop my gaze and stare at a worn spot on my bedspread.

"I'm worried about you." She reaches out to hug me, and I pull away.

"Sorry, it's just… I hurt my back." I stare at the floor.

"Did your Dad hurt you?"

"Yeah, he did," I mutter with a weak shrug of my shoulders.

"I wish I could do more." She reaches to put her hand on my leg but retracts it before I can pull away again.

"Dad's leaving for California to work for Grandpa Lee right after school gets out." I can't wait for him to be gone. Once he's gone, maybe

I can contact Michael and we can run away to Tennessee to his grandma, who might actually like me.

"Do you think you can last another week and a half?"

"I don't have any other choice."

Zoe calls me Thursday evening and tells me Mom said I could go to the dance if Michael wasn't going to be there.

"Michael doesn't mind skipping the dance so that you can get out of your house."

I wake up Friday morning thinking about the dance and seeing my friends. I crave something to be normal again. Hopefully Michael will write me a note and give it to Zoe so that I'll finally know how he plans to get me out of here.

I take a shower for the first time since Dad threw me into my bed frame. I wash my hair slowly; the shampoo runs down my back and stings the cut. I let the conditioner sit while I shave my legs. I accidentally nick my knee. I remember sitting in this shower the day they pulled me from school, looking at this razor. If Michael doesn't come for me so that we can run away, the razor is my only way out of this hell.

I dry off, carefully, avoiding my back. While I dress, I rehearse the apology that I hope Deckland and Kat will listen to. If I own up to keeping Michael's and my relationship a secret and remind them Dad is a jerk, hopefully they'll forgive me. I sit on the couch, flipping through my year book, my foot tapping nervously on the floor.

"What are you doing?" Dad's voice makes me jump, and my heart skips a beat.

"I'm waiting for Zoe to come pick me up and take me to the dance. Michael won't be there, so Mom said I could go." My stomach knots. I send a silent prayer to heaven that he won't hit me again.

"Zoe is not taking you anywhere. Why on earth would you think you could go to the dance?" His fists clench and unclench at his sides.

I look up at him, confused and terrified. He stalks off to find Mom. I hear him bellow at her in their bedroom.

"Emma, did you really tell Sarah she could go to the dance?"

"Yes. Deckland, Kat, and Zoe will pick her up." Her voice is raised but controlled. "They have all confirmed that Michael isn't planning on attending, and if he shows up, Zoe will bring Sarah straight home."

"She's not going to that dance with friends who didn't protect her in the first place. I don't trust a single one of them."

"Dave, the counselor said she needs to spend time with her peers."

"I do not want to hear about what that incompetent counselor said ever again." I can hear the growl in his voice grow deeper as he stomps down the hallway back toward me. "Sarah, go to your room, now."

"But they'll be here any minute," I protest. I look around Dad to Mom, coming in behind him, but she doesn't say anything.

"I am the head of this house and the priesthood holder, and you will obey the rules I put in place. Go to your room," Dad says, his teeth clenched, his face flushed. I can feel myself sinking. I knew going to the dance was too good to be true.

"If I can't go, can they at least take my yearbook and get it signed by my friends?"

"I think that is a reasonable compromise," Mom says.

"I'll think about it, now go."

I walk to my room and slam my door. I sit down with a huff. The doorbell rings, and I hear Dad speaking low and stern. I can't tell what he's saying, and in a few minutes my friends leave without me. I can't keep crying myself to sleep.

I wake up late the next morning, which is odd, because Mom never lets me sleep in. I hear one of the little kids running the vacuum cleaner.

"Where is Dad?" I ask as Mom pulls a plate of scrambled eggs and bacon out of the microwave for me.

"He's at work grading papers and planning for next week's field day," Mom says, returning to the dishes. "Did you sleep well?"

I ignore the question. "Did you let Zoe take my yearbook?"

Mom sighs, "No, Dad didn't feel it was appropriate."

"What? Are you fucking kidding me? First, I'm allowed to go to the dance, then I'm not. Then I give a reasonable compromise, and that's shot to hell as well. Shit, how long are you going to keep me imprisoned like this?" My eyes shoot fire at my mother, and I don't care. I've had it. "I'm on the verge of running away. I'd rather die than keep living like this, you stupid bitch! You can't stand up to him, can you? I got slapped and shoved around for trying to protect Ev, and you did nothing. He put a gash in my back, and you let him! You just look at the fucking floor or walk away. You're weak and pathetic. Why are you still married to him? I would never stay married to a man who abused my kids the way he abuses me."

I'm so angry my face is tingling.

"Do not talk to me like that, young lady!"

I step away from her.

"Dad cares more about what everyone thinks of him than he does about us. He doesn't love me. He hasn't for years. He's always calling me names. I'm going to make him pay for this!" I run down the hallway toward his home office. "I'm going to smash that stupid computer he cherishes."

Mom grabs me from behind just outside the office door. She spins me around and slaps me hard, and I spit and kick at her, stumbling backward against the wall. She crouches in front of me then raises her right hand high above her head.

I flinch, bracing myself for another blow.

"IN THE NAME OF JESUS CHRIST, I COMMAND THEE SATAN TO GET BEHIND ME!" she bellows.

I'm too stunned to say anything. What the hell was that?

She steps into Dad's office and grabs the phone.

"Hello, Bishop, can you please come over? It's an emergency... No, Dave isn't here."

AUTHOR'S NOTE

Before the mid-1990s, presidents of the Mormon Church often spoke of the dangers of mental health providers.[16] Former president and prophet, Ezra Taft Benson, offered extensive advice on overcoming mental illness. In "Do Not Despair," he cited the need for church members suffering from depression and suicidal ideation to repent, fast, and pray, to work and serve others, to take good care of their physical health, and to invest time and energy in personal relationships.[17]

---

16 Swedin, Eric G. "Psychotherapy in the LDS Community." *Issues in Religion and Psychotherapy*, 4, 25, no. 1 (2000). https://doi.org/https://scholarsarchive.byu.edu/irp/vol25/iss1/4/.

17 Ezra Taft Benson, "Do Not Despair," Saturday Afternoon Session, The Church of Jesus Christ of Latter-Day Saints, October 1974, video of sermon, 18:32, https://www.churchofjesuschrist.org/study/general-conference/1974/10/do-not-despair?lang=eng.

While some of the counsel he gave appears sound and encouraging, the issue lies in a man (or woman) with enormous sway and power presenting such counsel as *the* prescription to treat serious mental illness. Benson's counsel suggested that if employed correctly, righteous living will cure what ails you, implying that any failure in this method is user error.

President Benson was not the first prophet of the Mormon Church to promote the attitude that mental illness is a by-product of too little faith and too much sin. It's an attitude that gives birth to mistrust of mental health providers, and creates a stigma that shames and intimidates individuals with mental illness into an isolating silence devoid of treatment options. My parents, my father especially, was leery of the field of psychology, as well as any education or advice Brother Artus offered him to promote my well-being.

My mother's exorcism, or the casting out of devils in the name of Jesus Christ, is something the Mormon Church teaches can be done through the power of the priesthood. Since women are banned from "holding the priesthood" in Mormonism, my mother performed this right "In the name of Jesus Christ."

My parents failed to connect my outburst as a response to trauma and instead tied it to being possessed of some evil spirit controlled by Satan. While many religious sects espouse this type of practice, it is my professional opinion that doing so without treating the trauma causes much more harm in the long run. The approach is something known as spiritual bypassing, which simply stated means using some type of spiritual experience, ritual, or belief system to bypass the underlying mental, physical, or emotional cause.

PERFECT "MOLLY" MORMON

SUMMER 1997

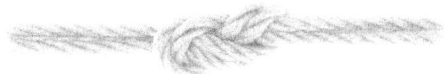

16 YEARS OLD

My life is ruined, and it's not because I had sex with Michael.

Bishop rushed over after Mom's failed exorcism. He sits in Dad's chair. Mom brought a chair from the dining room into the office for me. I don't know what I was expecting him to do to me, but so far, he's been pretty quiet.

I exhale loudly and look away. I don't want to talk to Bishop. Everything I had wanted to say, I had said to my mother. All the things I've been holding inside, biting my tongue to keep from saying, swallowing down and letting fester and rot inside me, had finally come blasting out.

Bishop speaks quietly since we both know Mom is eavesdropping just outside the door. "You know, Sarah, you have lots of friends, lots of people who love you. You might be angry at your parents right now, but I assure you, they love you. And when you can't feel any of that, your Savior loves you. He can always comfort you, no matter where you are or what's happening."

"Whatever," I reply. "I'm not allowed to hang out with anyone who still likes me. And you're wrong. My parents do not love me."

"I'm sure it feels like that sometimes. Humans aren't meant to be alone." Bishop places a hand on my knee, and I pull away.

And yet, there is nothing Bishop can do to change any of it. It's not any use to have lots of friends or people who love me when I'm being held captive in my own home.

Bishop keeps droning on, but this is easier to get through if I check out and occasionally look at him so that he thinks I'm still listening. He's not a bad guy, he just has no idea what he's talking about. I don't think Mom and Dad have told him all the things they have taken away from me when they thought I was not a virgin anymore.

"Okay, Sarah. I'd like for you to give some thought to what we've talked about today. Pray to your Heavenly Father. Ask for comfort, and pray that your family can work through this time together so that you can grow stronger as an eternal family, destined for the Celestial Kingdom."

His smile is sweet and hopeful. I think he knows that no part of the last hour was helpful, and he also knows that I'm not possessed by Satan. Mom tells me to wait in my room while she speaks with Bishop alone. He stands in the doorway and invites Mom into the office as though this isn't her house. I lay in bed dreaming about running away with Michael; my tattered black suitcase is packed and waiting. I'm ready to leave and never look back, I just need him to show up.

I hear Bishop leave, but Mom doesn't come check on me. It's Saturday, and I have a shift at Ed's, but Mom never comes to get me and I don't get out of bed. Eventually I fall back to sleep and have the same shit dream I always do about my running to Michael while Dad comes out of nowhere, his face scarlet, hands flailing wildly. I always wake up just as his hand is about to make contact with my face.

"Sarah?"

There's a soft knock at the door, and I can hear Mom in the hallway. I don't say anything, but she comes in anyway. I pretend to be asleep, but I give myself away when she touches my foot through the blanket and I flinch. She opens my curtains, and I shade my eyes with my hand and look at her. Her face is red from crying. "I think we've been too hard on you."

She sits on the edge of my bed, and I shift away from her. I don't think I could stand it if she touches me again.

"I called Zoe this afternoon. She is going to swing by Monday morning after Dad leaves for work and pick up your yearbook. She promised to take it around to your friends so that they can sign it." She waits, head cocked and staring at me like I'm going to thank her or something. For a second, I feel hopeful, and then I remember that she hasn't followed through on a single one of her promises so far.

Sandwiched in the pew between my Mom and the scratchy, carpeted wall, I sing along with a hymn meant to get me "in the right mindset" for the sacrament that I'm not allowed to take. Dad leans forward slightly to watch as Mom holds out the tray of tiny, torn pieces of white bread, and I put up my hand to reject it. It's not enough that I've been forbidden from participating; he makes sure that the tray is offered so I can signify to God and everyone watching to confirm the gossip that I am not worthy.

When the water is passed, we repeat the process, but when Dad leans forward to watch me reject the tray, he has a satisfied smirk on his face. The first speaker overflows with bubbly enthusiasm while speaking on the joy of repentance and what we can do to receive forgiveness from Heavenly Father. She doesn't say anything about how to receive forgiveness from an earthly father.

Sitting next to Mom in Relief Society is worse. The lesson is boring, and the women who are my Mom's age pretend not to stare at me, while the old ladies whisper about me. I know they are talking about me since old ladies don't know how to whisper quietly.

Monday morning, I go back to my room after family breakfast when Dad leaves for work. I don't get out of bed when I hear Zoe at the door, but I can hear enough to know that Mom gave her my yearbook. I don't get out of bed when she returns the book later that afternoon, before leaving for the senior trip. Mom knocks softly on my door, but I ignore her. She opens it and sets the yearbook on my desk. She looks at me laying in my bed, then walks back out.

I listen as her footsteps retreat, then get up and flip the book open. Most of the notes are from my band friends—Zoe probably didn't have time to bring the book around to get it signed by anyone else. Michael's note in the back cover says he had no idea, the day that he met me, that I would be the love of his life. I read it twice. There is nothing about him coming to get me, no plan, not even a hint. I know he won't come for me this week; he'll be in Disneyland with the rest of the seniors. I have to make it at least one more week in this prison.

When everyone is asleep, I climb out of my bedroom window and cross the desert wash behind my house. I walk for a long time in the dark. I don't really know where I'm going… I'm just going. When I come to a dirt parking lot half-filled with cars and pickup trucks, I walk inside the small building and have a seat at the bar.

The short, beer-belly bartender saunters over to me. "You're too young to be in here, sweetheart."

"Can I just have a water, and then I'll go?" I plead. I don't ever want to go home, but I have nowhere else that's safe.

The bartender sighs, "Sure." He fills a large plastic cup with ice and tops it off with tap water. "When you're done with it, you have to go, though."

"Thanks." I look around the room. There are mostly men, a few women, all of them staring at me. I recognize a few faces from Ed's, but there's no one here from church.

"I know you," one man says. "Aren't you a cheerleader?"

"I used to be, yeah."

"Hey, Lawrence, start up the jukebox. I think this youngin' is going to do a little cheer for us."

"No, thanks. I need to go home." My pulse quickens.

"Nah, you're here, just one little dance." He waves a $20 at me. "I'll make it worth your while."

I take another drink of my water, square my shoulders, and begin to dance. Several men catcall and whistle. I pull my T-shirt up, exposing my stomach. I let go and move, making my routine up as I go. After weeks of lying stagnant and numb, I can feel something; it's exhilarating. When the song ends, the man slides $20 in my jeans pocket. Another man pulls some bills from his wallet and hands them to me.

"Encore," someone yells over the clapping and whistling.

I spin and twirl, do slow hip circles and shimmy my shoulders. I bend low and touch the ground, rise slowly, and look up at Officer Jones.

I don't recognize him at first because he's not in uniform and he's not smiling. He grabs my arm and hauls me out of the bar while the men inside boo and protest. He puts his hand on top of my head and presses down so I don't bump into his car when he shoves me into the seat. He slams the door and walks around the front, punching the hood as he passes. I jump.

He opens the door and slides into the driver's seat, "Shit, Sarah, what in the name of God are you doing dancing in a bar?"

"What are you doing in a bar?" I spit back.

He faces me. "I happen to be a grown-ass man, and I'm not a Mormon. You, on the other hand, are a sixteen-year-old girl, surrounded by drunk men who won't ask for your age or your permission. Shit." He hits his steering wheel. "Shit! I could lose my job over this."

He turns the key in the ignition. "Buckle up," he orders, and drives toward my neighborhood. "Look Sarah, I know your life is hard, I know your Dad is an abusive asshole, but my hands are tied. I can't do anything without *real* evidence."

I sit quietly, watching the empty road, not able to say anything, not wanting to go home, not having any other place to go, afraid of what my Dad will do. Officer Jones pulls his car over to the side of the road just before reaching my house.

"You sneak back into that house. If I ever, and I mean EVER, catch you at a bar again, I will walk you to your front door and deliver you to your father. Do you understand me?"

The streetlight casts an odd shadow across his face.

"Thank you for not ratting me out. I promise, I won't sneak out again."

He leans toward me, holds my gaze for a few seconds and says, "I believe you."

School has been out for two weeks, and still no sign of Michael. As soon as Dad left for California, Mom lifted all of his restrictions and confided that, while she disagreed with his parenting methods, she had to do what he said because he's the priesthood holder. She tells me that I need to embrace my Savior's atoning sacrifice, and that if I do, I will find happiness and freedom from the burden of my sins.

The more "Mormon" I behave, the more freedom she'll give me. On the Sabbath, I wear my dress all day long. I only listen to music published by the church. I bear my testimony during every family home evening. As soon as Bishop lifts my punishments, I bear my testimony in church at every fast and testimony meeting, which is the first Sunday service of each month, even though it makes my stomach hurt.

My packed suitcase still waits in my closet, ready to go at a moment's notice. The last note I got from Michael was after the senior trip to Disney when Evelyn came home from school and shut my bedroom door behind her. She pulled a Pumbaa doll and a necklace out of her backpack and handed them to me with a folded-up piece of notebook paper. More of the same unfulfilled promises, and my hope has turned to anger. I let her keep Pumbaa.

When I tell Mom I'm angry with Michael, she allows me to call him at his father's house. She stands over my shoulder, approvingly, as I bear an outwardly enthusiastic testimony filled with insincere disgust and self-loathing, and I beg Michael to join the church. "I think you will be happier if you join the church and let Jesus heal you the way he has healed me." I pray Michael sees through my act, but he never comes to my rescue.

AUTHOR'S NOTE

My parents' discovery of my sexual encounter with Michael brought to fruition a loss of love and affection that was building since the onset of puberty. That, coupled with loss of access to my peer group and being singled out at church, was devastating enough that I did not hope to repair the relationship with my parents, nor was I given any encouragement to do so. I disengaged from my family and hung all of my hope on Michael's promise that he would come for me. Eventually accepting that Michael was not coming meant acknowledging a painful betrayal. Michael had been the one person who loved me as I was, no matter what, and then he abandoned me in my time of greatest need.

Out of options and faced with parents who oscillated between neglectful and abusive behavior, I became a "parent pleaser" as a matter of survival. I did my chores, kept my room clean, worked hard, and became the one thing I thought they could love: a perfect Mormon, a.k.a. Molly Mormon. I was neat and chaste, sang the hymns with gusto, read my scriptures daily, wore my Sunday dress all day on the Sabbath, volunteered when invited, bore testimony of the church's truthfulness, and for the icing on the cake, I "called" my sinner boyfriend to repentance. It felt deceitful but necessary for my survival.

In many ways, my efforts worked. Once my compliance was complete, my mother became more attentive and engaged in my life. Suddenly, I had at home what I had been craving my entire life, connection with my mother. Mom treated me more as her peer than as my mother, which meant that she shared her woes about my father, thereby validating my own.

My perfection soothed my father's bitterness toward me as well; an obedient daughter was easy to control, and a pious daughter confirmed his need to be viewed as "a good dad." Unfortunately, the trauma from his outward abusive behaviors destroyed what trust I had in him, and our relationship has never recovered.

PART THREE

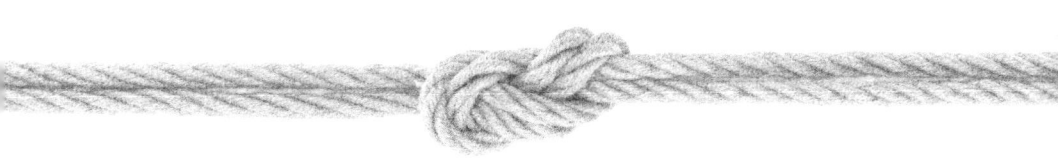

MEMORIES NORTH CAROLINA (TAKE TWO)

LATE 2014

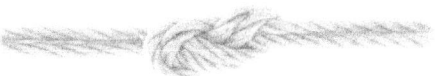

33 YEARS OLD

Boxes fill the kitchen, leaving a narrow pathway that my body barely fits through to maneuver. At least I already know where everything goes.

I'm grateful that the Army granted our request to move back to North Carolina for Mason's anesthesia residency. We still own our house here, and I have a ready-made support group. I'm not impressed by the hazing in medical training programs: long hours and a constant fear of failing imposed by supervisors who withhold approval as a matter of course. The academic portion was hard enough. I'm not sure I'm ready for two more years of Mason coming home stressed and exhausted with little positive reinforcement.

"Hello, Lady," Rita's smooth, caramel face and thick black hair appears in the doorway. I've missed how she knocks before letting herself in. "Do you need help unpacking any of this?" Some of the tension in my shoulders melts away... I might actually have a functioning kitchen before the end of the day with Rita's help.

"Yes, please. I feel like my kitchen is a scene from that show *Hoarders*. I'm not sure where to start."

She laughs. "Are you setting up your kitchen the same way it was before you left?" The sound of packing tape being ripped off a box breaks my moving trance, and I join Rita in opening the box closest to me.

"Absolutely!"

Rita's memory of my kitchen is better than mine, and we have the whole thing unpacked in less than two hours.

"That has got to be a record," I exclaim, handing her a water bottle.

"What's next?"

"Well, the kids are done unpacking their own rooms. Can you just take them outside and watch them play? I have four boxes left in my bedroom. I need to get those out of the way, or Mason is going to bang his shins into them again in the morning."

The kids are as thrilled to see Rita as she is to see them. It's my favorite part of coming back here, having a best friend two doors down. I climb the stairs to my tiny master bedroom at the back of the house and slide around the boxes by the door so I can open the closet. I hear Rita in the yard organizing the kids in a game. I open the first box to discover it's been mislabeled. The next box is full of shirts, still on hangers. When they're hung up, I pull shoes out one by one, pulling them back into shape before placing them in their spot inside the closet.

My yearbooks are stacked along the bottom of the box covered in a light layer of dust and dirt from the shoes. I wipe one off before tossing it on my bed and missing; it hits the floor with a small thump. I lean over to pick it up. A folded piece of paper falls from it.

Crossroads 1996-1997. I haven't opened that yearbook since I last saw Michael in El Paso a decade ago. I take a deep breath and open the back cover, knowing what I'll find. The ink is purple, the cursive perfect.

Sarah, what can I say? When I first met you at band camp, I had no idea that the little girl standing before me saying, "Hi, I'm Sarah Lee," would turn out to be the greatest love of all time. I'll be waiting for you. With every single moment that passes, I'll be waiting. I love you so much. Know that I'll be faithful. Make sure you read my senior dream. I love you. II Cor. 13. Class of 1997,

Michael David Iles.

I open the book. The cracked binding falls open to page 165.

Michael Iles: Big Dream – To do anything that makes a lot of money so I can buy a mansion & anything else my lovely wife & nine children want.

The words are that of young, untested love, and yet, they make my heart skip a beat every time I read them. They are all I have left of him. These two mementos, written when everything in our lives was falling apart.

I set the book to the side and unfold the paper I'm still holding. It is old and worn. I'm careful to open it without tearing at the fold lines. I haven't looked at this poem in years. I don't remember putting it in here. Tears slip from my eyes; my chest is heavy with grief.

He runs forth free, so carefree and wild, I'd love to travel the world on the legs of a child.

I shouldn't be sad, yet I cannot shake the emptiness I feel.

COLLEGE

SUMMER 1997-FALL 1998

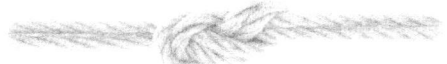

16-17 YEARS OLD

I've given up on hearing from Michael. After our last phone conversation, it's like he just vanished into thin air. Even though Mom lifted all the restrictions since Dad left for California to work for the summer, I am still incredibly isolated. I decide I'll spend the summer of 1997 working as many extra hours at Ed's as they'll let me and use the rest of my free time reading.

Lost in thought, feeling sorry for myself, and focusing on the familiar beep indicating the barcode has registered in the computer, I turn to bag the items while the customer writes their check to pay for their groceries—the repetitive scenario becomes my summer theme song.

"This is what I call a balanced meal." A bright voice interrupts my wallowing.

I look up, brow raised, and smile politely back at the dark, angular, and attractive face in front of me.

"I might have to disagree with you, there." I scan the bag of chips and soda bottle.

"Well, for a missionary it is." His deep brown eyes linger on me longer than my regular customers.

He's the right age with an appropriate amount of wholesome eagerness, but he's wearing cargo shorts and a T-shirt. Plus, he appears to be alone, which missionaries never are. "Are you a missionary?" Putting effort into carrying on a conversation isn't something I'm in the mood for, but I'm at work and "the face of the store" at the checkout line.

"Just got back." He shoots me a happy-go-lucky smile, which feels like he's trying to flirt. I ignore his efforts with a weak smile.

"Welcome home. Ed's IGA is happy to serve you. Your total is $3.27."

I reach for his money, and my eyes linger on the long scrape on his toned forearm. It's on the wrong side to be a self-inflicted wound. An image of the pink razor on the tub ledge flashes through my brain. He must notice me staring at it because he holds it up so I can get a closer look.

"Rappelling—it's awesome, but occasionally a tiny bit hazardous." I have no idea what rappelling is.

"Cool. Here's your change."

"Thanks," he cranes his head to see my name tag, "Sarah. I'm Curtis. See you around."

I do see him around. He comes into my line every time he's at Ed's, and we talk a little more. By now he has to have heard about me; any well-meaning gossip who sees him talking to me would warn him, but he's always friendly and eventually invites me to go rappelling with him. I'm expecting my Mom to say no, even though she's lifted the restrictions... he's 21 and I'm still only 16. It turns out "returned missionary" holds more powerful magic than "please," so I am granted permission.

Curtis smiles encouragingly at me. The bright summer sun beats down on us. At least the wind isn't too bad today.

"This is actually a pretty safe hobby as long as you follow all the rules and check your equipment, twice." His smooth Navajo cheek shines like a young child's, still too young to need a daily shave.

"Sure." I'm trying to stand still while Curtis tightens my harness. My legs tremble in anticipation of walking backward off the face of a cliff. He walks around me once again just to make sure everything fits correctly before nodding.

Curtis chuckles. "Try to relax. Remember, this is just a big boulder. We're going to learn here to help you get good and comfortable before we move on to anything more advanced. Besides, a little adrenaline might do you good."

I squint into his eyes, which are level with mine and nod. "Yeah, uh-huh. If you say so." I peek over the edge of the six-foot chunk of rock and swallow hard. A fall from this height would result in serious injury. The more I focus on relaxing, the more scared I feel, and Curtis keeps talking, which is very distracting.

"You know, I hate the way we treat people who don't fit into the Mormon mold," he blurts. I assume he's heard something about me. How could he not have in Snowflake? He finishes checking my harness then scurries down the sloped side of the boulder so he can be my brakeman in case I fall.

"What do you mean?" I call out over the edge. I look over my shoulder

again, determined to walk backward and try to ignore the new set of but-
terflies in my stomach due to the abrupt shift in topic.

"I had a good friend in high school who started her family early. She
lost her entire friend group as soon as people found out. And me, I hated
my mission, but I can't talk about it without people telling me I didn't
have enough faith or something. It's like we don't even believe in our own
doctrine." I've never heard anyone say anything about their mission that
wasn't positive.

"I get that," I say, my confidence lifting a little. "So, you really want
me to just walk off the edge of this thing?" I don't know him well enough
to know if I can trust him with my past.

"First, you need to sit into the harness. Keep your butt down and your
feet out. If you start to slip, I'll pull the rope and you won't fall. Just keep
your feet in front of you." He's repeated these instructions more than once,
and I appreciate his patience. I take a deep breath, close my eyes, and sit
backward. The heavy nylon rope slides in the 8 ring. I tighten my fist behind me, and as promised, I stop moving. I loosen my grip and walk slowly
down the flat side of the rock face.

"You did great!" His congratulations are enthusiastic, and I can't help
but grin from ear to ear in relief and pride. He disconnects the 8 ring from
the D ring and pats me on the back.

His dark eyes lock on mine and he says, "A person has value and is
loved completely in the Lord's eyes, no matter their mistakes."

I startle then examine his face. It's been months since I felt that acceptance
from anyone who isn't "perfect," not since Michael. I'm not sure what he expects me to say and yet, I'm surprised by the warmth of gratitude that fills me.

"Thanks, Curtis, I really needed to hear that." In my mind, I mull over
that it's been almost four months since anyone has been kind or gentle

toward me. It's attractive in a way that confuses me. It's not romantic, but more than friendship.

After so much time isolated and drowning in shame, surrounded only by people who won't let me grow out of the role they've pigeonholed me in, I feel liberated, appreciated, and seen. Curtis makes it okay for me to just be myself, but when fall comes, he leaves Arizona and heads to BYU in Provo, Utah. I start my junior year of high school in Snowflake. I find myself very much alone, again.

So far, junior year has been unbearable. It's only been two weeks, but Deckland is off in the Air Force somewhere and Zoe is two hours away in Flagstaff at college. Kat is here but pretends that I'm invisible. She's still mad at me for what she thinks happened with Michael, at least I assume that's why, but since she won't talk to me, I don't really know.

I had hoped Michael's brothers, Luke or Brian, might have a message from him, but neither of them came back to school this year either. There's no one I can ask where they went or how Michael is doing.

On top of all this isolation, my parents won't let me do cheer. They think I'm too busy, and they don't trust me to travel for school events anymore. I no longer belong in band either. Mr. Douglas began bullying me worse than any of the other students, just because I missed band camp due to family drama. Eventually, my parents have to get involved, and I join the orchestra. Mr. Douglas must have gotten into trouble because he shows up to my house with his wife to apologize to me. Apparently, Dad is the only man allowed to bully me.

High school is not the same without friends, band, or cheer. I've gotten used to being independent, but the loneliness hurts so much I almost miss being on house arrest.

I need out of this tiny town. I need to graduate early or something so that I can go someplace where no one knows me and start fresh. Mr.

Brundy, the principal, denied my request to graduate a year early. He doesn't think I can make up the second half of last year's credits as well as finish both my junior and senior year before May. He's probably right, but I don't care. I'm so desperate for change I pester my parents to enroll me in a correspondence high school, so that I can complete my senior credits through the mail while finishing my junior year at Snowflake High. They agree, probably because I'll be so busy with homework that I'll be home more often, but especially so that they can keep an eye on me.

With no social life and no extracurricular activities to consume my every waking moment, I knock out the remaining credits from sophomore year and all of my senior credits except math with American School of Correspondence before Christmas. In January of 1998, I begin applying for colleges and mailing tapes of me playing the flute to several "good Mormon schools."

A few months later, Dad whines as the acceptance letters begin rolling in with scholarship offers.

"She can't go, Emma. She'll just sleep around. Once you've had sex, you either hate it or can't get enough of it. Besides, she's not even old enough to buy Tylenol."

I thought my parents would be proud of me, but it only gave Dad something new to whine about and take away from me. He refuses to let me go. At 17, I need his permission to live in the dorms. "Think of all the returned missionaries; a promiscuous girl is a danger to them."

Mom takes his side, as usual. "Sarah, just take the scholarship at Northland Pioneer College. It's perfect… you can live at home."

NPC's proximity to "home" makes it my last choice, not my first. It's such a small school that I have to join the show choir in order to qualify for the full ride scholarship. I've never sung in a choir, ever. I'd stopped singing in front of people in the fifth grade when Dad told me I "sang through my nose."

"Joining show choir is a small price to pay for a free education, Sarah. Dad and I aren't going to go into debt to pay your tuition when you could go on a scholarship. That's why we paid all that money for flute lessons," Mom scolds.

I sigh. They're pretending like that's the only option.

"The other scholarships don't have show choir strings attached," I persist.

"You heard your father. The other scholarships are for schools far away, and you're not old enough or ready to live away from home," she adds for emphasis.

Realizing I never really had a choice shouldn't surprise me. NPC it is. I quit my job at Ed's and begin working at Arby's since the manager assures me that they will accommodate my class schedule at NPC. Maybe I can transfer to a university next year when I'm 18.

I sit in choir the first day of class, looking out for familiar faces, afraid that the rumors from high school will follow me here. Mr. Beaufort is in the middle of testing everyone's vocal range and assigning sections when a voice from the entrance bellows, "I'm here. Time for the fun to begin!"

I see a tall man with dark hair wearing bright yellow pants that shame the sun with a white T-shirt and burgundy suit jacket. His pants are tucked into his pointy-toe cowboy boots, and his felt cowboy hat has a feather sticking out of it. I'm as disgusted as I am intrigued.

Mr. Beaufort ignores him and waves off the laughter from students.

One of the tenors asks, "Hey, Mason, when did you get home from your mission?"

"Last week, Isaiah. Boston was great." His cheerfulness grates my nerves.

"That's enough chatter, Westbrook. You're a tenor if I remember correctly." Mr. Beaufort raises a brow and points for Mason to move to the tenor section.

"Yessiree, I sure am."

My lip curls under my wrinkled nose, and I cringe when he takes a seat across from me.

STICK SHIFT

SPRING 1999

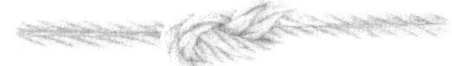

ALMOST 18 YEARS OLD

As soon as Dad discovers that he and Mason both served in the Boston mission, Mason receives the stamp of parental approval.

In Northland Pioneer College's show choir, I'm the only one in the class with any kind of dance experience. The student choreographer assigned Mason and me as dance partners because she knows I don't like him. She teaches us some weird version of the fox trot that doesn't really fit the medley we are supposed to dance and sing to. I'm mortified at first, and Mason is incapable of being serious. He laughs his way through the routine, not minding at all that he keeps stepping on my toes and spinning me with an ungraceful yank. For weeks, I try to talk myself into hating him, but disgust turns to amusement and intrigue to adoration.

Being the more experienced dancer in class, I stand in ballroom posture and show Mason where to place his hands for correct form. He purposefully pulls my right hand out of placement so that the audience will be able to see my face while we sing. Up and down our clasped hands go until my resolve cracks into a fit of giggles. Mason is unlike anyone I'd met before. Our little show choir may look awful, but at least Mason and I are having fun.

His suave pickup line for our first date is, "Do you like food?" Since I'm only 17, my parents require me to double date, so he brings his parents along and introduces them as his big sister and her boyfriend. I get over the weirdness of his parents joining us as soon as we get back to his house, where they leave us alone.

At the end of our first date, he pulls his guitar out and sings first to me and then with me. Apparently, the way to this girl's heart is through music.

My parents are thrilled when Mason asks me to marry him a few months after that first date. The fact that I'm still only 17 doesn't seem to bother them at all. He is everything they've ever dreamed of, and he's the only boy I've ever brought home that Dad liked. Another Mormon whirlwind romance success story, I guess.

I wish I could tell Mason the entire story about Michael, but my parents are right: If Mason knew what happened, he probably wouldn't want to marry me anymore. I really do love Mason, and I want him to love me for me, not the person he thinks I am. I feel guilty that our marriage is also my ticket out of my parents' home.

"Whoa, easy off the clutch, Sarah." Mason sits in the passenger seat directing my efforts to drive his touchy Chevy S-10. I hate his truck, but I have to learn how to drive it since it will be the only car we have after we are married.

"Press down on the gas until you feel the engine take hold, then slowly lift up on the clutch," he coaches.

Thanks to Zoe, I know how to drive a manual transmission, I just suck at it. Dad's 1966 Ford is a manual transmission, and at least twice I almost crashed it because I'm too short to fully depress the brake pedal. Zoe was as gentle a teacher as Mason is, but the clutch in her Colt was far easier to manage.

I grip the steering wheel, my knuckles white, and grind my teeth.

"Sarah, you look really rigid. You need to relax."

"I'm trying!" I shift back to first gear.

The truck lurches again before stalling in the dark parking lot. Tears form behind my eyes, and I let out an exasperated huff.

"Are you okay?" Mason leans in, his hand on my back.

I shake my head. "This morning, Dad punched Joey so hard he knocked him right out of his chair. Joey was being a smart mouth, but still."

"I'm sorry, Sarah." Mason is quiet for a minute. "I know what that's like. My dad has been violent with me and my siblings, too."

Every time something like this happens, we assure each other we'll raise our future kids without violence or fear. I'm comforted that Mason is as committed as I am to addressing serious problems without screaming at people. "That must have been really hard to see," he adds.

"It gets worse. The cops came by work today. At first, I thought maybe Joey told on Dad and they were looking to get a statement, but they weren't. They told me someone painted 'Sarah Lee is a slut' on the side of one of the high school buildings."

"Why would someone do that?"

I feel a twinge of guilt. I'm not ready to tell Mason about Michael. I haven't spoken to Jamie since my Mom called her mom about the prank. A searing pain explodes in my chest, and my vision begins to narrow. I push from my mind the images of Jamie standing above me at Ed's yelling "Michael is dead." I'm pretty sure Jamie is the graffiti artist, but I don't voice my suspicions to Mason in case I'm wrong.

"I don't know, I mean, I don't even attend school there anymore. I just…"

Mason turns the ignition off and leans over my lap, pushing the emergency brake pedal down with his hand. He sits himself back up, then wraps his arms around me and pulls me onto his lap. I sob into his shoulder until I run dry.

"You ready to try driving again?" Mason asks gently once I'm calm.

"No, I'm done for today." I lift my face from the crook of his neck, "Thanks, I feel better."

He leans forward to give me a slow, sweet kiss.

The truck cab lights up blue and red from behind. I climb out of his lap to let him slide over to the driver's seat.

I turn in my seat and squint at the bright lights, more irritated than concerned. "There are two cop cars behind us."

Mason opens the driver's side door and steps out.

"Get back in the vehicle," a voice booms over a loudspeaker.

I guess they're going to be overly dramatic about this.

Mason leaps back into the seat and rolls the window down while we wait for the officer to approach. I shift nervously in my seat; this guy is taking forever.

If Mason shares my annoyance, I can't tell. He addresses the cop with the same relaxed, friendly tone he does to everyone else. "Good evening, officer. Is everything okay?"

Sweeping his flashlight on Mason, then over to me, then down to our feet (most likely looking for booze), the young blond-haired officer says, "A gentleman in the building was concerned. Your truck was moving funny in the parking lot."

I lean forward so that I can see the officer's stupid grin. I roll my eyes and feel the slow simmer of annoyance at pious church members trying to protect our chastity.

Mason laughs. "I can see why he was concerned. I was just trying to teach my fiancé how to drive a stick. As you can tell, she needs a lot of practice."

The officer leans into the window a little and takes a long look at me.

"We needed a big, flat surface for her to practice on. The clutch is finicky." Mason maintains his pleasant tone, even though the officer acts like we are lying.

"It is hard to learn how to drive a stick shift from the passenger seat," the officer says. "You may want to find a different parking lot for your, uh… extracurricular activities."

"Will do," Mason agrees.

The cop steps away, and the flashing lights turn off. Mason starts the truck and spins his tires slightly on our way out. "What on earth do they think we'd be doing in the *church's* parking lot!" he exclaims. Leave it to Mason to assume no one would have sex in a car in the parking lot of the Church of Jesus Christ of Latter-Day Saints.

WEDDING DAY

JUNE 4, 1999

18 YEARS OLD

I sit alone in the bridal room of the Mesa, Arizona temple staring into the mirror. My blue eyes blink back at me. I'm stunning. My hair and makeup are perfect. The wedding dress that my mother has sewn fits flawlessly. I'm supposed to be giddy, overjoyed. Mostly, I just feel empty. Numb. Sad. Guilty.

I love Mason. He and I have fun together. He's one of my closest friends, but he doesn't know the real me. Hell, I don't even know the real me, anymore. I've spent the last two years of my life obeying Dad's orders, being followed by Mom, and pretending to be the perfect Mormon daughter in order to earn my freedom back. I'd fantasized about this day with Johnny, but he's in Amsterdam with an entire year left of his mission. I "Dear John-ed" him due to pressure from my parents about how amazing and "better for me" Mason was than "any of my other boyfriends."

I hear people moving around just outside the women's dressing room, and I think about running. I don't think I'll get very far, not in my gown. Not with Mason's and my extended family inside and outside the temple. I'm surrounded. Besides, I'd break his heart, and I don't think I can do that to him. He doesn't deserve to be hurt. My mind wanders to Michael. I ache for him, even though I haven't heard from him since that final phone call.

I play with a ringlet placed carefully in front of my right ear. The temple garment under my dress itches. I'm never going to get used to wearing this much fabric under my everyday clothing.

"Leave your hair alone, Sarah," Mom says as she walks back into the bridal room. "You don't want to ruin it, do you?"

"I'm pretty sure the temple veil will do more damage than my fingers," I snap back. I've been bitchy all week. Mom ignores me as she helps tie me into my Mormon temple clothing.

I don't understand the point of wearing this exquisite gown only to have it covered up by all the ceremonial clothing. After adjusting the robe on my right shoulder, Mom turns me around carefully so that she can tie the vibrant green apron around my waist without stepping on the hemline of my gown.

I look into the mirror again and crinkle up my nose. The vibrant green looks out of place against the stark white of my wedding gown. Mom ties the white sash atop the apron with the bow on the left side as instructed, then motions for me to bend down so she can add the temple veil to the costume.

Once again, I look into the mirror. I look ridiculous. There is nothing beautiful about all the extra fabric. I sigh. In wearing magic underwear, my wedding gown, the temple robe and apron, my wedding veil, and the temple's headdress, I would outlast any opponent in strip poker, but if this costume is what it's going to take to escape my prison, then so be it.

"You look lovely," Mom says.

I raise my eyebrows at her.

"Oh stop, Sarah. The temple clothes come off right after the sealing ceremony."

"Good to know," I countered. So much for the wedding I had always dreamed about. There would be no aisle to walk down, no wedding march, no fireflies, not even a "you may now kiss the bride" to complete the ceremony. The Mormon Church has commandeered everything else in my life, so why not this, too?

I let out a slow, resigned sigh. The temple matron, an elderly lady with snowy hair pulled into a tight bun, motions to my Mom that it's time. People speak only in whispers inside the temple.

Mom gathers up the back of my gown so that I can walk down the hallway to the sealing room. I steal one last glance in the mirror.

I mouth "goodbye" to my reflection, close my eyes, and let the images of the two other men I love—Johnny and Michael—hover in my memory before following the matron down the hall where I will marry Mason for time and all eternity.

LONG DRIVE HOME

AUGUST 1999

18 YEARS OLD

I'm tired and hungry. Mason and I have only been married for two and a half months. I'm not so sure I like this "goal" of attending the temple once a month until we have kids. Mason seems oblivious to the fact that I feel like standing in as proxy to baptize or marry dead people in the Mormon way is a chore rather than a date, and it's kinda culty. "As long as he's following the counsel of the prophet, it must be good. Screw creative dates that are fun and stick with repetitive rituals and ceremony," I silently mock.

Just thinking about it gives me the creeps. Finally, after three long hours, we're out of there and in Mason's S-10 heading home.

"Why do you do that?" The irritation in my voice is unmistakable after enduring the very long session at the temple. Going is supposed to make me more spiritual. It isn't working. If anything, it makes me bitchy.

"Do what?" he asks through a mouthful of sunflower seeds. His knee presses into the steering wheel, holding it in place while he spits shells into the cup in his left hand and spins the radio dial with his right. "Change the station before the song ends. It drives me nuts. The chords haven't resolved before you start searching for a new song." He glances my way and shrugs. "Hearing the first few seconds of the advertisement won't kill you, ya know?" I criticize.

He chuckles. "It might, you never know."

"Driving with your knee might kill us both," I retort. Mason's inattentive driving scares me. I've started inhaling sharply like Mom used to do anytime we passed big rigs on the highway after our car accident when I was six.

I'm feeling more irritable than normal after a trip to the temple. It's at least an eight-hour commitment when you add in the commute from the White Mountains down to the Valley. We've done it so many times that I've got all of my lines for the temple rituals down by heart and almost the entire video memorized. I can't shake the feeling that the temple ceremony is culty, with a secret handshake and series of code words in order to get into heaven. Besides, Joseph Smith taught that the way to know the difference between a messenger from God or Satan was to shake hands with them. Joseph had said if the messenger had lived on earth, died and been resurrected with Jesus, you would feel the messenger shake your hand. If the messenger was from God but hadn't been born yet, they would refuse to shake your hand. If the messenger was from Satan, then they would extend their hand for the shake but you wouldn't feel anything upon taking it.

In the temple video, Jesus's apostles Peter, James, and John, who have not yet been born, appear to Adam and Eve in order to teach them God's law. Adam knows they are messengers from God because Peter uses one of the secret handshakes taught in the temple. Adam can obviously feel the hand to know if the handshake was positioned correctly. It's a direct contradiction from what Joseph Smith said, and I feel like I'm the only one who has noticed or cares about the contradiction.

I told Mason about the discrepancy, and he said he didn't know what it meant either. He was more bothered by the fact that the creation story in the temple video didn't match the timeline in the Bible or the "Pearl of Great Price," and planned to ask someone the next time we went. I wanted to spend my Saturday doing something more fun, like going for a hike and picnic lunch, but we were demonstrating our righteousness by following the counsel from our church leaders to attend the temple often.

"Mason, stop. You are scaring me. There are too many twists and turns for you to be driving with your knee like that. Leave the radio alone and focus on the road for a change."

Mason moves his knee away from the steering wheel, sets his cup down in the cupholder and grabs a random country CD to pop into the disc player. Mason's love for country music has exposed me to a bunch of nasal, twangy, love songs.

The whine of country music is something I'm having a hard time adjusting to. "Thank you," I say, only slightly less irritated.

He reaches for my hand, and I take it. "Are you feeling okay?"

The way Mason takes the sharp turns so fast, veering the Chevy S-10 truck into the lane of oncoming traffic, leaning into his turns like a NASCAR driver, terrifies me. I usually close my eyes and count to 100 until we are out of the Canyon.

"I feel car sick when we go this way." I cross my arms across my chest and stick out my lower lip. He doesn't notice. If he knew how grumpy I feel after going to the temple, he'd just lecture me about how I'm not going "in the right spirit to feel the Spirit."

"I'll try to go a little slower," he promises. He made the same promise last month but forgot as soon as we entered the Canyon.

He is too caught up in the fun of driving through the death trap like it's a videogame to remember my discomfort. As usual, I lay the seat back and close my eyes. If I can fall asleep, I tend to do better. I'm almost asleep when a familiar tune sounds over the speaker. I jolt upright.

"Who is singing this?" I ask Mason.

"John Michael Montgomery. His version of 'I Swear' is way better than All-4-One's version. He was the original artist, I think," Mason answers.

I see the questions in your eyes

My heart skips a beat, and I hold my breath.

I know what's weighing on your mind

I lean forward and hit the skip button.

"What's wrong? I love that song," Mason asks, annoyed.

"I hate that song," I lie. "I don't care who is singing it."

I adjust the blanket and shift onto my side, my back to Mason so he can't see my face.

"Oh, okay. I didn't know that."

"Well, now you do."

I close my eyes as the warmth of a tear slides down my temple into my pillow. I wonder how Johnny is doing on his mission in Amsterdam.

NEIGHBORHOOD ADVENTURES

EL PASO, TEXAS
APRIL 10, 2004

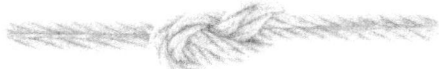

23 YEARS OLD

After almost five years of marriage and twenty months in the Army, Mason is finally going to begin his MOS—Army-speak for his job. Over the years, he's become my best friend, and we've settled into our marriage with ease. I'm so proud of him for graduating top of his class from Army nursing school in Tacoma Washington and am looking forward to our first real duty station in El Paso, Texas. We took some extra time off to visit family in California and Arizona on our move from the Pacific Northwest to west Texas, and Eric, our two-year-old, has been a champion sitting in the car for the better part of a week. All three of us are done with our move/

vacation and are ready to settle into our new home, grateful to finally be arriving at our destination.

"Here we are," Mason says as he pulls into the parking lot of a run-down outbuilding. Everything on Fort Bliss looks rundown and old.

"Mason, can you grab Eric and take him with you?" I snap the leash on the collar around the neck of our chocolate cocker spaniel, André, who is prancing on the pillows stacked high next to Eric's car seat, indicating the need to pee. The dog leaps from his perch and stumbles slightly onto the hot asphalt. He tugs against the leash, sniffing everything.

"Sure." Mason steps out of our gray Avalon, his arms above his head, his back arched as he reaches for the sky in a long stretch.

I allow André to explore the small parking lot while I wait for Mason and Eric to reappear with the keys to our new home. We haven't lived on post before, and I'm not too keen on the idea that they literally assigned you a house, as in, "Here are the keys. If you don't like the place… fuck you… this is the Army. You take what you get, and you don't throw a fit." I'm prepared to accept whatever is offered to us since we can't afford to rent off post. Mostly I'm just ready to be unpacked and settled into a new home. We'd moved three times in under two years. I crave stability more than chocolate these days.

"You ready to go see our new home?" Mason emerges from the housing office, exhaustion etched in the dark circles under his eyes.

"Keys, Mama, keys!" Eric exclaims, holding the keys in his little fist high above his head in one hand, his other hand clenched in Mason's.

André barks excitedly.

"For better or worse, right?" Mason offers.

I shrug. "Yup, let's go see this house."

We load Eric and the dog back into the car and drive the few miles to the duplex that is our new home.

"It's not too bad, is it? Sarah?" The home is larger than either apartment we'd lived in since leaving Lakeside, Arizona, for the Army. It has cafeteria stick-on tiles for flooring and a closed-in kitchen.

"It's very… white—walls, ceiling, floors," I finally respond. "Am I allowed to paint this place?"

Mason is squinting at a spot on the wall.

I look at the wall, but there's nothing there.

"Why are you squinting?"

"Because, it's white and bright," he answers with a stupid grin. "I bet we can have this place painted before the moving company delivers our furniture."

Mason grabs my wrist and tugs me into him, wrapping his arms around my back. I sigh and hug tightly. We stand there, swaying, drinking in the calm for a full minute. We have 48 hours before our household goods will be delivered.

By noon on the first full day, the walls are a warm beige and shaggy area rugs cover the ugly stick-on floor tiles. Mason removed the door to the kitchen to help the area feel more open. The warm light from a few floor lamps helps the place looks less regimented. It takes us only a day to unpack our household goods and about $600 to completely stock our pantry and refrigerator. In true Army family fashion, by the end of the first week we feel pretty settled, have met and made new friends, and Mason is ready to start work at William Beaumont Army Medical Center for the next three to five years.

Turns out Mason loves his job as a medical/surgical floor nurse, and I love his schedule. He works 12-hour shifts on a rotating schedule of four days on/three days off. I spend his working days getting to know my new Army sisters. Grace, Finn, Scarlett, and I met at church and have spent our free time exploring our neighborhood and the city of El Paso. We do everything together and soon feel more like family than friends. On Mason's days off, we leave Eric with one of them and go on a date, or less romantic, we work on the next step of preparing for the adoption of our second son Brigg. We are both anxious and excited to be adding to our family.

A few weeks before we left Washington, a pregnant woman from church, Jennifer, had called to ask some questions about her rights as a birth mother. She desired an open adoption and wasn't sure if it was even possible. It's fairly common for Mormons to seek counsel from other members of the church. Since Eric had joined our family, I had unofficially become an expert on all things adoption. I answered Jennifer's questions the best I could. It was a complete surprise when a few hours later she called back and asked if Mason and I would adopt her unborn child and honor her request for an open adoption.

As soon as we arrived in El Paso, we started the process of hiring a social worker to come to our duplex and do a home study. By the end of March, we had completed all the required steps in preparation for welcoming a second child into our little family. The baby was due in August, so Mason and I busied ourselves with setting up the nursery and shopping for baby stuff with whatever little extra we could squeeze out of an already strangled budget. Eric would turn three shortly after the baby would be born, so the timing was perfect.

Despite the anticipated stress of feeding another mouth, we were excited. Without even looking for it, we were going to bring another child into the loving, stable family we dreamed of creating. Mason was established in his new career, and my parents were hundreds of miles away in Arizona. For the first time in years, life felt happy, normal, and manageable.

In true military fashion, my new friends became closer than family in the two months since settling into our new home in El Paso.

"Finn, how much longer will Dallin be in Iraq?" I ask a little breathless.

Finn brushes the escaped dirty blond curls away from her face. "At least another ten months." Shortly before Mason and I moved in, her husband, Dallin, deployed to Iraq. Almost immediately, Finn had to have major surgery. That first Sunday at church, I volunteered to visit her in the hospital; we clicked immediately. As soon as she was given the clearance to be discharged, we started walking religiously in the evening with our young children.

"Is this pace good for you or do you need me to slow down?" I ask her. Even though Finn is 100 pounds overweight and theoretically still recovering from surgery, it's a struggle for me to hold a conversation while trying to keep up with her on our nightly neighborhood walk.

"You know I'll tell you to slow down if I need you to," Finn reassures me.

She is in much better shape than I am; she has an easier time keeping stride while hefting a toddler in a backpack than I have just pushing an empty stroller while Eric runs alongside. The infertility medications I took the first five years of my marriage have taken a toll on my mental and physical health. Finn's ability to out-walk and out-perform me is a frustrating reminder of how much my body has changed. I miss feeling fit. I just need to keep up so I can regain my strength.

"Mom, I need go potty," Kris informs Finn.

"Me, too," Eric chimes in.

Kris is a year younger than Eric, but six inches taller. The two boys are as close as brothers. They do everything together, including potty training. Just last week I snapped a picture of the two of them peeing in the toilet. When I asked them why they hadn't taken turns, they explained that going at the same time was faster and they needed to get back to their golf game. Their friendship reminds me of how close I once was to Susan Davis, before we burned down our bush fort.

"Kristoff, you went right before we left. We aren't even two blocks away from Miss Sarah's house. Can you hold it?"

"I pee-pee in diaper, go walk?" he asks, clinging his bony body to Finn's leg.

"I wonder if we could knock on some random person's door and ask to use their bathroom…" Finn's voice trails off as she looks up and down the street of identical duplexes.

Eric tugs on my pant leg, "Momm-m-m-m-m." He's prancing from foot to foot.

"I don't think we have time. We are only a block from the elementary school. I wonder if their playground is open," I suggest.

"Not helpful, Sarah."

"Hey boys, do you want to learn how to pee like we are camping?"

"Yes!" they cry excitedly.

I instruct the boys on how to "camping pee" by having them face the bush next to where we are standing. They giggle when I tell them they have to pull their pants down just a little bit, not so far that anyone driving by can see what they're doing, but far enough so that they don't pee-pee on themselves. The boys successfully water the bushes before yanking up their pants and running ahead of us, our route familiar to them.

We swing by the elementary school to check out the playground, which is surrounded by a tall, locked fence.

"Come on, Kris, let's look for a secret way in," Eric says as he tugs on Kris's skinny arm. Kris stumbles a bit then chases after him.

"Five minutes boys," I call after them.

"Only five minutes?" Finn asks.

"Camping pee isn't appropriate for moms on this neighborhood adventure," I sigh, feeling the need myself for a bathroom, "and I don't think I want to make new friends by asking to use their bathroom when my house is just up the street. Only a pregnant woman could pull that one off."

She laughs, and we watch the boys search in silence. They haven't found a secret entrance, but now they are shooting each other with their pretend machine guns and rolling in the grass to dodge the bullets.

"I wish I had their energy," Finn exclaims.

"I think you do. How do you keep that pace?"

"Dallin inspires me. If you think I leave you in the dust, just wait 'til you meet Dallin."

"How are things going for him?"

"He says good. He's discrete, but I know he's seeing a lot of stuff that's hard. He tells me he isn't in harm's way, but he's lying to try to protect me. He's a combat medic, so I know he's holding back. I'm grateful we invested in the satellite phones."

I've seen the bulky phones Finn is talking about. They're unreliable at best, but unreliable is better than nothing.

"I'm gonna need you to show me how to do the instant messenger thing on the computer if Mason has to go over there. We can't afford a phone like that."

"I can show you tonight if you like. It isn't hard to do. It's a good way to keep in contact with family since you live so far away."

"Mason's family doesn't talk. They aren't mad at each other… they just don't do phone calls unless there is a family emergency. We can go months without hearing from his parents, and they all think that's normal. My mom won't use the computer as long as we can talk on the phone every day, so I don't really need it unless Mason gets deployed."

"Makes sense. I'm looking forward to meeting your parents."

"They aren't coming for another six weeks."

My parents can't handle more than a couple of months between visits with Eric. El Paso was a six-hour drive from their home in Arizona, and since my siblings were older, they felt comfortable making a quick weekend trip every so often. Plus, I would probably make one or two trips to visit them in the summer, even though I didn't really want to.

"You don't seem very excited about their visit. I figured you would be excited to see your Mom considering how often you two talk."

"I'm very excited to see my Mom. She and I are really close. I'm not excited about seeing Dad. It takes me at least a week to recover my nerves when he visits. I'm not sure why, though, since he basically ignores me and plays with Eric the entire time."

"You should probably talk to someone about that. It's not normal to take that many days to feel better after someone leaves."

"I talked to the bishop about it once. He told me I needed to pray, read my scriptures, and forgive my Dad. He said my Dad didn't actually abuse me… was just trying to protect me. I think he might be right. My Dad slapped me a few times, yelled in my face once or twice, and pushed me to the ground once. That's not really abusive, maybe just a little excessive."

We hear Kris's piercing cry. His knee is red and bleeding. Eric is trying to pull him up from the rocky ground where he is sitting.

"Looks like it's time to head home," Finn says. I watch as she picks Kris up and helps him climb into her sling. Kris tugs at her shirt, searching for her breast. Finn is the only woman I have ever met who nurses her children so long; Kris is almost two. She's also the only woman I've ever met who is indiscreet in her nursing habits. Kris latches on and swallows loudly with his eyes closed. I worry about what my Dad is going to say when Finn whips her boob out in front of him to nurse her toddler. I secretly hope she weans him in the next six weeks.

Eric has climbed into the stroller and buckled himself in.

A cramp in my lower abdomen reminds me that I need to pee. I pivot the stroller and pick up my pace, attempting to speed walk the two blocks home with an unruly stroller. The front wheel spins out of control, causing the stroller to veer off the sidewalk. I nudge the front wheel back in line and notice a large black bird perched on the roof peak of the duplex across the street from me.

I smile, and it tilts its head to the side as if he's noticed I'm watching him. I step back around behind the stroller then look back up at the bird, but it has flown away. It's then that I notice the name plate next to the door of the duplex the bird had been on.

I lurch backward. A warm trickle escapes down the sides of my legs as I stare at the door.

It says: SPC M.D. Iles.

IT'S NOT MY FAULT

APRIL 10–11, 2004

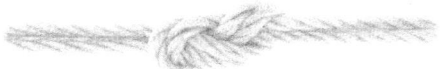

23 YEARS OLD

"Are you okay?" Finn's concerned face finally registers with me as I find myself standing in the middle of the street under the setting desert sun. "That looked like an absence seizure." She's looking at the puddle of urine I'm standing in. "You're white as a ghost. Do I need to take you to the hospital?"

I blink and shake my head.

"Do you have seizures?"

I shake my head again.

"Are you okay… Sarah?"

"I… I… I just want to go home."

Finn reaches out to me. I jerk back sharply, not wanting to be touched. Her hand retreats.

"Sorry, I thought I saw something, and it freaked me out. I'm okay, really."

I head home fast, wet fabric chafing between my legs. My face is cold and tingling. There is no way that's *his* house. No way. After six years of silence, I've lost track of where he might be, but I know that it can't be here. The chances that it's the same Iles are so minuscule, it's just not possible.

"Sarah, slow down, why are you jogging? I can't keep up with *you* now, not with Kris nursing."

I didn't even realize I was running. I stop and wait as Finn shuffles to me across the dividing road to our side of Steele Road, one hand clutching Kristoff's head to her breast, the other pinning his bottom to her belly.

"Sorry, I just want to get home and take a shower."

In front of my house, she loads a now sleeping Kristoff into his car seat without coming in. She closes the door gently.

"Call me if you need anything, seriously." I can tell she means it.

"I will. I just need a shower and sleep." I love Finn and how much she cares for me, but right now I just need to be alone so I can clean myself up and process this.

"Do you want me to take Eric? He's always welcome to spend the night."

She gives a weak smile and climbs into the driver's seat of her green Subaru Forester. It sinks under her weight.

"No, I've got him. He's pretty easy to get to bed." I shift uncomfortably in my wet pants, leaning toward my house where Eric is already waiting on the step. "Thanks for everything, Finn. I'll explain later."

She looks sharply into my eyes. "Call me if you need me."

I fight back the tears and wave.

She closes her car door and backs out of my driveway.

Eric grabs his plastic golf set as soon as we walk in the front door of the duplex. I close the door behind us and lean against it, clenching my jaw.

"It's not him, Sarah. You're being crazy," I say out loud.

"What, Mommy?" Eric drags his golf set behind him.

"Nothing, sweet boy. Mama's gonna go take a shower."

"Did you have an accident?"

"Yup." I try to keep my voice even so I don't upset Eric.

I walk past him, his golf club held high, ready for action, and lock my bedroom door behind me.

"It's not his house, Sarah, it's not his house," I chant as I remove my pants. The knee-length, white temple garment sticks to my wet legs. I've never felt comfortable in the Mormon underwear. It's always hot and sticking to me, and urine doesn't help any of that. Once in the shower, I soap up quickly, trying not to get my long hair wet. I don't have time for a full shower, not with Eric unsupervised.

I continue chanting my mantra as I pull on clean garments to wear under my pajamas and place my wet clothes in the washing machine. Eric is sitting on the toilet, waiting.

"Time for bed, kiddo," I say as I wet his toothbrush.

His thick black hair is sticking up in all directions and he smells like little boy funk. The creases on the back of his neck are covered in a light layer of rust-color desert dust. It's barely noticeable on his milk chocolate skin.

Adopting Eric soothed the pain of infertility. If I had married Michael, I wouldn't have Eric. Besides, there is no way that was his house. I hurry and get Eric to bed and flip off the light.

Once in my room, I sit on my bed, listening to the silence. The name plate said SPC M.D. Iles. I'm certain it did. I have thought about Michael every single day since we were forcibly separated. I have wondered about him, worried about him, ached for him.

I've wanted to apologize for so many things.

Dad had ruined his life. The last thing I heard about Michael was that he had been admitted to a long-term mental hospital. When Dad found out, he looked smug. "See, I knew it. I knew that boy was crazy. You should be grateful to be rid of him, Sarah."

I haven't cried over Michael since Eric joined our family. I am not about to start now. Raising my son was the distraction I needed to avoid the memories and nightmares of Michael.

After Michael, I fell into a dark hole. I didn't want to live. I could actually apologize to him now. I could say goodbye. God knows I need closure.

"I'm so sorry, Michael," I say to myself. "I went silent to protect you. I didn't know then that Dad was lying about throwing you in jail. I'm so sorry."

My whispered words break the dam holding back my tears. I let them come.

"It wasn't him!" I stand abruptly and march around the foot of our bed to the small computer desk nestled in the corner.

I flip on the monitor and wait for the screen to flicker to life. I've avoided looking him up on the internet for over six years. I navigate to the online white pages to search for "Michael Iles" in Texas. Only two entries

344

come back. One for Michael A. Iles and one for Michael D. Iles. I move the arrow on my screen to hover over Michael D.'s name and click.

I try to calm myself while I wait for the page to load.

Michael D. Iles
3150 A Steele Rd.
El Paso, TX 79904
(915) 556-8322

I inhale sharply.

My address, 3140 B Steele Rd., is 10 doors down.

I hear Mason come in the front door and move quietly about the house. It's Sunday. He'll want to take a short nap before we get out of bed and go to church. I hear him pour cereal into a bowl. I stand up from the computer chair and turn off the screen without closing the white pages. I stretch, not that it helps. My lower back aches, and my eyes are dry; I sat in that chair all night, even after I cried myself to sleep.

I creep past Eric's room to the kitchen. Eric is a grumpy little thing until an hour after breakfast, and I need time to talk to Mason. I have no idea how or where to begin, but I know that he doesn't deserve to have to deal with this.

"Wow, morning, beautiful. You're up early."

"Yeah, I didn't sleep last night."

He offers me the cereal box. I notice he's set two extra bowls and spoons on the table.

"No thanks, I'm not feeling very hungry."

"Are you sick?"

"No." I grab a spoon and run my thumb over the cold metal. What I really want to say is, "Can we move to Italy," but that's just ridiculous.

The way Mason tilts his head reminds me of the bird on the rooftop. I can hear the Raisin Bran crunching in his mouth as he chews; he's waiting for me to talk.

"Finn and I let the boys play in the field next to the elementary school last night after our walk. We wanted to see if the playground there was open to the public on the weekends. It's not."

"That sucks. We were always able to play in the school yard on the weekends growing up."

"Yeah, me too… anyway, we took Steele Road home from the school. I saw a bird…"

I hesitate. How do I tell Mason about my discovery?

Mason raises his eyebrows. "That's weird. There are no birds in El Paso. It must have crossed the border illegally."

I chuckle at his joke, then fall silent again.

"Sarah, is Eric okay?"

I nod.

"And you're okay?"

I nod again.

"Well, then… it can't be that bad." I watch Mason chewing obliviously; he has no idea.

"Michael lives ten doors down the street."

"Michael who?" he takes another big bite of cereal.

"Iles."

His brow lifts and his eyes widen. "*The* Michael Iles?"

"Yes."

Mason freezes, his spoon suspended in midair, his mouth open. "That's not a funny joke, Sarah."

I fight tears. "It's not a joke, Mason."

Milk drips from the spoon leaving splatters on the table. He is looking at me, but I can't read his face. I lean forward and push the bowl closer to him to catch the drips. Our pendulum clock ticks in the background. Finally, he lowers his arm and uses the sleeve of his fatigues to mop up the milk drips.

"Have you seen him?" His voice comes out strained. It hurts to see his discomfort on top of my own.

"I was reading the name plates next to the doors and his name was on it, so I looked him up on the internet and it's his house."

"He can't know you are here."

"Mason, we just moved here. The Army won't move us again for at least two years, probably longer. How are we supposed to avoid each other? We'll eventually bump into each other somewhere on post. Our kids will probably attend the same preschool next year... if he has kids..." My voice trails off when I see the redness in Mason's face, his teeth grinding.

"You seem to have put a lot of thought into this," he snaps.

I feel guilty even though none of this is *my* fault.

"What are the odds that we would be at the same duty station at the same time, much less the same neighborhood, on the same damn street?"

He winces. "Don't cuss, Sarah. You're smarter than that."

"I saw the name plate and peed my pants, literally. Finn thought I had an absence seizure or something. I've been up all night. Please don't yell at me."

"You're right, I'm sorry. It's probably not him."

"That's what I thought, too, but…"

"Yeah," he cuts me off short. "But you haven't seen him and now you have his phone number."

"I left the page up on the computer screen so you can see it," I offer, hoping that if Mason can see that I'm not trying to hide anything, it'll be easier for him to forgive me when he finds out what I've hidden in the past.

"You don't plan on calling him, do you?" Mason looks exacerbated. I can tell he doesn't understand; I'm not really sure that I understand, either.

"I don't know what I'm going to do. I don't have a plan. But I'd much rather have control over when and how we meet. I think a phone call saying, 'Hey, sorry for the shit my Dad put us through. I'm your neighbor… by the way, stay away,' is better than unexpectedly running into him in the commissary with our families and being like, 'Oh hey, Michael, yeah, I knew you lived here, surprise.'"

Mason scowls at my sarcasm. "Do you think he'll stay away if you ask him to?"

Michael was persistent in high school, but after my parents pulled me from high school, he wasn't there even when I desperately wanted him to be.

"I don't know him anymore, Mason. So much happened after we

stopped talking. Last I heard, he was in a mental hospital. I'm not even sure how he got into the Army. I don't even know what job he does."

Mason pushes his cereal bowl from him. "His job doesn't matter. He needs to stay away, and you're not allowed to call him." He crosses his arms.

I slam my fist on the table then stand and turn my back to Mason. "I'm going to go wake up Eric and get him ready for church." I walk away before he can respond. I hear his chair slide away from the table.

"So much for a nap before church," he mutters.

We finish our morning routine in silence and head to church.

Our ward in El Paso is home in the way that the Snowflake Mormon bubble never could be. Not that Mason and I ever really have problems (outside of infertility), but if we did, I know that here they'd be met with love and support by the church members instead of judgment and gossip. I get to be my real self here, and today my real self needs that love and support. I search for Grace's face as soon as I enter the building, with Mason and Eric trailing in behind me.

"What's up, girl?" she asks as I step into the pew in front of her. She always sits behind me so she can play with Eric during the hour-long sacrament meeting. "Finn said you might not be here today because you weren't feeling well."

"I'm more stressed than sick." I shift my eyes in Mason's direction, who is talking to a family across the pew from us, his purple suit standing out like a beacon of brightness in a sea of black suits and ties. "I just need a hug."

"I get it, girl." Grace wraps me in a hard, long hug and whispers, "No matter what Mason has done, it can't be as stupid as what Stephon has done." She's right. Mason is the epitome of "perfect husband." He never does anything "wrong" per se. Strict obedience and extreme faith protect him from actually having to experience anything hard.

Grace leans toward me. I laugh… too late. "Good point, I wouldn't get 'permission' to divorce him over this from the bishop or the stake president."

"That's good to hear. Too bad I haven't listened to them yet about Stephon."

"Isn't it a *sin* to ignore the counsel of your church leaders?" I wink at her.

"Which is a worse sin, divorcing my husband, the sex addict, or murdering him?"

"Murder?" Mason asks as he slides into the pew next to me. "I can't leave you two girls alone, can I?"

"We'll be proper ladies, now that you are here." I huff, turning my body away from him.

We turn our attention to the microphone at the front of the chapel as the bishop welcomes us all to church.

I tune the church leader out immediately. It's been the same talks, the same message I've heard for 23 years. My thoughts return to Michael. What am I going to do?

Eric and I load all my props from the children's church music class back into my bag. Since I hadn't slept, I needed something easy to entertain the 40 or so youngsters. "Fish Your Favorite Song" was a good go-to for this Sunday, since I hadn't prepped to entertain a group of young children.

"I got a snack." Eric holds up a box of frosted animal crackers with a wide toothy grin.

"Those look yummy!" I say ruffling his thick black hair.

"You ready to go?" Mason calls to us from the door of the children's room.

"Just about." I slowly untangle yarn from the small tree branch "fishing pole." The distraction of leading the music in Primary has left me feeling a little better.

A few minutes later, we step out of the cool building into the bright desert sun. I've never done well in the heat, and since going through the temple and promising to wear the Mormon garment, I tolerate it even less.

A bead of sweat trickles down my back. Mason has his hands clenched on the steering wheel, not turning the car on.

"Can you please start the engine? I'm dying in here."

He turns the key in the ignition and turns the AC knob to the highest setting. Hot air blasts my face.

He stares out the windshield, drumming his fingers on the steering wheel. "I'd like to drive by 3150A and see the name plate for myself, just in case you saw it wrong."

Irritated by his reasoning, I'm still glad he suggested it. I'd thought about walking by again on Monday evening with the girls, just to be sure, but was afraid Michael might be outside. Despite seeing the address on the white pages, it just didn't feel possible.

"I like that idea."

We drive past deep green lawns that are out of place in the arid desert back to our Logan Heights neighborhood in silence. Mason passes the turn for our house and drives the additional block to Ellerthorpe Ave.

We approach Steele Road a few moments later. My heart picks up speed, hoping that I had imagined this whole thing. I don't need my past haunting me like this. Mason doesn't need it either. We have enough to worry about.

The car slows to a crawl as I watch Michael, smoking a cigarette while watering his lawn. He looks older, smaller. A little girl with blond pigtails is playing in the driveway. I look away, praying that he doesn't see me, then realize it's unlikely since he has no idea I'm even here. He has a child, a wife; I think of the nine children we dreamt of having.

Cold dread fills my stomach.

AUTHOR'S NOTE

For years I felt deep shame for not responding well to Mason's emotional response to the discovery of Michael's residence so close to ours. I realize now that I was in a full-blown crisis, just trying to deal with my own emotional response. I had coped with the loss of Michael by staying busy with distractions and clinging to Mormonism as a way to keep my closest relationships strong. I understand how normal, yet unhealthy that was. During that phase of my life, I was living in survival mode with my main goal to be "enough" so people wouldn't leave me. The effort included maintaining a relationship with my parents, despite the abuse, and making sure I was a good Mormon wife so I wouldn't lose Mason.

With Michael, I had always been enough. Once I discovered his proximity to me, the desire to just be me overwhelmed my desire to perform for acceptance. The fear of losing Mason wasn't gone. It was overridden by the bond I had with Michael due to the unresolved trauma of my youth, or what is called a trauma bond.

One of the key characteristics of a trauma bond is the way it can negatively impact healthy attachments to those we deeply love. At this time in my life, my bond with Michael due to our shared trauma threatened the attachments I had with my husband and child.

CLOSURE

APRIL 2004

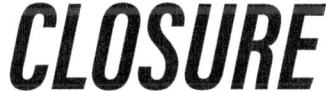

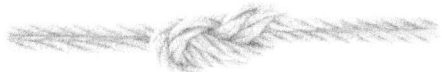

23 YEARS OLD

"No, Sarah, I don't think you should go over there and tell him you live here." Mason's voice is strained.

I wish he would just yell, do anything that would make me feel justified for being angry at him. Instead, he sits on our bed, shoulders hunched, looking defeated.

"I'll just pretend like he's not there," I say, not hiding my sarcasm, "and then one day when I'm all by myself, I'll run into him and it'll be like 'Oh, wow, long time no see.'"

Mason glares at me, his teeth clenched, his chin jutted forward slightly.

"Don't give me the stubborn Westbrook chin. That's not helpful."

"I hate it when you call it that. I'm not my father." Mason usually speaks fondly of his father, but his whole body cringes anytime someone compares him to his dad.

"Your mother does it, too. She sets her jaw forward and clenches her teeth. It's how I know she's not listening anymore and that all reason or logic has vanished."

"This isn't about my family. It's about us."

Guilt spreads like sewage in my chest. "You have no idea what happened in high school. My Dad ruined Michael's life, and he ended up in the psych hospital, all because of me." After Michael left the area without me, I heard rumors about his life falling apart.

"How is any of that your fault?"

My shoulders shiver just a bit as if shaking it off will somehow erase all the lies I had told that made Dad hate Michael in the first place.

"It's not my fault. Maybe I should call my Dad and make him apologize… oh, wait. He's not sorry. In fact, he'd do it all the same, all over again."

"Michael looks like he's moved on," Mason proffers.

"Like you and Jessie?" It's a low blow. Jessie broke up with Mason while he was on his mission. He sent her a Book of Mormon, inviting her to join the church, and in response she broke up with him in a "Dear John." He didn't talk about her much, but I know it still hurts that the end of their relationship was so abrupt.

"What do you mean?"

"I asked you once if you still cared for Jessie, and you said, 'In a way.' You're telling me that if Jessie lived down the street, you wouldn't want to go make sure she knew you were here and set up some sort of rules to keep our marriage safe?" I am aware as I'm saying it that the two relationships were completely different.

"Jessie didn't rape me."

I cringe. Michael didn't rape me. I never told Mason he had, but I did say I hadn't really wanted to have sex with him and wasn't ready for it. Mason understood that to mean rape. I had already married him without telling him I wasn't a virgin. I didn't correct him because it was easier not to. When he thought it was rape, he felt less betrayed that he wasn't my first, which is a big deal in Mormon culture.

"Mason, I just want to say sorry for what happened. I need to apologize. I need closure. I need to get Michael out of my head." Mason's reluctance feeds my anxiety.

"Do you think this will make the nightmares stop?"

I slump into the living room couch and look away. Every night since Michael and I were separated, I have dreamed about him. He was in my head when I married Mason. I had to work hard to stay focused on Mason and not imagine Michael during sex.

In my dreams, I try to protect Michael from my father. I run to Michael's open arms, but some force jerks me away before I get there. I wake up screaming his name, panting and crying. I never share the details of the dreams with Mason. I let him assume I'm trying to get away from Michael.

"I don't know," I finally answer, feeling my voice catch.

"Sarah, do what you think is right, but I'm afraid he'll break up our family."

I look down at the paper I've written a script on and begin to dial. My hands are shaking. I hit the wrong number and hang up, chest pounding so hard I struggle to breath.

Mason tugs my knee. "It doesn't have to happen today, sweetheart." The thought of putting this off another day makes me nauseous. I just need to do it. It would help if Mason wasn't watching me. It reminds me of my mother watching my every move after being pulled from high school.

"I have to," I plead. "I won't be able to sleep until this is finished."

I hit the *talk* button on the phone again and dial, more slowly this time.

"Hello?"

I haven't heard his voice since the summer after sophomore year. I close my eyes and feel his hand on the small of my back, leading me in a dance at the Jazz Band fundraising dinner. I open my eyes and blink away the memory.

"Is this Michael? Michael Iles?"

"Yessss." He draws out his "s" in anticipation.

"This is Sarah Westbrook. I mean Sarah Lee."

"Bullshit. Tell Sawyer *this* isn't funny. He's gone too far this time." Michael's best friend Sawyer loved pranks. He was also one of the few people who had been happy for Michael and me to be together.

"I haven't talked to Sawyer since your mom screamed at you for bringing me home years ago. This *is* Sarah Lee." I'd never considered that he wouldn't believe me.

"Fuck off. I don't know how much Sawyer paid you to say that, but

I'm not in the mood, damn it." Mason leans forward on the bed, listening and watching my reactions. I try to stay even and hope that Michael will just listen to me.

"Michael, it's me, Sarah. Please, just listen."

"And what does *Sssarah Lee* have to say?"

Irritated at Michael's continued disbelief and now his sarcasm increases my nerves. I look up at Mason who shrugs his shoulders and opens his hands as if silently asking me *now what?*

"My husband joined the Army in 2002. We moved to El Paso at the end of February. I saw you out watering your lawn a couple of hours ago. A little girl was playing in your driveway. A woman with dark hair who looks pregnant was standing in your front door." I try to hide the pleading in my voice.

"Holy shit, is it really Sarah?" Relief floods through me.

"Yes."

"Fuck, no way. I don't believe it." Despite the hostile edge to his tone, he sounds more like the Michael I remember. I ache a little, realizing for the first time how much I have missed him.

"Twenty dollars and a Neon," I say.

I can hear the chatter of a child's voice in the background on his end of the phone. He's silent.

I wait, holding my breath, wondering if he'll remember giving me money for dinner and promising to buy me a car someday.

"God, it really is you." I want to reach through the phone and touch his cheek. I close my eyes and envision his vivid crystal blue eyes peering back at me.

"I live ten doors down the street. I didn't mean to… I mean, I didn't know you lived here. You know how the Army is, assigning houses. I didn't choose this." I sound so stupid. I push the script away and rest my forehead on my hand.

Michael's voice cracks, "You have got to be fucking kidding me. You say you live down the street?"

"Yes, 3140-B Steele Road. Your house is one duplex away from the elementary school."

I can feel Mason stiffen next to me. Our address was definitely not on the script. "Michael, are you still there?"

"What do you want?" his voice is barely above a whisper.

"I want to come by and talk to you. I have some things I'd like to tell you in person."

"Now?"

Mason and I hadn't discussed a time for this, but I can't see that it matters when.

"I can come now if that works for you, or later. Do you want to talk to your wife first?" I wonder if she knows who I am, if the story she got is as off as the one Mason got, if she'll want to be a part of the conversation like Mason does.

"No, come now."

I hear the click of the line disconnecting. I turn to Mason, whose hand is still on my knee.

"He wants me to come now." My voice trembles.

"Might as well get this over with. I'm not going to get any sleep today before work, so go." He sounds resigned… beaten, but I can't not go. Not now that he knows I'm here.

I stand, dropping the phone onto our bed. Mason stands as well. I turn to walk out of our room, when he grabs me from behind and turns me around.

"I love you, Sarah. No matter what, I love *you*." He looks distressed and old somehow. I ignore the desperation in his voice. I can barely manage my own emotions, much less his right now.

I sink into his arms. "I love you, too. This will all be over soon," I promise.

We walk hand-in-hand to the kitchen. I grab a cup and get a drink of water. We hug again and then I walk out the front door. I look down the street toward Michael's house. He is already in his front yard, pacing and kicking at something on the ground. I turn back to look at Mason, who gives me a weak smile. Eric's face peeks out from behind Mason's knees.

"Can I go with Mommy?" he asks Mason.

"Nope, you get to take a nap," Mason says, swinging him up over his shoulder. He looks back at me and mouths, "I love you," again.

I love him. I want to get this entire thing over with so we can go back to our normal life.

The late afternoon sun has lowered enough in the sky that the heat is tolerable. I have two blocks to figure out what I'm going to say to Michael.

"You can do this, Sarah," I mutter to myself. "Apologize for Dad trying to have him thrown in jail. Explain that you didn't know Dad was lying about his ability to throw Michael in jail because you didn't know how all that legal stuff worked. Tell him you stopped trying to reach out because you were keeping him safe. Tell him you learned that he had joined the

Army from Zoe, and that's the last you had heard about him. Tell him you didn't know where he was until last night. Tell him you hope he's happy, then say goodbye."

I run my list over again, inside my head this time, hoping I'm not leaving anything out.

"Closure, Sarah. You want closure. You are doing this to get rid of the dreams, to finally love Mason with your whole heart. Mason deserves you to be his and only his. It's like breaking up with someone you aren't actually with. You can do this."

I look up and see Michael standing with his mouth open, staring at me as I approach. I'm almost there. I stare back at him. He's shaved his head, most likely to keep it in Army regulation for his job. As I get closer, I notice his eyes are slightly bloodshot. He looks tired, worn down and old, much older than I am. Much older than Mason.

I step onto his lawn. "Hey," I stammer. My rehearsal over the last few minutes escapes me, and I have no idea where to start.

"Oh my God, I love you. I just want to kiss you."

My knees feel weak. I take a step backward as Michael opens his arms and reaches toward me for a hug. My heart splits open, filling my chest with warmth. I have to bite my tongue to keep myself from saying "I love you" back.

I shake my head and glance over to his front door. The dark-haired pregnant woman is standing behind the closed screen door, her arms crossed in front of her, her bushy eyebrows drawn together.

"You probably shouldn't say that," I warn.

"You're right, I'm sssorry." He slurs the "s" of sorry, his narrow shoulders slump. "What did you want to tell me?"

360

"I want to apologize, for everything. I didn't know, Michael, I didn't know. Dad said he found a loophole in the law and that if I tried to call you again, he'd call the police so they could arrest you. He said you'd serve a minimum of twenty years in jail. I didn't want you to be thrown in jail."

"That's the ssstupidest shit I've ever heard." His face reddens, and spit escapes his mouth as he low punches the air at his side.

"I know," I stammer. I'd expected him to just understand, he knows how my Dad is. "I know now that he lied. I didn't know that then." The more nervous I am, the more I talk with my hands. "Hell, he dragged me into the police station and made me admit I had lied to them this one time before I met you and that I had ditched school with you to make out and have sex. He made me do *community service* for it and told me the police had sentenced me to it." I drop my hands.

"Of course, you didn't know, Love."

Hearing him call me that is thrilling, but my gaze rests on the pregnant silhouette behind the screen.

"You can't call me that. We are both married."

"You're right, I'm sssorry. I just don't know what to sssay. Sarah, I love you so fucking much."

I look away, down the street toward home. Mason is sitting on the ground, his back supported by the outside tan stucco wall of our duplex. At least he can't hear Michael's proclamations.

Michael follows my gaze and squints at Mason.

"Looksss like your husband is making sssure I don't do anything questionable."

A flash of anger rises to my face. "I don't need him to babysit me. May I borrow your phone?"

"Sure," Michael says. He steps into his house, sidestepping his wife, whose pregnant belly blocks the doorway. I study her puffy face, her arms folded over her chest, until Michael closes the door and blocks my view. I turn back and glare at Mason, wishing he could see me.

A moment later, Michael hands me his phone, and I dial my number furiously while staring at Mason. Mason lifts the cordless receiver up to his face and sets it back on the ground. I listen to my own voice asking me to leave a message.

"You don't need to watch me," I growl into the receiver as I hand the phone back to Michael. My irritation at Mason seems to have calmed Michael's nerves. He stands more confidently in front of me now, blocking my view of Mason.

"Everything okay?" he asks.

"Yes," I snap.

"Sssorry, I didn't mean anything by that." He seems more hopeful. "You are absolutely gorgeousss, even when you're mad at me. You're stunning."

I raise one eyebrow at him, indicating that I've noticed his change in tone, and he just smiles gently at me. I don't like how good his attention makes me feel.

"Please don't say stuff like that to me." This is much harder than I expected.

"How are you, Sssarah? Are you happy?" I think of Mason, of Eric, of the new baby on the way. I am happy, but I didn't come here to talk about that now.

"Ummmm, yes, of course. After us, I quit my job at Ed's and started working at Arby's."

"I know. Zoe told me."

"Really? I figured you didn't know because you never stopped by." I don't tell him that I watched, waited, suitcase packed, for him to never come for me.

"I didn't want you to get into any more trouble either, and then I spent sssome time in the psych ward trying to put my life back together. I lossst my purpose, which is why I joined the Army, to get away from it all and ssstart over." I knew that he had spent some time in a psychiatric hospital. It's part of why I felt so guilty, but now that he brought it up, I don't know what else to say about it. I'm not ready to explore his discomfort, just say sorry and move on like I'd promised Mason.

"What happened to your brothers? They weren't at school when I went back junior year. I missed them." I really had. Luke and Brian had been my friends, and while they got annoyed with how often Michael and I were making out, they were supportive of our relationship.

"They went back to Phoenix to live with dad."

"Why?"

"It's what was best for them. Tell me more about you."

"Ummm, I graduated a year early 'cause after us, school sucked. Everyone said I was pregnant, and then when I didn't get fat they said I must have had an abortion. The rumors were awful. Dad wouldn't let me go away for college. He said I wasn't eighteen and therefore not old enough to buy Tylenol. He also said that if I went away for school, I would have had sex with every boy I met, so they made me stay home. I went to Northland Pioneer College, you know, NPC, in Taylor?"

He cocks his head to the side, his face full of pity. "Then what happened?"

"Well, I met Mason and we got married a few months after I turned eighteen."

"Did your Dad like *him*?" There's an edge to his voice; I know what it feels like to not be good enough for my Dad.

"Well, yes, but only because Mason served his mission in Boston, like Dad, and Mason hates the color green, like Dad."

"So that's what it would have taken?" Michael's eyes grow dark, his tone bitter.

"Dad didn't like Curtis at all either."

"Curtis?"

"A returned missionary I sort of dated the summer after you disappeared and the summer before I met Mason. We were mostly just friends. Curtis taught me how to rappel. Actually, he was my only friend. After us, Deckland, Kat, and Cassidy wouldn't talk to me. No one would. Dad called all of them and chewed them out. The 'good Mormon' kids wouldn't touch me because their parents were afraid I'd be a bad influence. It was lonely." Talking to Michael like this is still so easy. I never felt like I had to worry about how I look for him to care. I still don't.

"It was lonely for me, too."

The ease and familiarity of our interaction unsettles me. Michael's intent focus on what I'm saying, the way his body moves, how he makes me feel like everything I'm saying is okay… it all draws me back to him. The longer I'm with him, the more I realize how much I still love him. I need to end this, or I'm going to say too much.

"I need to go, Michael. Mason needs to work tonight. I just wanted to come by and tell you how sorry I am for everything that happened. I wish it could have been different. I really do." I'm not sure if I feel any better, if I can put this behind me now. I just know that Mason's been sitting there waiting by himself for long enough.

"I'm sorry too, Sssarah. I have thought about you every day. You visit me in my dreams. I sssee you doing dishes in our home, our children playing on the floor. I imagine how beautiful you are pregnant, how ssstrong you are in childbirth."

"I can't get pregnant," I blurt, immediately wishing I hadn't said anything.

He looks at me for a long time. "You will make a wonderful mother sssomeday."

I think of Eric's chubby little hands and sweet smile.

"Do you still love me?" he asks.

"You know I can't answer that." I feel like I've said too much already.

"Which means you do. If you didn't, you would have just said no." His bleary eyes are pleading.

We look at each other, saying nothing. I blink back tears. He extends his hand toward me but drops it back to his side before making contact.

"I need to go, Michael. We can't talk, we can't hang out. If you see me in the stores or at some post event, please just ignore me. I'll do the same, okay?" My voice cracks. Saying goodbye physically hurts.

"Isss that what you want?"

"It's how things have to be. We can't hurt our families. This isn't their fault."

"I know, but isss that what *you* want?" My heart skips. I'm losing control of the conversation, which means it's time for me to go.

"What I want doesn't matter."

"Will you at least hug me goodbye?"

I stare at him for several seconds, then finally step forward, my arms open. He wraps me in a tight embrace, buries his head into my hair and inhales deeply.

"God, I love you, Sarah Lee," he whispers, then presses his lips onto my ear and kisses me softly through my hair. I loosen my grip, and he tightens his. "Just another moment. Pleassse don't leave me like this."

I pull away. "I'm sorry, I really have to go."

He drops his hands to his side. His tears break me.

I have to control myself; I can't do this in front of him. It will just make things worse.

"Goodbye, Michael."

I don't wait for a response. I walk past him then step onto the sidewalk. I don't turn back, I just walk forward. I can see Mason get up. My vision blurs from the tears as I walk farther away from Michael.

I let the tears fall freely. When I make it home, I pass Mason and walk straight into our house.

He follows me into our bedroom, where I collapse on the bed.

"May I hold you?" he asks tentatively.

I nod, unable to speak.

He climbs onto the mattress next to me and pulls me into his body. He holds me, my back to his chest, and he just lets me cry.

Several minutes later he asks, "Did you get the closure you were looking for?"

AUTHOR'S NOTE

Trauma changes the way our brain functions. I use the term "trauma
bonded" to describe the phenomenon that occurs when two people experience a shared traumatic experience that creates a level of loyalty and
connection due to the changes in their neurology. This type of bond can
supersede healthy decision-making by driving those who share a trauma
bond to sacrifice almost everything to meet the needs or desires of the
person they are bonded to.[18,19]

I have witnessed this type of unhealthy bond in my veteran clients
who share war-time trauma, in individuals who share trauma from natural
disasters, and in myself and Michael due to our forced separation and the
abuse and manipulation of my father.

No matter how harmful meeting Michael's physical and emotional
needs is for me, I have an underlying feeling of obligation to do so in order
to protect him from harm, including the harm he creates for himself due
to his own trauma responses. Because of our shared traumatic experiences,
I have an instinctual need to aid him in his healing process. It may not be
logical, but it is very real, very carnal, and incredibly unhealthy.

A trauma bond is also a term I use to describe the type of bond a
person forms with their chronic abuser. This type of trauma bond is created in relationships with a narcissist or with a parent or spouse who has
a borderline personality disorder. Those who are in a captor situation (i.e.,
Stockholm Syndrome) or within domestically violent relationships are prone

18   Levine., P. A., & Kline., M. (2007). *Trauma through a child's eyes: Awakening the ordinary miracle of healing: Infancy through adolescence.* North Atlantic Books. Pages 73-74
19   Herman, J. (2015). *Trauma and recovery.* Basic Books. Trauma and Recovery pages 74-95 and 200

to developing a trauma bond. In such cases, it is normal for the victim/survivor to have difficulty setting and maintaining boundaries and leaving the toxic relationship.[20,21]

I believe both my parents are on the personality-disorder spectrum (which is a common phenomenon we call "the perfect storm"). Combine that familial dysfunction and the fact that I was held "captive" in my own home, I also share a trauma bond with both my parents. For me the effect presented itself as an inability to say no to uncomfortable visits, maintain healthy boundaries within our communications, and a visceral need to please them and gain their approval.

20   Levine., P. A., & Kline., M. (2007). *Trauma through a child's eyes: Awakening the ordinary miracle of healing: Infancy through adolescence.* North Atlantic Books. Pages 73-74

21   Herman, J. (2015). *Trauma and recovery.* Basic Books. Trauma and Recovery pages 74-95 and 200

HOSPITAL

APRIL 12, 2004

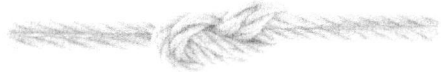

23 YEARS OLD

Seeing Michael sucked away all of my emotional energy.

"I have to leave for work in about thirty minutes, Sarah. Are you going to be okay?" Mason asks, the concern in his voice is tender but still grates my nerves.

"I'll be okay. I'm exhausted. I need sleep more than anything." I feel instant regret knowing neither of us has slept much the last 36 hours. I peel myself off my bed, needing to move until the internal jitters work their way out of me. I follow Mason into the hallway and rummage in the cabinet above the dryer, searching for the canister of Pledge dusting spray.

"I bet you could sleep at Finn's place." I understand why Mason would want me to go be with a friend tonight, but I doubt Michael will come over since he has a family to take care of. Besides, I just want to be alone.

"No, I'll be okay. I promise."

"Eric took a late nap for about an hour while you were talking to Michael. Are you going to walk tonight with the girls?" The chance of seeing Michael again tonight feels incredibly overwhelming.

"No, I told Finn I wasn't feeling 100% yet, so we are going to wait until later this week. I'll stay up late watching *Monsters Inc.* with Eric."

I follow Mason into the kitchen, needing to be close to him. I ache for the reassurance that he still loves me… that he will continue to be the rock I can count on no matter how much shit life throws at us. He presses start on the microwave to warm up leftovers and starts packing himself a midnight lunch.

His eyes have bags under them, and he moves as if weighed down by something heavy. "Are you going to be okay, Mason? You worked last night and didn't sleep at all today."

"I'll be fine. Our floor is full. I won't have time to notice how tired I am or have a second to think. I need a break from thinking." He closes his sandwich, smashing the bread together in his jerky movements.

His words stab at me. I feel guilty even though I haven't done anything wrong.

"Are you ready to tell me how it went?" He pushes his sandwich into the baggie, which rips from the extra force.

I owe this to Mason even though I don't feel ready to share. Air passes loudly from my lips. "I told him I was sorry for what my Dad did. He asked about how my life was. I gave him a basic rundown. He asked me if

I was happy. I told him yes. The conversation was a lot longer than that. It was awkward, it took a while."

He turns away from me, opens the fridge, and puts the mayonnaise back in its place. "Why did you hug him?"

I flinch. It is a fair question. He has every right to ask. If I had hugged any other man, it wouldn't have bothered him. I know he trusts me. It's Michael he doesn't trust.

At least Mason hadn't had to hear Michael's profession of love that came with the hug. That would cause him more worry and pain than he is already feeling. It was bad enough that Michael's wife had heard everything standing just behind the door.

"He asked me to." Mason stares at me, waiting. "I think he's looking to heal, too, you know?" I add. "He held on a little longer than I wanted him to, but…"

I let my voice trail off. There is no way I'm going to give Mason more details. I made sure *my* behavior was appropriate. Michael's behavior is his and his wife's business, and if Mason knew that Michael said he loved me more than once, it would only make him mad. He needs to think clearly for work tonight. My goal is to just put this day behind me and pretend everything is normal 'til the pain subsides. It shouldn't be as hard as when I was in high school, since I have Mason and friends who still love me.

Mason kisses me on the forehead, his warmed dinner in one hand, his lunch sack in the other. I hold the carport door open for him, and he steps out. He places his dinner on the roof of the car and turns to me.

"I would feel more comfortable if you kept the car tonight. That way you can go to Finn's if needed or leave… you know, if Michael tries to come over or something."

I concede. I ask the neighbor to sit with Eric and drive Mason to the hospital.

The alarm on my nightstand chimes. I roll out of bed. I had fallen asleep quickly but had dreams that I was married to Michael and couldn't find Eric, which made for a restless night.

I stretch, then fall back onto my soft pillow and groan, the spring sun peeking through the gray curtains.

"Mommy, can we go get Daddy?" Eric's voice cracks as he climbs into the bed next to me.

"Yes, go potty in the big boy potty and go get your shoes on. We're going to go to Kris's house after breakfast so Daddy can sleep, baby." He bounces off the bed and slams the master bathroom door behind him. I yank the covers off me and slide my feet into flip-flops. Eric follows me to the carport and climbs into his seat. I smile at him as he struggles with the straps and wait for him to commandeer the buckle; his toothy grin smiles up at me with success.

Smiling back at him, I wonder how Michael would have handled my inability to get pregnant. Would he have been okay with adopting a child? Would he have been able to love a child that wasn't biologically his, the way Mason does?

The phone rings inside the house but I ignore it, not wanting to be late for Mason. He must be exhausted after two night shifts with no sleep in between. I slide into the driver's seat and pull the door closed, then turn the radio up and sing along to the music on the short drive to WBAMC.

Ten minutes later, I pull into the staff lot and help Eric unbuckle.

"Eric, where are your shoes?"

He shrugs, "I took them off."

Feeling anxious to get to Mason, I have Eric climb onto my back, crossing my arms behind me to support his bottom and grip the back of my pajama pants to keep them from slipping down. We enter the hospital through the basement doors. I lean down so Eric can push the elevator button. The doors open within moments, and we step in. Once again, I lean over so Eric can push the button for the seventh floor.

He chatters about playing golf with Kris.

The moment I make it out of the elevator, Brandon, a tired-looking coworker informs me, "You just missed Mason, you must have crossed in the elevator." I step backward feeling confused.

"That's weird. He normally waits for me here since Eric likes to say hi." Mason changing his routine is usually a bad thing.

"It was a long night. We are completely full and have some rough patients right now. Hi, Eric." Brandon extends his hand for a high five.

Eric releases his grip on my neck and holds his hand out. "Sucker!"

Brandon laughs and reaches under the counter to fetch the bucket full of stickers and dum-dum lollipops. "Here ya' go, little buddy."

I bounce Eric back up onto my hips, pulling my loose pants up. I've lost some weight since I started walking with Finn most evenings.

"Thanks, Brandon." He gives me a curt nod, then checks the chart in his hand and walks away.

I pin Eric's hands to my neck with my chin, to stop him from pulling the wrapper off his lollipop and getting sugar in my messy bun. "Don't open your sucker until after breakfast, kiddo."

I turn around and almost walk into the patient standing behind me.

"Oh, I'm so sorry, I didn't see you there," I say before registering the patient's face. I feel a jolt of panic grip me.

"Michael," I exclaim, stepping backward. "What are you doing here?"

"How did you know I was here?" he asks at the same time.

"I didn't. This is where my husband works." I'm acutely aware of Eric on my back, watching. ·

"Oh God, I hope he wasn't the one who put the catheter in my dick." Michael's face contorts with concern.

I shimmy Eric around to the front and wrap my arms protectively around him. "Why. Are. You. Here?"

"I had a few drinks before you came over last night, and then once you left…" He smiles a little, does he think that's funny?

Then it clicked. All his slurred words… he'd been drunk. But that doesn't explain why he's a patient on the med/surg ward.

"So why are you here?"

"Can you come talk to me in my room?" He gestures down the hall behind him, like he's inviting me into his home instead of my husband's workplace.

"No." My confusion is turning into annoyance. "I have Eric."

Michael scrunches his face.

"Hi," Eric says, rocking on my hip.

"I thought you couldn't have kids…" Michael waves at Eric. "Hi."

"I can't." The heat of jealousy licks at me as I think of Michael's pregnant wife.

"Then, who is this little cutie?" I hold Eric tighter, and he leans in to put his head on my shoulder.

"My son."

Michael doesn't question this; he crinkles up his face then shakes his head and sighs loudly. "I lost track of how much alcohol I'd had. I drank too much and passed out." He shrugs. "Megan called an ambulance. They had to pump my stomach. Sarah, I don't want to live in a world where you aren't with me." He hasn't changed at all, always so intensely romantic, so extreme.

"That was stupid of you." I'm not going to let him blame me for his choices. He was drinking before I even got there.

I leave Michael and his IV pole and his pain alone in the hallway.

Four minutes later, I shield my eyes from the morning sun as I come out of the building, shifting Eric back to my back, keeping one hand under him. Mason gives a little wave. I search his face for clues to see if he knows Michael was on his unit last night. All I see is tiredness and a weariness about him.

"I tried to call you and tell you not to come up to the floor," he calls out to me, pushing himself off the hood of our Avalon.

My heartbeat picks up, worried that he knows Michael was there. He must not have wanted me not to run into him. I shift Eric on my back and mutter, "Why didn't you wait on the floor for me like normal?" I demand.

"I wanted to get home and go to bed as soon as possible. I'm exhausted."

That could be true, at least in part. I still have no idea if he knows. "How was your night?"

He takes a deep breath lifting Eric off my back. "Busy. Much of our staff is deployed so the medical and surgical floors are combined." He gives Eric a big tight hug. "How are you, champ?"

Eric lifts the purple sucker he managed to unwrap up to Mason's face. "Sucker!"

Mason gives him a weak, tired smile, seeming unable to muster the energy to respond more. He starts to put Eric into his car seat. "Last night was crazy. I didn't sit down once, not even to eat my lunch."

If Mason is hiding anything, he's hiding it too well for me to tell. I drive my exhausted husband back home, unable to stop fidgeting in the driver's seat. What the crap was Michael thinking, drinking like that and then blaming me? Clearly, he has a problem. A big one. He drank in high school but nothing that caused him to end up in the hospital.

Once we are home, Mason comes up behind me and wraps his arms around my waist. He kisses my neck and I lean my head into his cheek. "Everything go okay last night?"

"Yep, we watched a movie."

He kisses me on the cheek and heads to bed, leaving me with my thoughts of Michael in his hospital gown. I need answers. I didn't handle seeing him in the hospital well. I mean, what he did *was* stupid, but people do stupid things when they are hurting. Did he try to drink himself to death on purpose? He has a wife, a daughter, and another child on the way. He loves kids. He seemed okay when I left yesterday. I know this isn't my fault, but I can't help but wonder if it's partly because of me. The whole point of going to see him was for both of us to have closure. I wet my pants just seeing his nameplate. Maybe it made things worse for him because he was blindsided, maybe he just needs more time with this. I decide to go see Michael at the hospital while Mason sleeps. I apply a bit of eyeshadow and mascara, I'm not really one for makeup, but if I'm going to see Michael, I'm going to look at least one step above toddler mama.

On the way to Finn's, Eric plays with his fingers in the back seat, and I continue to wonder what my next step is going to be. I promised Mason this was over, but I didn't expect to see Michael again, and I certainly didn't expect that he'd try to drink himself to death over *me*. If I caused him to drink too much, I *have* to do something.

Finn's kitchen looks like something has exploded. She has an apron on, and she's baking something that smells wonderful. Her giant black lab, Helaman, is sitting nearby, waiting for her to toss him something.

"Wow, you're ambitious today."

She laughs and brushes her wild bangs away with a floured hand. "I am."

"There's a friend from work in the hospital. Could I leave Eric for a bit so I can go say hi?" I hope my voice sounds normal.

"Works for me. Eric will entertain Kris, so I can homeschool the teen in peace. Take as long as you need."

The goal is to get past the nurses' station without being noticed by Mason's colleagues. The hospital is buzzing with activity, so it's possible, but the moment I am out the elevator I see Michael's blond-hair daughter being towed behind his wife, who looks exhausted. I lower my head as she lightly brushes up against me on her way into the elevator.

"Sorry," she says without looking at me. Her voice is soft, sweet, but strained.

"No worries," I say automatically.

The room assignment board is at the nurse's station. Michael's room is just a few doors down on the left. His door is open, and I'm relieved to see that he's alone.

I knock on the open door lightly.

"Come in." His voice sounds tired.

He looks up from the book he is reading and makes eye contact. A slow smile crosses his face. "God, you are beautiful." I catch myself before I smile. I can't let him distract me.

"Michael, we are married," I scold.

"I don't care. It's true. I love you, Sarah, more than anything or *anyone* else."

I fight the urge to roll my eyes, remembering how over-the-top and romantic Michael has always been. I stare at him, not wanting to make this worse for me, him, his wife, or my husband. I need to keep the boundaries clear.

"I think I saw your wife leave on the elevator I arrived on," I say, hoping the thought of his wife will redirect him.

His face flattens a bit with the mention of her. "Yeah, she just left, so you probably did," he shrugs.

"Your daughter is beautiful. She looks just like you."

"Savannah? Yes, she does. She is my light."

I stiffen, remembering him going on and on about the significance of what a name meant. Savannah's name has rich history, a place where love is found and nurtured and able to withstand the storms that life will throw at her. He had wanted to name our future child that.

He looks at me differently today than he did last night. There is less desperation in his eyes, but more sadness.

"What happened last night, Michael, after I left?"

He flushes and sits quietly for a long moment, then looks away. "I told Megan that I loved you, that I would always love you, and that I wanted to be with you."

I stared at him, disgusted. He. Did. Not. Poor woman. That is a horrible thing for him to say to her. I realize a part of me feels that way too.

"She threw plates and mugs at me, screaming about how she was my wife."

I gasp. Their daughter shouldn't have to live with that.

"I told her she had been my second choice."

I suck in my breath, not believing what I was hearing. How could he be so insensitive?

He shrugs and drops his chin to his chest. "Things between us have been bad for a while." He says it so matter-of-factly, as if that makes his words okay.

I look at him, my body longing to curl up next to him in his hospital bed and talk for hours like we used to. Pushing down that impulse, I say, "I'm sorry to hear that. I had hoped that wherever you were, you were happy."

"How could I have been happy, Sarah?" His eyes are desperate and yearning as he adds, "I wasn't with you." He looks down at his sheet. "All I have ever wanted in my life is to be with you." My face flushes, partly because I'd wanted to hear those words since 1997 and partly out of anger because he never came to get me.

"But why the alcohol? You can get kicked out of the Army for that."

"I just told my staff sergeant that you came by, and I wasn't expecting it. I told him it took me to a dark place, and I drank more than I thought I did."

"Is that what happened?" He's avoiding eye contact. He's been in a psychiatric hospital before, so it's not a leap to think there was an element of intent in his actions.

"Mostly, yes. I wanted to die, but not kill myself. I don't know if I can live in a world where you don't want me." Part of me does want him.

I look away. A soft knock on the door breaks our attention for a moment.

"Good morning, Specialist Iles. How are you feeling this morning?"

"Better, thank you, Susie." Her flaming red hair makes my favorite day-shift nursing assistant unmistakable. Mild panic sets in, seeing someone I know complicates things. Susie works with Mason.

"I need to take your blood pressure and vitals, then I'll be out of your hair." Susie smiles politely before her eyes widen a bit as she sees me and recognition crosses her face. "Oh, hi, Sarah."

I hurriedly answer her unasked question. "Michael is my neighbor. I just came by to check on him," I say, hoping I don't sound guilty, offering information she didn't ask for.

"That's wonderful. Don't you just love that about the Army. Family away from family. I hope Mason is getting some good sleep. I hear he was hoppin' last night."

"He practically passed out the moment he got home."

I reassure myself the rotating schedule gives me two weeks before

380

Mason and Susie will see each other again. Hopefully she'll have forgotten about this by then. She removes the blood pressure cuff from Michael's arm then wraps the cords around it and places it in the slot on the wheeled machine. "Have a great day, Sarah, and give Eric a kiss from me. I sure do love that little boy."

Susie closes the door behind her.

"How did you know I was here?" he asks as if forgetting seeing me earlier.

"I didn't. My husband works here, remember? We only have one car, and I was picking him up after his night shift when I bumped into you."

"I bet he hates me."

I don't explain to him that Mason thinks Michael is an opportunistic rapist. "He's not a fan, that's for sure. He doesn't trust you and thinks you'll hurt me."

"I would never hurt you." He always was professing his undying love, telling me he'd take care of me and he'd be there for me, but when I desperately needed him to make good on his promises, he failed to show up.

My brow wrinkles. "I waited for you to come get me. You never ever came. You abandoned me, left me in that hellhole to rot."

"I'd never hurt you." Michael looks incredulous.

"But you did." I remember the tattered black suitcase I'd kept packed and hidden in my closet for months, believing that he'd come for me.

"I was just as trapped as you." He wasn't, though. He got to go stay with his dad, he had his brothers and friends. I was alone for months.

I shake my head. None of this matters now, and as I look at him in that hospital bed, I can't pretend that I've fared worse than him. It's pretty obvious my life is more stable than his.

"Michael, you need to move on. Your daughter and unborn child need you. Your wife needs you."

"Stop lecturing me. You have no idea what I've gone through the last seven years. I want *you*. I love *you*. *You* will always be the woman I love more than life itself."

I can't process his words. All of this is making me feel jumpy and itchy. I need to leave. It was a bad idea to come. This is making everything messier.

"I need to go." I grab the pen from the clipboard hanging on the foot of the hospital bed and write my phone number on his copy of the Fort Bliss *Monitor* folded on the bedside table. "If I can help you work through some of this, we can meet in a public place. Just to talk."

"Don't leave me, Sarah. I'm yours, I've always been yours. You have my whole heart."

I see an 18-year-old Michael in that bed, floating on a cloud of romantic ideals, always extreme, oblivious to the reality we live in.

"I'm married. I'm happy, we are adopting another child in August." I think of Mason, home in our bed, sleeping, and start to back away.

"Do you love me?"

I back into the light above his bed. "Loving you was never the problem, Michael. We can't hurt them. Mason. Megan. You know that."

I hear him as I walk away, down the hall, "I'll call you when I get out of here. Goodbye, my princess."

AUTHOR'S NOTE

Looking back on that day in the hospital with Michael is like watching a tragedy unfold. I can clearly see all the mistakes I made. I struggled because I didn't understand the significance of the trauma bond I shared with Michael, or how that bond would drive my behavior, despite the cost to me or to the people I love the most in this world. It has been a journey, but I have come to understand that no matter how wonderful my marriage, no matter how many beautiful children Mason and I have, no matter how many letters come after my name, when interacting with Michael, I will forever be guided by my scared, irrational, and traumatized 16-year-old self.

TO THE RESCUE

APRIL 2004

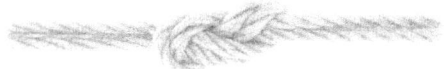

23 YEARS OLD

"Hello, Sarah. It's me, Michael."

Eric stares me down with his large toddler eyes as he slowly reaches back into the snack cabinet and scurries out of the kitchen with his ill-gotten package of fruit snacks. I prop the handset of the cordless phone between my shoulder and ear.

"Is your husband home?"

I bristle; the question alone is inappropriate. "Maybe."

"That means no. Look, I'm out of the hospital. I didn't handle either of your visits very well."

I allow my irritation to seep into my tone. "You told me you loved me and that you wanted to kiss me with your wife standing right there, and then you go and drink yourself to oblivion and almost die."

"Sarah, please don't yell at me. I really need to talk to someone who understands. I was wondering if you'd, I don't know… maybe we could go talk somewhere, where Megan isn't right behind the door, listening in."

"How is that going to help?"

Mason wouldn't understand. Church standards do not make room for women to be alone with men they aren't married to, and I already risked enough, sneaking a visit in the hospital.

"I have so many questions. I don't want to cause any trouble, but I need answers. You name the place, I mean if you're willing."

I'm not sure I am willing. The first meeting on his front lawn, I had done most of the talking. Michael didn't ask questions or tell me about what he went through, and he obviously didn't walk away feeling like he had closure. I didn't want him to get worse.

"It has to be in public. I'm not going to be alone with you." I feel like I owe him another chance, but I also owe it to Mason to set clear boundaries.

"How public? Like can it be public but not crowded?"

"That depends, what do you have in mind?"

"We could drive to the top of Trans-Mountain and sit at one of the picnic tables at the lookout."

The lookout is right next to the highway. Everyone passing by can see it, but the conversation would still be private.

"Sounds fine. When?"

"I'm free now." His desire to see me so soon is unnerving. I'm not sure

I'm ready to see him, but Mason won't be home for hours, so the timing works.

"I can go in about thirty minutes. I just need to get Eric ready to come with us so things stay kosher. You wanna walk to my place and I can drive?"

"Who's Eric?"

"My son. The child on my back, remember?" It's hard to hide the annoyance in my voice.

"Not really. I was pretty out of it for a couple days after they pumped my stomach."

"See you in a few."

"Sounds good. Sarah, I really need this, thank you."

I am annoyed, seeing Michael's name on the caller ID. In the four hours at the lookout yesterday, Eric perfected his rock-throwing techniques, and Michael talked a blue streak about nothing of substance, never mind healing.

I answer it anyway.

"Sarah, I really miss you. Do you think we can talk again?"

Every one of these contacts is another secret from Mason.

"Michael, I really can't. I have dinner plans at Denny's with some friends. Besides, what else is there to say?"

"Things with Megan are really rough. She's been hostile since you showed up."

Guilt burns in my chest.

"I just need to talk to someone who won't lecture me about leaving the past in the past."

I picture him in his hospital gown. Harsh words won't help him heal, neither will meeting with him. It didn't matter how much I wanted to help him, I knew I wasn't the person.

Cheryl and Donald wanted to meet for dinner tonight to discuss what's needed to be in the letter of reference for our upcoming adoption.

They get straight to business when we meet up. "We are really honored that you asked us to write a letter of reference, but there's something we need to tell you first."

I wait, feeling a trickle of sweat slide down the back of my neck.

"We were investigated by CPS for a freak accident with James when he was two. It was awful; they took all of the kids out of our home, and we had to fight to get them back." Cheryl stares into her untouched Cobb salad, her thick bangs dangle in midair.

"We sued the state for wrongful separation and won." Don pushes a packet of paperwork across the table.

Eric grabs the lemon slice Cheryl is holding out to him and shivers as he licks it.

"We wanted to talk to you and Mason together, we just didn't have enough time before Donald deploys again. You're welcome to share the court documents with Mason," Don said, tilting his head toward the papers he'd just given me. "You and Mason will be awesome parents to whatever child comes into your home, and we'd love to show our support with a letter. We just want to be sure that a letter from us won't do more harm than good."

I glance at the top document, which shows a judgment in their favor.

"What a painful nightmare. I'm so sorry, I had no idea."

"We ask that you and Mason keep this between us."

"Of course." I reach for Cheryl's hand; she hasn't made eye contact with me since she started talking. "I'd be honored to have a letter from you. You haven't done anything wrong. The state doesn't run background checks on references, just on the adoptive parents."

She squeezes my hand, and the color begins to return to her cheeks. "That's good to know, if you are sure… I'll have it for you at church on Sunday."

"I'm sure, so Donald, do you know yet where you are going for deployment?" I ask.

Cheryl finally picks up her fork. "I won't know where he was 'til he gets home, if then," she says, her mouth full.

"Does this spot work better for you, sir?" I hear the waitress seat another family one table away from mine.

"Yes, much better. Thank you."

Michael's voice.

I look past Michael's back to the familiar birthmark on his daughter's face. I'd mentioned I was coming here when he called; it hadn't occurred to me that he might show up like a stalker!

I pick at my meal while Cheryl busies herself rearranging Eric's food.

"Are you okay?" she asks me, "You've barely touched your food."

I can't concentrate on anything other than trying not to look at

Michael. "Yeah, I just feel a little off. I'm grateful we got to do this, though. Thank you for making sure Eric eats his dinner."

She smiles. "He sure does love sucking on lemons."

Donald slides out of the circular bench and stretches. "I'm going to go pay."

My gaze falls on the back of Michael's head. I can't wait until Cheryl and Donald leave so I can confront him.

Cheryl picks up her paperwork and waits for me to follow her.

"I'm going to give Eric some more time to eat. I'll see you tomorrow for our first Pilates class."

I watch through the window until they leave the parking lot before I grab Eric and what's left of my dinner and join Michael at his table.

"What the hell are you doing here?" I demand.

"I'm just enjoying dinner with Savannah Collette." He smiles.

"Liar. You knew I was coming here." I open my hands in a dramatic sweeping motion.

He shrugs. "Good to see you." He smiles playfully. "Can we talk?"

I have about an hour before I need to go pick Mason up from the hospital, but if I don't talk to Michael, I risk his coming to my house.

"Fine," I concede.

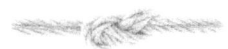

I feel guilty and anxious about meeting Michael yet again. We've been talking for almost two weeks and have gotten nowhere on Michael's healing. When he called from work, explaining that he and Megan had fought and he didn't know what to do, I suggested marital counseling. He scoffed at it the same way Mason had scoffed at it when I asked him if he would be interested in going to counseling with me. Both men had said counseling wasn't helpful in *this* situation, but neither had really defined what "this" was.

Mason has two speeds: troubled and spiritually "right." If anything troubles him, he prays himself back to spiritually right and moves on. The only counseling he's interested in is from the Lord.

"Mason, how late do you think you'll be tonight?" I ask while stuffing an extra set of clothing into the diaper bag.

"I'll probably be home by nine. We're meeting at the church building to work out a plan to take better care of the families with deployed dads." Mason was called to the Elder's Quorum presidency shortly after we moved here. They're constantly trying to figure out how to fill in for the deployed dads. I love that he's trying to dial into the needs of the wives in the ward, but he's oblivious to what's happening with his own.

I hand the ready diaper bag to him. "Tell Hank thanks for picking you up, and thanks for taking Eric with you. I need the night out with the girls, kid-free." I look away, hoping he doesn't sense that I'm lying.

I'm fairly confident Mason won't ask me questions about "girl's night." Mason never talks to Finn. I mean, he'll go to his priesthood meeting and talk *about* her, but that never leads to action. I imagine that conversation will go something like, "How about the Willis family?" And Mason will say, "She and my wife are close, they are doing great." They'll move onto the next family and will eventually determine the women of the ward have things covered.

Michael keeps asking to meet and talk because he needs "healing," but the previous times were a whole lot of speculation about how great life would be if we'd only ended up together. We talk about other things, too.

I feel so drawn to him, but at the same time, I'm confused and angry and hate the hold that Michael has on me. I hate what I'm doing to Mason. Every time we meet, I swear to myself that it's the last, and within days, I'm making plans to meet him again. I can't stay away from Michael's ability to make me feel heard and valued.

Mason is a good listener. He lets me talk for hours about anything, but there isn't much of an exchange; if he responds, it's to lead me back to what we are taught at church. Half the time I wonder if he's even paying attention.

Michael comments on my "insightful critical thinking skills" and takes time to think about my perspective before responding, and he validates my feelings. Mason and I live a "to-do list" guided by the rules of the Mormon Church and its promise that doing so will result in a happy marriage. Michael and I connect. I've tried to talk to Mason about the lack of emotional connection, but it hasn't changed anything. How do you teach someone to *feel?*

Hank honks out front. I watch Mason wrestle Eric into Hank's son's car seat before they pull away.

I park my Avalon in the Walmart lot and take one more look at myself in the rearview mirror, satisfied with the little bit of makeup I applied for my "girl's date." I'm supposed to meet Michael by the building so we can drive to the Trans-Mountain lookout together. The lookout isn't on the way to work or church, and Mason is terrified of heights, so even if he was looking for me, he wouldn't be likely to go there.

A familiar truck slows to a stop in front of me. Bishop Highlands leans over his girls to call out the open window to me.

"Hi, Sister Westbrook, do you need a ride somewhere?"

I walk toward the small truck just as Michael's red Ford Escort pulls up behind him. I hope Michael figures out not to approach me until the little truck is long gone.

"No, thanks, Bishop. I'm just waiting here for a friend to pick me up." Adrenaline surges through me; if the timing was just a little different, I'd be caught.

"Great, just wanted to make sure. Have fun." Bishop drives away as his girls wave goodbye.

Michael also waves as he passes me and circles an aisle of cars before driving back around. He slows to a stop and looks around as if he's being followed.

"That was sneaky," I tease as I slide into the passenger seat.

He reaches his hand over to squeeze my knee. He waits for me as I fumble with the seatbelt before pulling forward. "You look absolutely beautiful."

"Ummmm, thanks. My blue jeans and T-shirt are what I plan to wear to the ball tonight," I joke.

"You'll outshine even the most sparkly gown in the room for sure." He slows to a stop and raises my hand to his lips, kissing it softly before pulling onto the access road. My heart skips a beat, and I pull my hand away. "I'm sorry. I didn't mean to make you feel uncomfortable," he adds.

"It's fine. So, what's up with Megan?"

"She was so upset, she threw a picture at me. The glass shattered, and later Savannah stepped on a piece of it and cut her foot. Honestly, I don't know how much more I can take. It doesn't seem to matter what I do. It never makes her happy." Mason and I have never fought like that; we promised each other to parent differently than our parents had. What a nightmare.

"Wow, is Savannah okay? How bad was her foot cut?"

"Not bad. Nothing a daddy kiss and Band-Aid couldn't fix. I don't like the insane way she fights all the time, but I'm an adult, I can deal with it. Once her craziness starts hurting Savannah, though…" His voice trails off.

"I can't even imagine what I would do if Mason did something like that. I'm sorry, Michael." Mason is even-tempered to a fault. In a way, I wish he would engage but not to the point of violence. I just want him to feel with me, instead of standing by half listening while playing solitaire on the computer.

Michael places his right hand back on my knee and squeezes it gently again, sending jolts up my thigh. I reach for his hand and squeeze back.

"I'm really sad that your marriage isn't as happy as you had hoped. Truly, it breaks my heart." I'm grateful that Eric has never been exposed to that kind of volatility.

"Thanks, Sarah. I can't help but imagine what it would have been like if we had been allowed to stay together."

"I'm sure we would have fought. I'd cuss at you. I'd tell you that you were an overly romantic idiot…"

He doesn't laugh. Instead, he turns left into the Trans-Mountain Overlook parking area, next to one of the covered picnic benches and parks the car. He releases his seatbelt and turns toward me.

"We would fight, and I'd think your cussing was the cutest thing ever. And after the fight, I would apologize because I would be wrong, and then I'd hold you and promise to do better and kiss your tears away."

His voice is solemn. His blue eyes have tears in them, and his sadness pulls in my chest as I'm reminded of what it feels like to have someone show such emotion over me. I release my seatbelt and brush a tear off his cheek. He clasps my hand to his cheek and kisses the palm.

"God, Sarah, I've missed you. You are who I dream about, who I want to spend my life with." This isn't where I wanted the conversation to go, but the pull of that warm familiarity of Michael's adoration is overwhelming.

I wrap him in an awkward hug, the center console digging into my hip. He kisses my ear through my hair. I pull away a few inches, and we look at each other for a few moments.

"I love you, my Sarah."

"I love you, too."

Michael leans forward and I allow him to kiss me; I don't have the emotional energy to turn down the loving acceptance I've craved or to fight the building arousal.

He climbs over the console and supports his weight awkwardly above me.

"God, I've missed this. I've missed you, Sarah."

I ignore the tug in my stomach, the urge to stop. I lift my hand to the back of his head and pull him toward me. We kiss, and soon, our hands are exploring. I find comfort in the familiarity of our intimacy. The voice in my head telling me to get away falls silent.

I have crossed a line that I can never come back from.

RED ROOF INN

APRIL 30, 2004

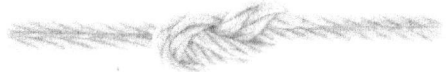

23 YEARS OLD

"Five eighteenth maintenance company SSA, how may I help you sir or ma'am?" Hearing the disinterested formality eases my nerves slightly.

"Is Specialist Iles available, please?" I try to match the official tone.

"May I ask the nature of this call, ma'am?" I'm jumpy, even though I was prepared for the regimented questions from the soldier on duty.

"I'm calling to discuss his recent lab results." I'm relieved that the words come out as smoothly as I'd rehearsed.

"Of course, ma'am, please hold." I hear the receiver clunk on the desk and listen to the muffled noise of the warehouse Michael works in.

"This is Specialist Iles, how may I help you?"

"It's me. Look, what happened yesterday…" My facade breaks and I fall silent, not able to find the words.

"I know," he whispers. "We went too far." His willingness to take ownership for his part is relieving. Maybe we can figure out a way to be friends without the physical stuff.

"We need to talk. Are you free tonight? Mason will be at the Fathers' and Sons' Campout with Eric this weekend." Even as I ask, I know that more sneaking around can't be the answer, but I can't help myself.

"Yeah, I get off at 1700. I'll tell Megan I'm gonna hang with Sergeant Spencer tonight. What time do you want me to pick you up?"

I add another Pull-Up to Eric's backpack and toss the tiny sleeping bag into the pile of camping gear. I pace the living room and check off all the packing items that Mason will need for his overnight with Eric. I've been over the list that he left me at least five times, but it's not distracting me from my nervous energy. Eric sits on the floor in front of the television with the Nintendo controller in his chubby hands, leaning his whole body into Mario's moves on the screen.

I can't figure out what to do with myself. I haven't curled my hair since adopting Eric. I apply makeup as I wait for the curling iron to heat up. Section by section I curl my chestnut hair into ringlets. It reminds me of prepping to cheerlead for a football game when I was in high school. Still two more hours until Mason gets home.

I decide to do dishes… again. I pull the apron over my head before seeing that the only things in the sink are Eric's two plastic cups. I sigh and wash them anyway. I sit on the floor and pull everything out from the cabinets, wipe them out, and refill them.

I walk back into the living room and pick up Eric's discarded socks and set them on top of his Crocs. I glance at my watch again. I sort through all of Eric's clothes for the things he's grown out of. Finally, I hear the carport door slam shut hard.

"I'm in Eric's room," I call to Mason.

"Man, that wind is brutal. It about took the screen door off as I came in. Is everything ready to go?" Mason kisses my forehead.

"Yep, I made you a pile in front of the front door since the kitchen is so narrow."

"Did you remember Pull-Ups?"

"Yes, and I bought you some new matches." I lead Mason out of the bedroom and into the living room. The anticipation is making me a nervous wreck. I hope he doesn't notice.

"Eric, it's time for us to go camping! Put your shoes and socks back on." I watch Eric on the floor in front of the couch, nagged by thoughts that it's not too late to back out of tonight.

I show Mason Eric's backpack and sleeping bundle before he goes to change out of his uniform.

"Eric, let's go potty so you can go with Daddy."

"Yay," Eric yells, finally abandoning the Nintendo. I grab his Crocs and socks and follow him to the bathroom.

"Here ya' go," I say to him, handing him his shoes. He grabs his Elmo doll and sleeping bag and pulls on his backpack.

"Wait, I want to take your picture," I say to him, grabbing the camera from the kitchen table. He grins at me until he hears the click.

I hand the camera to Mason as he passes me. "I want pictures of Eric's first campout. You ready to go, buddy?" Eric nods. We load the gear before I load Eric into his car seat.

Michael's red Ford Escort drives past. He's still in his uniform. He stares straight ahead. Gratefully, Mason doesn't notice since his head is still buried in the trunk, playing Tetris with the camping gear.

"I think I have everything." He closes the trunk just in time for another gust of wind to unsteady our stance. "This wind is going to make sleeping in a tent interesting. Thanks, Love, for making sure everything was ready to go."

I stand on my tiptoes to kiss him. "Have fun with Eric. I'll see you tomorrow afternoon." I wave at Eric as they drive away, a little less anxious now that they're on their way.

Twenty minutes later, I hear Michael honk from my carport. I swallow a flash of irritation. I hate being honked at. The least he could do is knock on the door and come in. He's probably not getting out because he doesn't want to be seen. He honks again. If he doesn't want to be seen, he should stop honking and drawing attention to himself. I grab my purse and rush out the carport door.

"You look amazing!" he says, as I slide into the passenger seat of his car. He begins to back out before I've buckled my seatbelt. "Where are we going?"

"I don't know," I snap. "Sorry, that came out harsher than I expected." I'm irritated at him for honking. I'm also uncomfortable with the enthusiasm of his compliment, especially since Mason didn't even notice. Mason never notices. I'm angry at myself for putting in the effort to look good.

"Are you cold?" He looks at my folded arms. "You can be in charge of the air conditioner." It's hard to feel negatively toward him when he's cognizant of my discomfort.

"Just nervous, I guess." I'm worried; the more we do this, the easier it's getting.

"What are you nervous about, Love?"

I startle at the term of endearment. Isn't that what Mason just called me?

Michael kisses my hand, and we continue to drive toward the freeway.

"Can we just drive for a bit?" I'm having a hard time focusing, and his constant touching and kissing my hand doesn't help.

"They went camping, huh? I'd especially love camping with you. That's one of the things I've dreamt about. Us camping, you know?"

I find this hard to believe.

"I've imagined us doing all kinds of things. I've dreamt of coming home and seeing you doing the dishes, your shirt wet from leaning against the counter. I've imagined you on your hands and knees picking up Legos or Barbie dolls. I've envisioned you reading to our children. All of it Sarah, I've held you in my heart every day."

The tender images of his fantasy soften my irritation. I've longed to be noticed.

We look at each other. He smiles at me before turning his attention back to the road. I watch him check traffic over his shoulder before merging onto I-10 West.

"Yesterday was…"

"Incredible!" He interrupts. "I felt more love for you and more connected to you than ever before. It's like we've never been apart."

I was going to say, "nice." I was also going to say that we can't do this anymore, and that we need to find a way to be friends without hurting our families. I look down at my clasped hands. Feelings of shame make my chest feel cold and hollow. The intensity of my arousal surprised me, as does the desire to do it again.

"It's just… we're married to other people."

"Sarah, I'm going to be honest with you. Things between me and Megan haven't been good for a really long time. We're on the verge of divorce."

Before this mess with Michael, I never imagined there was any possibility Mason and I would have a reason to discuss divorce. "I don't have those same struggles in my marriage. Mason is wonderful to me, and we're really happy, at least I think we are." I don't know how Mason will react when he finds out how I've been betraying him.

"You think?"

"Well, I doubt he'll want to stay married to me after he finds out what we've done."

"Are you going to tell him?"

"We are supposed to be adopting our second baby in just a few months. There are so many things going on in my life right now. I just don't know."

"I plan to stay with Megan 'til after the baby is born. After that Sarah, I'm free to be yours. We can work things out, come up with a custody plan that meets everyone's needs. I will love your children as if they were born to me, and I know you'll love mine the same way."

His fantasy is both intriguing and disgusting. I don't want to end my marriage, but I can't seem to stay away from Michael. This is all so overwhelming.

"This is all just really fast. I need time to think."

Michael gives me a reassuring squeeze on the leg. "Take all the time you need."

I look up as Michael exits. "Where are we?"

"We're at the west edge of the city. I'm just turning around, and we can keep driving back the way we came."

We drive in silence for a few miles. I see him glance at me a few times out of my peripheral vision. I keep my eyes glued to a smudge on the windshield.

"Sarah, when we kissed yesterday, it sent electricity through me. It was like I was alive again for the first time since 1997. I want more of that."

"So do I," I confess in a whisper. I bite the inside of my cheek. I hadn't meant to say that out loud. I promised myself I wouldn't go there with him again.

Michael's face lights up. He reaches for my knee and squeezes, then leaves his hand there and caresses my lower inner thigh with his thumb, igniting the familiar heat of arousal.

"Sarah, we were bonded in '97. You were to be my wife. As far as I'm concerned, you are more of my wife than Megan, and I'm more your husband than Mason is. I know no one else sees it that way, but we were meant to be together. What we have is different. It would be wrong *not* to be together. Our parents broke us apart. We never did. We need to honor that commitment."

The anxiety flip-flops my stomach. Michael's touch on my leg and his romantic declaration excites a craving that deepens my shame. I crave the way he worships my body, crave his complete devotion to my pleasure. I need to feel close to him as much as I need to get away from him.

"You're intoxicating," Michael says. "What do you say? Are you ready to be mine, again?"

I close my eyes. I swallow hard and ignore the jumping frogs in my stomach. "I think so."

Michael exits the I-10 and pulls into the parking lot of the Red Roof Inn. While he registers and pays for the room, I alternate between panic, excitement, and wondering how things have gone this far. I hesitate at the elevator doors.

He places his hand at the small of my back and leads me forward. It feels so familiar.

I pause at the open room door while Michael waits for me. I'm not supposed to be here. My heart is racing, and I'm overwhelmed with desire. This is happening so fast. I can't think. Michael pulls me into his arms and kisses me passionately on the lips, moving down my neck. I kiss him back. I feel like I'm floating above my body. Detached, but still connected, somehow.

Michael pulls me to the bed, kissing me while sliding his hands up my shirt to unclasp my bra and caress my breasts. The more aroused I become, the less my conscience nags at me. I tug at his shirt, pulling it over his head and toss it to the floor.

He leans back and smiles, then slowly pulls my shirt and garment top together over my head. He pulls my bra away from my skin and gasps.

"You haven't aged at all. You are as fit and as beautiful as the day I met you." His words soothe the ache from a lifetime of body shame. I wrap my arms around his waist and pull him into me. I feel the warmth of his chest spread against mine. His heart quickens against my sternum.

He pushes me backward onto the bed, unzips my pants and slides them down over my hips, stopping abruptly. He steps back off the bed.

"What the fuck are those?"

I look down at my garment bottoms. The underwear goes down to my knees, concealing the flesh meant only for my husband, protecting me from sin.

"These are my garments." His focus makes me feel ridiculous; I want him to stop looking at them.

"Do you have to wear them?"

"You are supposed to wear them day and night after you have gone through the temple." I just want to take them off or pull my pants back up.

He shakes his head. "You, my princess, are too beautiful for these pioneer panties."

He peels them away from my body, kissing my belly as he does so.

As my garments are tossed aside, I feel sorrow for Mason. He deserves better than this. He deserves better than me.

I close my eyes and sink into Michael's touch, away from the pain.

AUTHOR'S NOTE

As I wrote these chapters, it was hard not to scream at my 23-year-old self. How could I not see what was happening? It's so obvious. Just say no!!!

It's normal for individuals who are bonded in trauma to feel obligated to the person with whom they share the bond, even in a way that is damaging to all other relationships.[22] I was isolated, in that I did not yet have the skills to reach out to someone for help, and I was filled with shame. I felt very similar to how I felt at 16. The need to be there for Michael was compulsive and overwhelming, as was the need *for* Michael and the unconditional love and acceptance he offered. Unfortunately, this left me feeling like an affair was inevitable.

---

22   Herman, J. (2015). *Trauma and recovery*. Basic Books. Page 200

CONFESSIONS

MAY 2004

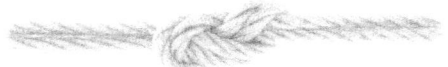

23 YEARS OLD

I fight the nausea back with a long swallow of ice water. It's been five days since Red Roof Inn. Mason deserved for me to tell him of my rendezvous that same night, but I lost my courage. The camping trip had been a failure. He and Eric returned home around nine o'clock. They couldn't keep the tent staked down in the high winds, and Eric was terrified by the quaking fabric.

I had screamed when Mason walked into the bathroom unexpectedly just as I was climbing out the shower. For a moment, I thought he was Michael. He was so frustrated about the torn tent and toddler fears that he went to bed without noticing my swollen, bloodshot eyes.

I tried to tell him again the next night after I pushed his hand away when he groped my breast, but he rolled to his side and wallowed in disappointment. I decided to wait until he would have a few days off to process the bad news.

My secret is a festering distraction. The house is a mess. Eric has been playing Mario Brothers for hours. Today is the day. It's the end of Mason's work week, and he'll have four days to work through his initial response. He walks in the door at 7:30, as usual.

"Hey, gorgeous, how was your day?"

"Same-o, same-o." I don't make eye contact. "Your dinner is in the microwave."

"Thanks. Is Eric ready for bed?"

"Almost. He'll be ready for story time by the time you're done eating."

I walk down the hall to check on Eric's progress and get out of view of my husband. I can't sit and chat with him while he eats like I usually do. The shame is eating at me, and I'm a jumpy mess. Eric is standing on the stool brushing his teeth. His pajama bottoms are twisted around his waist, making the seam skew to the right.

"Hi, Mama! I did it," he exclaims, holding his toothbrush out to me so that I can do the mommy go-over.

I take the small toothbrush from his small hand. "A child *always* blames himself for their parent's divorce," my Dad had said hundreds of times. I run my fingers through Eric's crazy hair and smile into his sparkling brown eyes. Will he remember how completely I love him? Or just that I ruined his family?

"Open up, kiddo," I say. The toothbrush shakes in my trembling hand as I count out the swipes. He clamps his mouth shut around the toothbrush and swallows. "You did a good job tonight, brushing all by yourself."

He grins, jumps down from the step stool, and races down the hall. He grabs *Ten Apples Up on Top* and *Would You Rather Be a Bullfrog* and settles onto the couch to wait for Daddy to finish dinner.

"Did you have fun with Mommy today?" Mason asks him from the dining room.

"No, she cried a lot."

I gasp, shocked he noticed.

Mason immediately looks at me for answers.

"Later," I mouth at him.

Eric continues to talk about his day, and fear fills my body. I have to tell Mason. I have to. I have been so stupid. I have ruined our family over Michael's neediness. And I guess mine. Everything seems to shift into slow motion as I wait for the "talk."

I look at my exhausted husband. He works so hard and tries to be there for everyone, including his son, even though he's tired and achy and most likely wanting to find out why his wife has been crying. I have no energy for all this sadness that is rising in me. We might not be able to adopt our second child. I have been a horrible wife, and I feel nothing but awful and guilty.

I leave the two to have their time together and go back to the dishes.

"Do you want me to read it forward or backward?" Mason's voice sounds tired.

"Backward!" Eric cheers. Mason opens the books to the last page and begins reading from the last word of the story to the first. Eric squeals with laughter while I wash Mason's dinner dishes.

Eric comes into the kitchen for a goodnight hug and kiss before Mason tucks him in.

"Thanks for doing the dishes. You usually leave that job to me," Mason says, giving me a hug from behind.

I spin in his arms and take in the smell of his starched fatigues, wondering if it will be the last hug I get like this, ever. Sadness has never felt so cold, so dark, or so lonely before.

"We need to talk about Michael."

Mason's body goes tense in my arms. "What about Michael?"

He waits for me to find my words, but I'm not ready for him to let me go; once it's out, I can't take it back.

"The worst has happened." I can't seem to bring myself to use the word *sex* or *affair*.

He lets go of me and takes a few steps back.

"What's the worst?" All the color drains out of his face.

Pain screams through me. "Please don't make me say it."

"I think I need you to."

"Mason, please," I beg, ignoring the urge to lie.

He waits.

I look away. "I slept with him. I don't even know how I got to a place that it happened, but it has."

Mason says nothing. I can hear him breathing a little harder. I look up only slightly and see him clenching and unclenching his fists.

"I'm sorry. I didn't want any of this. I didn't want to hurt you, I swear. I will make sure our divorce is amicable. We have to, for Eric."

His eyes narrow and he tips his chin up, a signal that he is digging in.

"We made a solemn covenant, together, in the temple, before God. I am not divorcing you."

My head whirls. "What?" I look over at him. He remains immobile. "Why not?" my voice cracks. "I cheated on you."

"We are *not* getting divorced," he says belligerently.

I flinch as tears rise in his eyes. "I'm... sorry." It's a weak response, I know this, I just don't have any words that can begin to make this better for him.

He heads for the door, and before closing it, he says, "I need a minute." He turns and walks away, closing our bedroom door behind him.

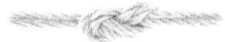

Bishop had made an emergency appointment to see us after Mason called him last night. I'm not sure what to say. Mason and I have barely spoken about the affair in the 23 hours since I told him.

"Good evening, Brother and Sister Westbrook," Bishop Highlands says, his voice gentle and inviting. He motions for us to sit in the chairs crammed into the tiny office, against the wall opposite his desk and shuts the door behind us.

I haven't been in the painted brick office in the month since he was called as bishop, and with the last bishop, I'd only been in for brief conversations about routine business. Not much has changed with the transfer of leadership. The brick is still stark white, the AC still rattles, the same picture of an overly white Jesus in red robes hangs on one wall with the picture of the Prophet and his counselors on the opposite one.

Mason pulls out a chair for me and squeezes my hand.

"Would you mind if I start with a word of prayer?" the bishop asks.

411

Mason and I fold our arms across our chests and bow our heads. I try to listen to the familiar requests of having the Spirit with us and such, but my mind wanders, playing through possible directions this conversation might take.

"In the name of Jesus Christ, Amen."

"Amen," Mason and I echo in unison.

"So, what brings you in today?" Bishop supports his chin on his thumb, his middle finger curls under his nose.

I stare at his hand. I'm not ready to be here. I'm not sure I'll ever be ready to be here. I'm my 16-year-old self again, numb, waiting for the bishop to decide my fate.

Mason squeezes my hand again, bringing my mind back into the room. The only way out is to start talking.

"I had an affair about two weeks ago. My high school sweetheart happens to live ten doors down the street from us, and I allowed things to go too far."

Bishop sits back in his chair; the air suddenly feels heavier. "I see." His face pinkens. He looks to my husband. "How are you and Mason doing?"

"We are fine." Mason says, an edge to his voice.

Bishop raises an eyebrow.

Wanting this over, I jump to the parts I know the bishop needs to hear. "Mason helped me write a letter to Michael asking for no more contact. Mason and I are going to work through it."

We all sit quietly for an awkwardly long time; I get the sense that this is the first "serious sin" the brand-new bishop has had to deal with. He'd only been a member for six years, and he acts like he doesn't know where or how to start.

Finally, he says, "I'm glad to hear that you're both committed to working on this." He clears his throat. "I'm humbled, Mason, that you are willing to love and support your wife. I know you must be working on pain of your own. The Lord will comfort you and give you strength to endure while holding Sarah up. The atonement is not just for sin. With Christ, you are never alone. You know that, don't you?"

He says it more as a statement than a question, but in my periphery, I can see Mason's head bobbing slightly, the tension in his jaw less noticeable.

Bishop clears his throat again. "The Lord cannot look upon sin with the least degree of allowance. You no doubt already know and feel that this is a serious transgression. I can see, Sarah, that you are also in pain. I'm encouraged to hear that you have already cut communication and are ready to engage in the repentance process."

This is so similar to the time that my parents dragged me into the bishop's office to confess. It's like they are reciting some lame script.

"The first step is coming to me today, doing just what you're doing. The second step is to hold a disciplinary council. This is uncomfortable, but ultimately will help you heal and experience the change that will free you."

This doesn't surprise me. I knew this was the process.

"I'll speak with my counselors and executive secretary and get back to you on when the disciplinary hearing will occur. In the meantime, I'd like to meet with you weekly to see how you are doing." He leaned in toward me with warm concern. "Do you have any questions?"

I shake my head, relieved that the cadence of his voice indicates the meeting is coming to a close.

"This won't be easy for either of you. I promise, it will be worth it.

Let's close with a word of prayer. Brother Westbrook, would you be willing to say it?"

Mason offers a really long prayer, which I don't hear. Instead, I feel empty, numb. I try not to think of the last time I'd been forced to confess to having sex with Michael. I try not to think of the humiliation and public shaming that followed with my Dad. It doesn't matter what punishment they give me; I'll do whatever Mason wants in order to keep our marriage intact.

The night I told Mason, he had yelled at me for about two minutes, and then apologized for losing his temper. He told me that I needed to write a letter to cut ties with Michael and that I needed to confess to the bishop after church on Sunday. He supervised the letter writing and then hand delivered it himself. I'm grateful that he found Michael in his carport, smoking alone, and that Megan wasn't there.

I've been on autopilot since then, and I can't seem to snap out of it. I didn't want to write that letter. I did it Mason's way because it would make Mason feel better. I owed him at least that. I wasn't ready to talk to the bishop, but Mason made the appointment. So here I am, confessing to a man I barely know, who knows nothing about my history with Michael or my parents. It's all happening too fast. I haven't had any time to think. I've been doing whatever Mason says when he says to, even though I'm not sure if that's what he really wants or expects.

I sit alone in the bishop's small office with four men whose faces and names are just about the only thing I know about them. The air conditioner is weak, and the air is heavy; this whole process is weighing me down. It's been a week since my "confession."

"Good evening, Sister Westbrook. Would you mind if we start with a prayer?"

"No" isn't really an option. Mormons start *everything* with prayer.

Brother Albrecht, Bishop's first counselor, asks the Lord to guide the men's decision regarding my worthiness status in the church. I swallow the dismay of being completely helpless in this room, resenting that the only qualifications any of them have to judge or help me in this situation is that they happen to be Mormon, male, and chosen. These four men hold complete power regarding my membership in the church, which is where all of my friends are, and where my marriage is. It doesn't really matter what "restrictions" will be placed on me, or that the content of this meeting is supposed to be "confidential. " It will only take a few weeks for most of the ward and my entire social network to know I did *something* bad enough to confess to the bishop.

"In the name of Jesus Christ, Amen." Brother Albrecht closes his prayer, his German accent barely noticeable. I don't know what he did for a living before retiring; he seems gentle, but has a fiery temper. He came to visit Primary once to talk to the children about paying tithing. When he left, the Primary president had to do some damage control to convince the children that they didn't have to give God all of their money via the bishop, only 10%.

I don't know much about Brother Taylor, Bishop's second counselor. He's a lieutenant colonel in the Army. His children are perfect angels in Primary. They never wiggle in their chairs and always answer requests with "ma'am" or "sir." Mason was at a military function that Brother Taylor also attended and came home complaining that his language was not becoming of a Lord's servant.

I know the executive secretary and "recorder" for the council, Brother Allen, a little better. He's also an Army officer, and Fort Bliss is his first command opportunity. He works with Air Defense Artillery, having been a former department manager at a local sporting goods store. I chatted with his wife a couple of times at ward luncheons. She doesn't speak English well, which gave cause for a miscommunication that ended with both of us giggling. She was very kind and invited our family to their modest home for dinner once. Brother Allen received us well and thanked me at the end of the evening for helping his wife feel welcome in America.

Bishop Highlands glances at the paper on his desk several times while addressing me.

"Sarah, serious sins often require the assistance of loving church leadership in order to work through the repentance process. The purpose of this disciplinary council is to help you receive forgiveness from the Lord, but we also want to help you earn forgiveness from Mason, to strengthen you as an individual, and to strengthen your marriage and your testimony of our Savior, Jesus Christ."

Mason and I are fine, because he is a good man and truly loves me. They don't need to worry about that, but I don't say anything. I bow my head in submission.

"We want to help you regain peace of mind and avoid transgressions in the future. With that in mind, is there anything you would like to share with your brethren this evening before we deliberate on how we feel best to proceed?" His face was warm, his voice soft.

"Well, shortly after Mason and I moved here, we discovered that my high school sweetheart lived just down the street. Michael and I had a lot of unresolved issues, so I went to his house to meet with him to gain closure and set some boundaries about what to do if we met in public and stuff… anyway a couple weeks later, he and I had an affair," I say.

"It doesn't sound like your meeting went very well, does it?" Brother Taylor's voice is controlled, gentle.

"Actually, the meeting went fine, but he ended up getting sick and hospitalized. I went to the hospital to check on him. Things didn't go well after that."

"Why did you go visit him in the hospital?" Brother Albrecht leans forward in his chair, his bushy gray eyebrows furrowed.

I felt the judgment of the eyes on me. The room grows hotter. "I was worried about him."

"Did his wife know of your visit?"

I don't trust the gentleness of the men's voices.

"No."

"Did Mason know?" Bishop asks.

"He was at home sleeping when I went."

Bishop said the council is one of love. I shift in my seat under the interrogation. At least Bishop Blythe had told me he understood why I was so upset by being pulled out of high school.

"Where did you have this *affair?*" The word "affair" leaves Brother Taylor's lips with an airy quality. He rolls his eyes then looks at me in quiet disgust.

"At the Red Roof Inn." I swallow. My throat is dry, and I'm sweating from the heat building in the room.

"So, you and this man planned to go to a hotel to sleep together?" The aggressive change in Brother Taylor's posture and tone startles me.

"Not exactly. We just went for a drive to talk."

"And where was Mason during this drive?"

"Brother Taylor," Bishop warns. We glance around at each other and after a few moments, Brother Taylor relaxes his shoulders and asks the question again, the breathy quality of his voice returning.

"Where was Mason during this drive?"

"At the Fathers' and Sons' campout."

My vision narrows at the collective gasp of all four men. I blink hard, I think I might pass out. I swallow again, but it doesn't help. I need out of this room. I need water and fresh air.

Bishop softens at my distress. "Thank you, Sarah. We would like to speak with Mason for a moment. Can you send him in?"

I stand up and yank the door open, cool air from the foyer rushes into the hot office.

"They want you now," I say to Mason.

I guzzle water at the fountain outside the children's classrooms. My stomach churns, the water sloshing uncomfortably. I sprint for the bathroom, vomiting water and the remnants of my barely touched dinner into the sink.

Hot tears blur my vision. I choke back a sob and chase small chunks of pasta around the bathroom countertop with a paper towel. Despite a now empty stomach, I heave again while I lift the vomit-soaked paper into the trash can. I splash cold water on my face and flick handfuls of water on the porcelain to rinse the sink.

I wait on an uncomfortable, ugly, flowered couch in the foyer for Mason to be finished with his "interview." I close my eyes. I want to run away with Michael. I wonder how his grandmother in Tennessee is doing. Would she still be a safe haven for us after an affair?

It took the bishopric about 30 minutes of discussion to decide my fate. Brother Taylor makes sure that I know that sexual immorality is a major offense against the laws of God. He backs that up with a verse from Doctrine and Covenants 42 about those who lust being cast out and tells me that the language is aimed at men, but that the same standards apply to women. Then he quotes Alma 39:3–5 from the Book of Mormon. He slows his speech and emphasizes, "Know ye not, my son, that these things are an abomination in the sight of the Lord; yea, most abominable above all sins save it be the shedding of innocent blood or denying the Holy Ghost."

Wait! Do they *really* think my affair is the second worse sin of all time? How the hell does my sleeping with Michael *once* even come close to cold-blooded murder?

The bishop delivers my sentence. I am to be disfellowshipped for one year. I am no longer allowed to take the sacrament because I am "unworthy." I am no longer allowed to lead music in the Primary, though no rationale for this was given. I am no longer allowed to offer prayers at church, which means every auxiliary leader and teacher will be "confidentially" informed that they can't invite me to take a turn offering group prayers. I am, however, encouraged to continue to pay my tithing and wear my garments with a promise "from God" that those two actions will keep me safe from further contact with Michael. I am required to meet with the bishop every Wednesday evening so he can check on my "progress" in the repentance process.

Bishop cancels our first meeting due to a family emergency. The following Friday, Mason gets orders to Iraq. He will be serving with Finn's husband, Dallin, in a marble hospital in Baghdad. Mason joins me for the first follow-up meeting with the bishop to inform him of his impending deployment.

"I want to make sure that Sarah stays on track while I'm away," Mason says.

After meeting with his counselors again, Bishop Highlands explains that they prayed about our situation, and God prompted them to tell me I need to move home to live with my parents during Mason's deployment in order to keep Michael out of my life.

"God didn't tell them that!" I yell at Mason. "God knows that it would be better for us to get divorced than for me to live with my father again. Besides, what about the baby? Our home study and legal pathway won't work if I move. There is no way we can afford another home study, and no social worker is going to recommend us for placement if I live with my parents."

"I know, Sarah. I don't understand the council either. Let's pray about this together," Mason pleads, his hands spraying water droplets all over the kitchen floor from the dishes.

"You can pray. It doesn't matter what God tells you, I'm staying put." I stomp down the hallway and slam our bedroom door shut. The latch doesn't catch, and the door ricochets back at me. I slam it again and twist the lock. I drop my body onto the chair in front of our computer, open my secret email account and compose a message.

I didn't write that letter. Mason made me. He's deploying in June. I will give you the key to my house, and you can come and go as you please. I love you. I'm sorry for putting you through this hell.

I hit the send button, sign out of the account, and wipe the computer's history. So much for "inspired men talking for God." Scripture reading, wearing garments, and paying tithing didn't keep me from becoming Michael's neighbor in the first place. Giving endless hours of my personal time to the church didn't stop Mason from deploying in our greatest time of needing to be together. These rules, this church, this doctrine, it's all bullshit.

AUTHOR'S NOTE

Acting before thinking is a common response to anger, and anger is a common response to any negative emotion that hasn't yet been processed.[23] The suggestion that I live in Arizona under my parents' watchful eyes triggered panic and fear. Mason's very calm suggestion that we pray about it, instead of matching my outrage, gave rise to more fear. I was terrified that Mason would side with the bishop, and I would find myself back in an intolerable hell that I couldn't survive a second time. In a moment when I was feeling incredibly triggered, betrayed by my church leadership, in some ways betrayed by my Heavenly Father, and irrationally anticipating being betrayed by my husband, I reached for the only person who had once promised me a way out.

---

23   Linehan, M.M. (2017). *DBT skills training manual.* Guilford. Pages 10-12 and 357

LOSS

MAY/JUNE 2004

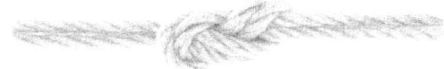

23 YEARS OLD

It only took a couple of hours to convince Mason that I was absolutely *not* going to go to Arizona to live with my parents while he was deployed to Iraq. Honestly, I had been so adamant, he knew he didn't have a choice.

Since then, we've functioned with an unspoken agreement to act like nothing bad has happened and have fallen back into our regular routine. I acknowledge his determination to "make things work" by avoiding any topic having to do with Michael, even though I know returning to "normal" so quickly and not talking about it is a ticking time-bomb. Maybe we can work this mess out when he gets home from deployment.

Eric wriggles next to me on our oversized sofa watching Disney movies, while I fold laundry. The phone on the end table rings, causing me to drop a wrinkled shirt mid-fold and bump into Eric. I lean across him trying to reach the handset and miss.

"Mommy, you're smashing me." Eric leans to the side to look around me with his dark chocolate eyes. "You're in the way, I can't see Wazowski or Boo." He grunts and pushes me off him with his elbow.

"Sorry, kiddo." He's watched *Monsters Inc.* at least a dozen times this month alone and still going. He loves the sound of Boo's squealing laughter.

The phone rings again. I stand up on the couch and reach behind him this time, avoiding the folded laundry piles on the floor in front of me. My hand freezes midair. It's Michael's warehouse on the caller ID.

"Hey, babe."

"Sarah, I can't talk," Michael whispers.

His voice is upset. My heart skips a beat. Something is wrong.

"Megan hacked into my secret email account. She's read everything. The poems I sent you and your last message about giving me a key to your house when Mason deploys."

I feel cold.

"How bad is it?"

"Well, you didn't leave anything to the imagination about our relationship. It's bad. She printed all the emails and brought them to my commander, and worse, she called my mother." The last time I saw Michael's mother was when I accidentally called her Mrs. Iles and she kicked me out of her house. From what Michael has told me, the years have made her more hostile and unforgiving.

"Sweet Jesus, God."

He's so quiet on the other end, I can just imagine what he has to go home to. "I'm sorry, Michael. Will they'll kick you out of the Army for infidelity?"

"Nah, that almost never happens."

Relief sweeps over me. At least our affair won't ruin his career. "What can I do?"

"Do nothing, Sarah. I love you. I'll reach out when it's safe again."

Sticky desperation fills my lungs. I don't want to lose him… again. "I love you, Michael. I love you."

"I love you too. Don't worry, we'll figure out a way to be together. When does Mason leave?"

"In about three weeks, on Father's Day."

"My chain of command will probably contact his chain of command," he says.

"Okay," I reply. "Mason's superior already knows about us, so it should be fine, unless he sees the emails." I flush thinking about telling Michael that Mason wouldn't understand. It would just crush him.

I hear the garbled intercom.

"That's my commander calling for me. I have to go. I love you."

I set the receiver back on the end table, my hands shaking.

"Mom-m-m-m," Eric demands. "Are you mad?"

"No baby, just have frogs jumping around in my stomach." I swallow the acid that has risen in my throat.

He shakes his head. "If you ate a frog, it would be dead, not jumping in your stomach. And it would taste gross."

I ruffle his thick black hair. "Good point."

I slump sideways on the couch, waiting for the wave of dizziness to pass.

Michael does call twice more to give me updates. His commander broke with traditional ultra-parental Army HR tactics and returned the printouts of the emails and told Michael that his private business would remain that way as long as Megan stopped making an issue of it. If anyone contacted Mason's commander, we never heard about it. Michael's mother, on the other hand, was furious that the Army didn't punish Michael in some way, issue a counseling statement for his file, or charge him with adultery.

In stark contrast with Megan's rage, Mason's calm demeanor is unnerving. After my confession and disciplinary council, we don't talk about the affair at all, and he seems mostly back to his normal self. He doesn't ask for details about my second visit with the bishop, either. I ask him how he's feeling, and he just says, "Jesus forgives and forgets. You've confessed and are working on repentance; it is my responsibility to forgive and forget like the Savior did."

He means it, but I can sense that he's still hurting, and I wish he'd talk to me. Megan may be a bit crazy, but I think I'd prefer that over the way Mason acts like nothing happened. At least Michael has evidence that Megan cares.

My anxiety calms down once Michael tells me he's shredded the email printouts and closed out his account permanently. I delete my secret email account too. It would devastate Mason to see that I'm not as repentant as he thinks I am. Twentydollarsandaneon@hotmail.com is juvenile, anyway. I feel guilty that I'm only pretending we've cut ties, but I've also stopped caring.

Mason has two weeks of leave prior to his deployment, during which we are going to Arizona to visit his parents. Before leaving, we visit Alltel Cellular and purchase a flip phone for me so I won't miss any of his calls when he's gone.

When we arrive home, I set the new phone on the counter and take Eric to the potty.

"Who is Thomas Gunderson?" Mason calls to me from the living room.

"No idea, why?"

"He called while we were gone."

I help Eric pull his pants up and release him so that he can go play with his toys. I come back into the living room to find Mason scowling at our home phone.

I am starting to feel uneasy. I walk up next to him and look at what he is looking at. "What's the matter?"

"Nothing, I'm trying to figure out if I know who this Thomas guy is."

"It's probably a wrong number, but if it bothers you, call him back."

He moves the phone out of my reach. "I think I will." He picks up the receiver, scrolls through the recent calls and hits the talk button when the name Thomas Gunderson shows on the display.

The cell phone rings. I giggle when I see our number on the caller ID.

"Hello, you've reached Thomas Gunderson," I answer jokingly.

"Dork." Mason hangs up the phone. We'd both forgotten that we used the cell phone in a test call to our home phone.

"They must not have changed the name for caller ID from that number yet," I yawn, feeling more tired than usual for this time of day.

"Mystery solved," he declares. "Do pancakes and scrambled eggs sound good for dinner."

I cringe. I don't *hate* pancakes, but I'm not a huge fan of them either.

"You do the pancakes, and I'll do the eggs."

"Deal."

We bump into each other in our narrow, alley kitchen. After the first accidental bump, we hip-check each other playfully. I drop an egg on the floor, and it splatters my foot.

"Now look what you did, clumsy," Mason teases, reaching for a paper towel.

"That was *totally* your fault!"

Mason leans down to wipe the egg off my foot and mops the mess off the floor. I step around him and grab a dinner fork to beat the eggs. We dance around each other in our narrow kitchen, each working on our half of dinner. I watch Mason pour the pancake batter onto the electric griddle. I love the way we play. I'm overcome with gratitude—and almost immediately overcome by guilt.

"You know, Mason, we make a good team."

He looks down at me, smiling, with a spatula in his hand. "What makes you say that?"

I pour the whipped egg over bacon grease and shake salt and pepper into the pan.

"Your pancakes will be ready at the same time as these eggs. Warm breakfast for dinner is much better than cold breakfast for dinner." I glance back at him. There are so many other things that make us a great team, I don't understand why I keep risking it.

He slides the wide spatula under the first pancake and flips it. The smell of pancakes wafts into my nose. My stomach jolts. I set my spatula down and steady myself on the counter.

"Sarah, you're pale." He places his hand on the small of my back.

I nod and take a deep breath in through my nose, then push Mason to the side so I can throw up in the sink. I reach over and unplug the electric griddle.

"I don't know why, but the smell of pancakes is making me sick." I lean over the sink and retch again.

"Wow, that came out of nowhere."

After rinsing out my mouth, I mutter, "I'm going to step outside."

"Sure, do you want me to bring you dinner?"

"No, please. I'm not hungry anymore." I retch again, but nothing comes out. I go out to the carport. I take a great gulp of air, but I can still smell pancakes. Our neighbor, Jamal, is outside mowing his lawn. I wave to him, then retch again and walk farther from the house. The hot breeze bites my face but carries the smell of fresh-cut grass. The nausea subsides.

Mason brings me a glass of water. Jamal cuts the engine and crosses the carports.

"Y'all okay?" he asks.

"I think so," Mason says, concern still etched on his face. "She was fine all day, then threw up in the sink while we were making dinner."

Jamal smiles as if he knows something we don't know. His wife Shanice comes up behind him.

"Everything good here?"

"Oh yeah," Jamal's inflection indicates he's excited for me. "Sarah was fine all day, then puked 'cause of the smell of food."

"Oh, my Gooood! Girrrrrl, you're pregnant!" Shanice wraps me up in a huge bear hug and jumps up and down. "I just knew you'd be able to get pregnant someday. Your skinny ass needs some widening up."

"I'm what?"

"She just threw up," Mason says dismissively.

Shanice crosses her ebony arms across her chest and leans back on her feet. "It's called *morning sickness.*"

I look up at Mason and shake my head. He and I haven't had sex for over a month… not since before Michael.

"Hang on, I got you girl." Shanice runs inside her home, screaming, "Praise the Lord Jesus, Sarah's having a baby."

"Where is she going?" Mason asks Jamal.

"She buys pregnancy tests in bulk and hands them out like candy on Halloween."

A minute later she comes back with a skinny white foil envelope containing a single pregnancy test in one hand and her phone in the other.

"Hang on," she says to the caller. "Sarah, take this, and let me know in the morning what it says. I gotta take this call." She winks at me and does a little dance on the way back inside.

"Well, I hope congratulations, if not, feel better soon, Sarah," Jamal says before returning to his lawn mower.

I look up at Mason.

His mouth hangs open. He looks back at me. "When was your last period?"

"I… I don't kn… know exactly. It's written on the calendar hanging on the fridge."

We stare at each other for a long time. I'm reluctant to go look at the calendar.

I'm two weeks late.

After dinner and bedtime stories, I open the little foil packet and dip the test strip in pee. Two pink lines. I stare at the strip, light-headed, waiting for the new wave of nausea to pass before I open the bathroom door and hand the strip to Mason, who is waiting just outside. "They're right."

"How is that even possible?" Mason asks.

I chew on my lower lip, wondering if this will change Mason's decision to stay married and work things out. "I have no idea. It's Michael's baby, though."

His Westbrook chin juts forward, lips pulled tight. "No, it's not. The baby is mine."

"Shhhhh, we need to talk more quietly, or we'll wake Eric." Still light-headed, I lean against the hallway wall.

"Michael doesn't get to be the one who fathers your baby," Mason says in a forceful whisper.

My temples begin to throb. "Mason, I'm sorry, I don't know what else to say."

"The baby is mine."

"Mason, there's no way the baby is yours. I'm sorry."

"The baby is mine." His arms are folded across his chest, his face set in anger.

"Stop saying that! You sound like a robot. How am I going to tell Michael? What do we do?"

"We don't tell him, or the baby, or anyone else."

I feel defeated. "Mason, that's wrong, and it's not fair to the baby." I look up at Mason's dark features, there's no way that Michael's frail frame would produce children that could pass for Mason's.

"As long as you don't tell him, no one needs to know."

"The baby has a right to know the truth about its parentage. So does Michael."

"Michael gets no say in this," Mason snaps. For the first time since he found out about the affair, it doesn't feel like he's trying to reign in his feelings. "I will love the baby as if *I* am the father, just like I love Eric. The baby will never know the difference. Sarah, we've tried for a baby for *five* years. I get this, not *him*." He looks so desperate, clinging to my hands, his voice pleading.

I pull my hands away. I don't understand. Mason and I started trying to have a baby a couple months after we got married. Years of infertility treatment and three surgeries later, we've never even had the whisper of a potential pregnancy. Once Eric joined us, I didn't need a biological child. I love being Eric's Mom. I can't imagine that I'd love a biological child any more than I love Eric, and I'm sure I'll feel the same way about the baby we're adopting. Oh shit…

"Mason, do you think we should pull out of the adoption? I'll have two babies, less than nine months apart. Is that fair to either baby?"

"I'm going to bed. Don't tell Michael you're pregnant. I forbid it." He walks away from me.

"You are *not* my father. You do not get to forbid me from doing *anything.*"

He turns around to face me. The dim light in the hallway casts odd shadows on his face, but I can see the tears in his eyes.

I pace the floor, running through my to-do list and counting the rings, knowing someone at the nurse's station will pick up after the third ring. Everything about the Army is regimented.

"William Beaumont Army Medical Center, Med/Surg Unit, how may I help you, Sir or Ma'am?"

"Hey, Jeff, it's Sarah. Is Westbrook free to come to the phone?"

"Let me check… hey, are you free to take a phone call from some crazy lady?"

"I am if she's a crazy hot lady." I hear Mason's laugh in the background. It's the same joke every time I call.

"I think she's decent," Jeff chides.

"You need to get your eyes checked." Mason's voice grows louder, "Why, hello beautiful."

"Hey, I'm calling because I can't read your handwriting on this packing list. Do you remember what it says underneath 'socks and garments?'"

"Umm, is it scriptures?"

I squint at the list. "I think so. Your handwriting gets worse the longer you work in the medical field."

"I'm just trying to fit in."

"Ha! Very funny. Love ya."

"Love you, too."

I set the cordless receiver on the kitchen table and continue to cross the packed items off our list. Today is Mason's last day working at the hospital before he deploys. As soon as he gets home, we are leaving for Arizona to visit his parents before Mason deploys. Eric is a good traveler; still, the six-hour drive will go faster if he sleeps.

I grab the cell phone. I haven't used it since we bought it. Mason thinks it's a good idea to test the signal in Arizona, so I know what to expect if Eric and I decide to visit any of the grandparents while Mason is gone. I doubt we will, especially now that I know I'm pregnant.

I'm both excited and devastated by my pregnancy. I feel icky shame every time I think about the baby. The OB clinic scheduled me for my first appointment a month from today. Mason will be gone by then. The clinic also assured me that if I got pregnant spontaneously, there is no need to come in for early scans. They also assured me that menstrual-like cramps are normal in the early weeks of pregnancy as my body adjusts to being pregnant. I'm tired all the time, my boobs hurt like hell, and I've stopped eating breakfast entirely.

I grab the cell phone and tiptoe down the hallway to peek into Eric's room. He's still asleep. I smile at his angelic face and pull the door gently closed behind me. I cross the hall into my bedroom for a quick nap and toss the flip phone into my open suitcase.

I lay back on Mason's pillow and pull the velvety throw over me. Despite feeling exhausted at my very core, I cannot sleep. I can't shake the feeling that I need to tell Michael about the baby. "Just rip off the Band-Aid, Sarah," I say to the ceiling. I didn't agree to keep it a secret, but I also haven't said anything to Michael yet. I don't want to fix lies and deceit with more lies and deceit. I was hoping Mason would change his mind. He hasn't.

He is as adamant as ever that he can love the baby as if it is his, and I believe him. He is a wonderful father to Eric, who idolizes him. I place my hands lovingly on my lower abdomen. I love you little one. I close my eyes and revel in the miracle this pregnancy is. It defies the odds. The last doctor I saw for infertility told me it would be nearly impossible for me to get pregnant without medical intervention. He never explained why and I didn't ask. I have "unexplained infertility." And yet, here we are.

Will he have Michael's blue eyes? Will he stay blond like his father, or turn brunette like I did? I hope the baby gets my nose. I flip again. It's no use… I can't nap any more than I can keep a secret of this magnitude from both Michael and our child. I know what I need to do, and I'm not going to sleep well until I do it.

I look at the cell phone perched atop my folded clothing. Thomas Gunderson… the caller ID will say Thomas Gunderson. I reach for the flip phone and dial my home phone number just to be sure. Sure enough, it has not yet been updated to my name. I sit up and look at the clock. It's 4 p.m. Michael usually gets home between 5 and 6:30. I climb out of the bed and pack Mason's scriptures from the nightstand. I zip my light gray suitcase closed and wheel it out to the front door with the other suitcase and diaper bag.

I hear Eric's sleepy voice call my name, followed by his footsteps down the tiled hallway. I put on a movie for him.

"In here, buddy. I have your sandwich," I say once he comes in. "Here you go, kiddo." He reaches his hand out to take the sandwich from me without taking his eyes off the screen.

I use the time to do my hair and a bit of makeup and eat a few saltine crackers to take the edge off the nausea. When the movie ends, I call out, "Time for golf, Eric."

"Yay!" He sprints back to his bedroom and returns just as quickly, tugging his sunbaked, plastic golf set behind him. He lugs the set to the front lawn and sets up his targets.

I pretend to play along while I watch for Michael's car to pull into the carport. It's a Friday, so I expect he'll be home closer to 5. I look at my wristwatch: 4:45.

"Mama, get it." Eric demands.

He points at his golf ball bouncing down the street.

I step off the curb and into the street only to freeze at seeing Michael's red Escort pull into his driveway. He walks around to his front door, pauses, and looks my way. We stand still, staring at each other for several seconds.

"Mom! Mama!" Eric is holding out his hand. I toss the ball back to him and step back onto the sidewalk. I look down the street just in time to see Michael's screen door close behind him. I glance at my wristwatch: 4:50.

I'll call in him in 10 minutes. I try to distract myself by hitting a few golf balls for Eric. I keep checking my watch, but time moves so slowly. What is he going to say? Eric gives up on my lack of enthusiasm and sets up rocks on our porch as targets. His plastic ball hits them but doesn't knock them over. Eric's frustrated grunts come in intervals, his face pinched in concentration.

Finally, it is 5 p.m. I dial Michael's phone number.

"Hello," Megan answers. I try not to think of Megan's baby as I consider the one growing within me.

"Hello, this is Major Gunderson. Is Specialist Iles available?"

"Yes, ma'am, he just got home."

"Who is it?" I hear Michael's voice in the background.

"I don't know, but she's a Major."

"Major Sealy is a man."

"I said I don't know."

I shift uncomfortably, hoping Megan doesn't ask me questions. I don't have any other ideas if she does.

"Hello, ma'am?" My heartbeat quickens as I hear Michael's voice, clear and official.

"It's me. This is my new cell phone number. We need to talk. Can you step outside?"

"No."

I hear a click and the line goes dead. I tell myself he's just waiting to talk until he's alone. I keep the phone in my pocket, hoping he'll call me back soon, mapping out what I'm going to say when he does. But he doesn't call. Mason walks in the door right at 7:30. By 8:00, we are on the road to Arizona.

Mason sleeps the entire drive. I wouldn't be able to sleep if I tried. I don't understand Michael's newfound silence. He's always been able to step away from Megan or find a way to call me back. My anxiety about it rides with me all the way to Arizona.

The cell signal at Mason's parents' house is surprisingly good, but I still don't hear from Michael; I can only conclude that he doesn't want to talk to me. I'm not 16 anymore. I'm not going to cry myself to sleep every night waiting for him, but I still hurt.

I haven't said much so far this trip, and no one seems to notice my unusual somberness. Mason and I had agreed to keep the pregnancy a secret until after my first doctor's appointment, and aside from Michael abandoning me again, I can't think of much else.

Two days later, the cramping turns violent. I double over in pain and stumble into the bathroom. There's blood in my garment bottoms. I reach my hand down and catch a clot the size of a small dessert plate, followed by a gush that leaves me dizzy.

"MASON!" I scream.

I hear him take the stairs two at a time. He bursts into the bathroom, looks at me, then down at my hand. As he takes a step toward me, I close my eyes and feel my body fall forward.

Something cold splashes on my face. I open my eyes and see Mason.

"Good girl, keep looking at me, don't close your eyes."

I'm on the bathroom floor.

"Mason?"

"I think you're having a miscarriage. We need to get you to the hospital."

No one questions my silence during the remainder of the visit. I feel cold and heavy. I can't stop crying. My abdomen aches for the baby that is no longer there.

"Six to eight weeks."

"It's fairly common this early on."

"She is young."

"You can try again."

The words aren't comforting, but everyone around me keeps saying them.

Mason does all the driving on the way home and leaves me to my thoughts.

I am numb. Michael still has not returned my call.

A week later, Mason deploys. I watch Mason shrink in my rearview mirror as I drive away from Biggs Airfield. In less than three weeks I lost Michael, my status at church, my baby, and now, Mason.

I jolt upright on the couch. I must have fallen asleep when I came home from Biggs Airfield.

BANG, BANG, BANG. "SARAH! I'll kick this damn door in if I have to. OPEN UP! I know you are in there." Finn pounds on my door.

I pull myself off the couch.

BANG, BANG, BANG.

"I'm coming!"

I open the door to see Finn standing on my front porch, alone. My heart lurches. I was supposed to pick Eric up at her house on the way back from dropping Mason off.

"Where are the boys?"

"With Grace. Good God, you scared me, Sarah. Shit, you look worse than I did when Dallin left."

Something in me cracks.

"I miscarried my baby last week in Arizona." The words come out in a whisper, then a guttural wail escapes me, carrying the weight of my emptiness.

"Oh, Sarah, I'm so sorry." Finn wraps me in a hug. "That's right, girl, scream it out."

She holds me until my anguish goes numb.

EL PASO, TEXAS

FEBRUARY 2005

23 YEARS OLD

"Good God, I've fucked up my life," I sigh as I plop onto the couch in Jim's office. "I'm not even twenty-four, and I've already destroyed my marriage."

Jim has been my counselor since shortly after the affair. When I scheduled the appointment, it was because I'd had two panic attacks that landed me in the emergency room, thinking I was having a heart attack.

Mason had deployed to Iraq weeks after I cheated on him. Five weeks after that, I took custody of Brigg. There was no way I was going to add to Mason's stress by telling him I had been in the ER twice, especially since there wasn't anything actually wrong with me.

"How is Brigg doing?" It's the first question Jim asks me every time; otherwise, I hijack the entire session whining about what a difficult infant he is.

"Sleep is optional, right? Because that kid never sleeps. I'm serious, he sleeps maybe three hours a day in fifteen-minute increments. One of these days, I'll come for my session and just take a nap on your couch."

"Sounds good to me. I'll catch up on paperwork while you snooze."

I laugh and feel my shoulders relax. I tilt my head side to side; my neck pops.

"How are you and Mason doing?" It's Jim's regular second question since Mason had returned from deployment last month.

"Well, he does better getting up with Brigg at night than I do. He finally believes how hard it all is, now that he's experiencing it for himself."

"I meant, how are *you and Mason* doing?"

I don't want to talk about how Mason and I are doing.

"Mason seems content that my 'disfellowship-ment' from the church is punishment enough for my affair. He doesn't seem to understand how much pain I'm still in. He's never been good with feeling his feelings, much less anyone else's. He has two emotions, angry and content, and since anger is 'evil' he avoids it like it's an adult poopy diaper with c-diff."

"That's a unique comparison, can you say more about that?"

I pick at my thumbnail. "Mason only yelled at me for *maybe* five minutes when I told him about the affair. Then he turned his anger off and devised a 'solution.' As long as I check all the Mormon boxes for repentance, he'll forgive and forget, just like Jesus."

"It sounds like you are hurting because Mason can't connect with you emotionally."

I pull the depressed corner out of the decorative pillow then set it back in its place on the couch. "I guess."

Jim raises his eyebrows. "Why do you think Mason can't feel with you?"

"No one in his family knows how to emote. All the Westbrooks are very monotone, emotionally speaking." I shrug my shoulders.

"That sounds very lonely." Jim's voice is gentle.

I drop my gaze to the floor. "Anyway, I have, like, six months to go before I've fully 'repented.'" I lift my fingers in air quotes. "I don't think being excluded from participation in church is a good way to get right with God, but that's the Mormon's prescribed 'path to repentance.'"

"Your bishop doesn't seem to understand the emotional impact this is having on you either."

I tap my heel rapidly against the floor. "That's a Mormon Church issue. *My* bishop is actually pretty chill. Mason's just happy I put my magic underwear back on. As long as I do what it takes to get back on the 'path' like a good, repentant Mormon, he's happy."

Jim cocks his head to the side, "Are *you* happy?"

I know he knows the answer to that is "no," but I don't understand *why* I'm not happy.

"Mason is a good man. He provides for our family, he's kind to me, he listens, he helps with the kids and household chores. I have no reason to be unhappy. Besides, since Brigg joined the family, I'm too busy and exhausted to think about anything other than Brigg."

"It's okay to be unhappy in your marriage, Sarah, even when things seem to be perfect at first glance."

"I love Michael. And I love Mason." My shoulders fall. "I'm not supposed to love two men. I can't seem to let Michael go."

"Where do you think that comes from?"

443

"Your 'what and how' questions are annoying." I press my middle fingers into my temples.

"Yeah, I get that. They are annoying, especially when you don't feel like you have enough emotional energy to do anything different."

"Good, then can I claim a *Maslow Hierarchy of Needs* deficit on this one? Seriously, I'm so sleep deprived I can hardly see straight. The kid screams twenty hours a day, sleeps for a total of three hours, and spends the rest eating just so he can puke it all up and start over again."

"You asked me to challenge you when I thought you might be exaggerating. Are you?"

"Damn it, Jim. Yes, okay, I'm exaggerating. He probably cries closer to twelve hours a day. I'm so fucking used to it that I can actually sleep through his screaming. Grace took him from me yesterday for three hours so I could rest. Finn is coming today for three hours so I can sleep, and Scarlett is going to take him tomorrow."

"I'm glad your Army family is taking care of you as much as they can. I'm sure Brigg's needs are getting in the way of healing your relationship after the affair."

"Maybe. Brigg can't hold anything down either. I feed him an eight-ounce bottle, and he pukes up ten!"

"Exaggerating?"

"Not that time. I've started walking around with a puke bowl. He sucks his formula down, then vomits it up within minutes. I poured the puke back into the bottle to show the pediatrician, and there were leftovers in the bowl."

"I'm going to trust that you need to talk about Brigg today. How much are you exaggerating to the doctors about his struggles?"

I know his words aren't an accusation, that Jim is genuinely curious, but I still feel exposed. I look away.

"Give me a percentage, Sarah. How much are you exaggerating Brigg's symptoms?"

"No one pays attention to me unless I exaggerate. It's been like that my entire life, Jim. If I don't exaggerate, I get ignored. When I do exaggerate, I'm 'looking for attention.' It's a lose-lose. It's always been a lose-lose for me."

"It must be dehumanizing to feel like you have to lie to be noticed." Jim's voice is soft.

"I get accused of lying even when I tell the truth."

"I know. You've been lying and exaggerating your entire life to be noticed. It's normal for people, children especially, to crave attention. We need it to develop appropriately. Seeking healthy attention isn't a bad thing."

"Tell that to my parents *and* my in-laws," I retort bitterly. Still, it makes sense, and I mull over what he just said.

"I'm going to ask you a question, Sarah. It's a hard question, but I think it's important for you to hear in order to get Brigg the care he needs and heal your relationship with Mason. Are you ready?"

Jim waits for me as I take several slow deep breaths in and out for a full minute.

"I'm ready."

"How much do you think your exaggeration of Brigg's symptoms is impeding his care?"

My cheeks feel hot. I'm trying to control my tone, but I can hear that my voice is raised. "I need help for Brigg, as much for myself as for him. Why would I get in the way of that?"

"I just want you to consider how many doctors aren't taking you seriously because they can tell you are exaggerating."

The wind rushes out of me. I feel the hot sting of shame rise within me, and I break. Silent tears spill onto my cheeks. Jim sits back in his chair and waits for me. I sit without speaking for several minutes.

"You're right, Jim. They aren't listening to me. They aren't helping Brigg because they don't believe me."

I look up, and Jim nods. I'm afraid to say more. He waits for me. I hate silence. I know he knows I'm still holding back. He's waiting for me to say something.

"I don't know how to avoid exaggeration when I feel worried. I…" my voice trails off.

"You're hiding behind the exaggeration because you don't feel like the truth is enough," Jim offers.

"No, it's because I'm not enough. I'm only important when I'm the 'hero,' only noticed when the story is 'fantastic.' I'm not enough unless the story is better than I could ever be. I've never been enough unless I'm living my life the way the Mormon Church says I'm supposed to, which is completely impossible. According to everything I've been taught, people who aren't Mormon only *think* they are happy and have no idea what they are missing."

"But you aren't happy, and Mason doesn't see it."

"He doesn't even know how to look for it. If I check the Mormon boxes, it means I'm happy. I'm always failing, Jim—at everything. I ruined my marriage, and now I'm ruining my kid."

Jim helps me create a system for staying honest with the pediatrician for Brigg's upcoming appointment. I journaled Brigg's symptoms for two days. I've also taken a video of him with my camera that I plan to show the doctor so they can see how bad the breathing issues are. My goal is to speak less, listen more, and stick to the script, literally. I've written everything out, and I plan to just read it. I need to prove that I'm being honest in order to feel heard.

I've never met Dr. Bowen. In military medicine, you rarely see the same provider twice in a row. He seems nice enough. I read him my list of symptoms. Brigg is laying in the chair next to me, sucking down his bottle. As soon as he pulls the bottle out of his mouth, I push the bowl in front of his face. Brigg vomits everything he's just eaten and more. Then I show Dr. Bowen the video of Brigg struggling to breathe, which happens several times a day.

For the first time in my life, the doctor listens to me. He even watches the video more than once. Dr. Bowen has Brigg admitted, and within three days, he has life-saving surgery and referrals to several specialists to keep him stable.

The morning of discharge, Dr. Bowen says, "You came prepared to meet with me. The information you provided saved your son's life. You are his hero, Mrs. Westbrook."

I don't feel like a hero, at least not the kind I'd always wanted to be growing up. Mostly, I feel relieved to have answers and a plan to care for Brigg. I've learned a valuable lesson. My son needs me to be straightforward in order for *him* to get the attention *he* needs. I vow to figure out how to stop exaggerating, how to stick to the truth, especially when I don't feel heard.

PART FOUR

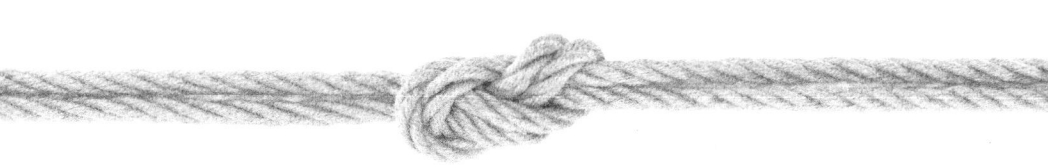

EYE MOVEMENT DESENSITIZATION AND REPROCESSING (EMDR) THERAPY

SAN ANTONIO, TEXAS
2013

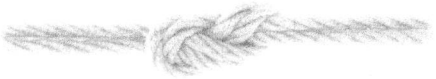

32 YEARS OLD

A heavy weight presses me down onto the cold exam table, squeezing me. I push a large hairy hand away off my chest and manage to get to my feet. I scan the Fine Arts building and see Michael. I run toward him. We make eye contact. He turns and walks away—disappearing.

Desperate to get away from impending doom, I search for Mason. I don't see him. I see no one, but when I turn around, I see my father looming in the distance, growing closer.

"You are an embarrassment," I hear him roar, his voice carrying in the wind, sending chills. I try to flee, but he reaches me before I make it past the double doors. He shoves me into a wall of spikes that pierce my back.

I scream out in pain and see my mother off to the side, standing there.

Her eyes lock on mine. "Give your father another chance. He loves you." I want to protest, but when I try to speak, nothing comes out.

"You slept with a louse, you filthy slut." Dad slaps my face.

I punch and flail. Something warm grabs my forearm and pins it to the fabric beneath me.

"Shhhhhhh, it's okay. I'm right here. I'm not going anywhere."

I open my eyes and realize it is Mason who is holding me. I am not in Snowflake. I'm in my bed in San Antonio. It's just another nightmare.

I melt into him. He slowly lays me back down. I turn away from him and curl into the fetal position. My body quakes, my heart still racing.

He molds to my back, holding my upper body firmly to his to soothe the tremors.

This therapy office isn't as welcoming as Jim's was. There is a lot more medical equipment and cheap furniture covered in vinyl that creaks under me when I move.

"Why do you minimize what happened to you, Sarah?" Dr. Lopez-Martin asks gently.

I'm only a few months away from graduating with my master's degree in Mental Health Counseling. At 32, you'd think I'd have a handle on the nightmares and intrusive thoughts of Michael already.

"What do you mean? I'm not minimizing, I'm in therapy, dealing with it." My foot taps anxiously on the ground. I don't have time for therapy. EMDR is supposed to cure you in two sessions, according to my professor, anyway.

"You share your life history like you're reading a list, with little emotion." He tilts his chin, inviting me to explain.

"I worked through all this history with Jim, years ago." I allow my irritation to seep into my tone. "That's not what I'm here for. I haven't slept well in years; I was told EMDR could help me get rid of the nightmares."

"Yes, EMDR may help with that, but EMDR is not a magic wand. Like any therapy, there is a process, and this process starts with talking." He pauses, and I refuse to say anything. "You tell your most traumatic moments without feeling, as if they don't affect you. That is very concerning to me."

"Okay, but how is talking about this going to help me sleep?" I'm not trying to be argumentative or resistant. I sit with clients, hear their stories, and become so overwhelmed with memories from my childhood that I can't function when I get home from work. My professor warned us that our unresolved trauma might rear its ugly face as we all started our supervised practicum. I had been sure I would be fine since I'd spent almost three years working with Jim after the affair in 2004, but I was only getting a few hours of sleep at night due to the nightmares.

I sigh in resignation. "I'm too tired to talk about it again. I need to get over it and just get on with my life now." As soon as I say this, I know how wrong I am.

"I hear you. I also know that you understand feeling a wide range of emotions is vital for healing. You know this, you told me about a client you saw last week who felt like anger was a sin, and once he was able to identify it as a tool, he made significant progress in treatment. What feelings are *you* running away from, Sarah?"

"If I start feeling the emotions again, I'll lose my mind. I keep them 'locked up' on purpose."

"You need to separate your feelings from your clients; that is appropriate. I'm concerned that you keep them locked up and hidden away from those closest to you. You and I need to better understand what that is about so that I can more effectively guide you through EMDR. We have to have a therapeutic alliance in order for your brain to trust the process; otherwise, all you will be doing is moving your eyes funny while I talk to you."

"If you say so. I'm not sure I'm able to do that right now." I fight back tears. Sticky shame that I cry over the smallest things rises in my throat.

"Willing or able?" He raises a bushy eyebrow as if to challenge my motivation.

"Probably a little of both." My shoulders slump, and I wipe at my face.

"You said your Dad over-disciplined you; I wouldn't call what you described 'over-disciplined.'" His statement feels like a hot prodding iron to my belly button. I grit my teeth, thinking of Dad screaming in my face, his raised hand threatening. The image pushes me back into defense.

"What would you call it?" My sarcastic tone is meant to warn.

"You're almost finished with your master's in counseling. If you were your patient, what would you call it?"

I glare at him. "I know I'm supposed to say 'abusive,' but it's more complicated than that. I lied about being kidnapped. It didn't happen in a void.

In some way, I think I deserved what I got. Dad never beat me until I had sex…" My voice trails off as I realize I just blamed myself, the victim, which is exactly what an abuser seeks in order to gain control over another person.

There was a reason I had lied, and it wasn't from a place of malice. My home had not been a place where telling the truth would have been safe for me. I was fucked either way. I lied in an attempt to lessen the intensity of the impact of discovery. I shifted the blame to others, in the same way my parents modeled for me my entire life. Dr. LM sits quietly, studying my unsettled fidgeting, allowing the silence to be my teacher.

"You said that whenever your Dad comes to visit, you can't function. You have panic attacks, suffer anxiety, and you withdraw from life around you. You said it takes you several days after he leaves for things to return to normal, is that right?"

"Umm, yeah, it used to take just a day to recover. Last time it took me over a week." My voice is calmer now, almost contemplative.

"No one deserves to be abused, Sarah. There is no excuse for a parent to beat their child, to isolate them from their entire world, to hold them captive in their own home." The gentleness of his voice makes me feel uneasy.

"Fine, so he abused me, but it's not like the stories I listen to with my adjudicated teenagers. I've never experienced anything *that* horrific."

"How does comparing your trauma with theirs help you?"

"Am I comparing?"

Dr. LM looks up at me over the thick rim of his dark glasses but does not respond. Silence is his strongest therapeutic tool.

"Ugh, yes, I'm comparing. I feel like a pussy. Some of my clients were neglected and abused from the time they were little. I got abused for just a couple of years."

"*Just*? Can you say more about the use of that word?"

With a slight smile, he watches me scowl. He's right. What my parents did may have been more subtle, but it had been chronic, like my adjudicated teenage clients. I let out a long, low sigh.

"Can I answer that next week? I didn't recognize I was using comparative suffering. I know it's not useful. I'll get back to you on what that means for me."

Dr. LM nods. "Of course. How often are you having the nightmares?"

"Almost every night. I catch myself looking over my shoulder during the day, too. I haven't seen Michael in over a decade, and I still look for him everywhere I go. I hear his voice when I'm tired, and then I panic that Dad is going to beat me or take my kids. I know it's irrational. I'm a good mom, and there is no reason anyone would try to take them from me, except that Dad is so critical of everything I do with my children. I think he wishes Eric was his. He thinks Eric is perfect, and he always wanted more children. Brigg makes him uncomfortable. He has no sway over Brigg at all. Brigg doesn't give a fuck what anyone thinks… he can't, he's not aware of very much of what is going on around him."

"Why do you think your Dad wishes Eric was his?"

"Dad always wanted more kids, and Eric is easy to love and a champion wrestler. Dad loves to have a child he can brag about. Besides, Dad has 'teased' about taking Eric in the past, but it doesn't feel like he's joking."

"That's… interesting and a bit unnerving."

I shrug it off, not willing to examine it further.

Dr. LM seems to follow my lead. "At our first meeting, I suggested you might have PTSD. Have you given that some thought?"

I had, and I didn't like the prognosis if I didn't get my symptoms under control. "The diagnosis makes sense. It explains the flashbacks, the hyper-vigilance, and the intrusive memories. I also read the articles you gave me about prisoners of war and the one on complex PTSD. It fits. I don't like it. It makes me feel weak, but I agree." I recognized myself immediately in the literature, but it had taken me all week to admit it to myself.

"Good, I'm glad."

"That's great!" I smirk.

"I apologize, I did not intend my words as an 'I told you so.' I said it because now that you better understand how the complex trauma is impacting your daily life, we have the ability to start helping you work through it, or at least lessen the intensity of it so that it no longer interferes with your daily life."

I hate being the patient. I already know a lot about all of this, but being on the receiving end feels overwhelming. I know I'm an intelligent woman, but I feel foolish for not being able to use my knowledge to heal myself. I take a deep breath in and focus on his bushy unibrow as I blow the breath out slowly, just as he has taught me to do, until my heartbeat slows and my defensiveness dissipates.

"Look, Dr. LM, I've read about EMDR. The thing that makes me most nervous about it is no one knows why it works. I just don't see how holding vibrating paddles or wiggling my eyes is going to get rid of my nightmares or chill my hypervigilance. It just seems too easy."

He chuckles at me. "It really does, doesn't it? Don't think the EMDR alone is going to be a cure-all for all the trauma in your life. Look at it as a possible tool to help you experience the hard things with less intensity. It takes the edge off of the panic response so that we can really begin to focus on the trauma bonds you are experiencing."

"The what?" I ask. I know counselor lingo, but "trauma bonds" is a new one for me.

"The bonds created when people share trauma."

"You mean like Stockholm Syndrome?" A wave of nausea makes me dizzy. To think I have *that* type of a connection to my father makes me want to bolt out of this office.

"Not exactly. Your discomfort around your father makes sense. It's also completely normal and expected based on your history of abuse and emotional neglect."

I wipe the cold sweat from my forehead and nod, indicating I'm ready for Dr. LM to continue his explanation.

"I'm referring to the bond you share with Michael. The fact that you went to him when you became aware of his pain and vulnerability, foreseeing that it would harm your relationship with Mason and threaten your marriage, yet not feeling like you could stop it, even though you wanted to."

The room begins to close in around me and grow incredibly hot.

"That you threw 'caution to the wind' per se," Dr. LM continues. "You got the closure you were seeking when you discovered you were neighbors and finally got to apologize; however, despite knowing the risks, you chose to be there for Michael so that he could accomplish healing, and when your efforts failed, you increased the frequency and intensity of the destructive relationship."

He's right. Part of me felt driven to protect my marriage, but I couldn't abandon Michael, who was still emotionally wounded.

"It wasn't forced. I didn't feel coerced." I breathe through the confusion.

"Can you say more about that?"

"I went with Michael because I loved him, because I *wanted* to be with him. I wanted us to heal together. I didn't want to hurt Mason or Eric, I just… it's just so fucking complicated. I don't know how to explain it."

"It is common for individuals with c-PTSD to self-destruct as they try to maintain relationships with those to whom they share a trauma bond. Did you want to stay married to Mason?"

A wave of heavy guilt for what I've put Mason through threatens to consume me. Even though Mason and I have struggled to connect emotionally with each other for years, my affair had never been about his shortcomings or about my not wanting to be with him. "Yes, of course. I love Mason, and we were happy. I love Michael too, and I hate myself for that. No matter what I did, one of them would be hurt, and that kills me inside. I don't know how to stop loving Michael. I don't think it's possible."

"In our work, we like to say, 'what fires together, wires together.' Usually, we mean our brain likes to do what it has always done. It's hard to break old habits, especially those charged with strong emotion."

My nose scrunches up, not sure why Dr. LM has shifted the conversation. I'm fascinated by the implications that neuroscience has in psychotherapy. Learning how the brain functions and what that means for behavioral health feels empowering.

"Well," Dr. LM continues, "those who experience shared trauma, bond in a way we are just beginning to understand. It's one of those things that we know happens, even if we don't know why. You and Michael share the trauma of what happened to both of you in high school. The choices you made that led to the affair in 2004 demonstrate that you share a connection, much deeper than love. I would describe it as more instinctive and primal, and not entirely healthy. It's like your brain is hard-wired to respond to Michael in a specific way, no matter the consequences. It's similar to how soldiers behave toward those with whom they experienced combat with."

"So, like war veterans, I am willing to go to any extent to protect Michael?"

"Not only protect. It's much more than that."

"Are you saying I would go to any extent to meet his needs and desires despite what that means for myself and everyone else around me?" I ask.

Dr. LM nods. "Almost like you feel overwhelmingly compelled."

"Is that why I still can't seem to be completely honest with Mason about what happened? Because I'm still trying to protect my relationship with Michael?" I sit back, grateful for the comprehension, but disgusted by my devotion to a man I don't want to love.

Dr. LM gives me a full smile for the first time this session, my reward for working toward a paradigm shift. "It seems odd, doesn't it, and yet we know that trauma often changes the way we think, feel, and behave. What happened in 2004 was strongly influenced by the unresolved trauma from your high school experience. Does that make sense?"

"Yes, I think so. I need some time to chew on and digest all of this information. It's easy for me to pass blame to my father for the affair, which isn't helpful, even if he's responsible for most of the trauma I experienced in high school."

"It's easy to blame someone else and avoid reality when we are ashamed of ourselves," Dr. LM says, apparently reading my mind. "Your homework this week is to study up on trauma bonds. I want you to identify how your thoughts, feelings, and behaviors are influenced differently with Michael than with other people in your life whom you love and who love you in return."

TUTU SHIRT

ARIZONA/TEXAS
SPRING 2018

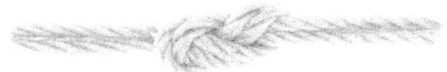

37 YEARS OLD

"Mom, will the airplane crash?" The concern in nine-year-old Kaydee's voice is unmistakable. Our oldest daughter and fourth child, Kaydee, got Mason's hazel eyes and large smile. Other than that, she is the spitting image of me, right down to her tendency to be outspoken and anxious.

"Airplanes don't crash very often, Sweet Girl." I reach toward her to give her a reassuring hug, and in true Kaydee fashion, she leans away from me with an impish grin and fake scowl. She knows what she wants and embraces "my body, my choice" with sass and exuberance.

It's family tradition for the kids to spend a week with my parents around their eighth birthday. Kaydee was excited for her turn to have a week alone with Grandma and Papa Lee. She was even more excited that

I was letting her miss a week of school to go at a time that worked best for Grandma's work schedule. Due to military moves and Brigg's hospitalizations, we were behind on Kaydee's visit. Secretly, I was grateful. My Dad treated girls differently than boys, which had become more and more noticeable the older Kaydee got when my parents visited us.

Eric's smart-ass comments earned him a laugh from Papa; Kaydee's earned her a scolding. The only reason I am comfortable with her going is because my Mom, who is pretty good at keeping the peace, is taking a week off work and has a plan to keep everyone entertained. Kaydee is anxious about the plane ride, but I am anxious about the visit itself. Kaydee will be the first girl to go. My gut aches with nerves, which I ignore by keeping overly busy, but my family notices when I snap for the smallest offenses.

Kaydee and I have been attempting to pack her suitcase for hours. Kaydee does nothing fast. She is meticulous and intentional in her choices, unless she's uninterested, then she'll do the bare minimum (if that) and move onto another task.

"Kaydee, I love your Tutu shirt, too, but it's very hot in Arizona where Grandma lives. The long sleeves and extra fabric might be uncomfortable for you."

"I don't care. It's my favorite shirt, and I'm going to wear it with my favorite sparkly pants."

Her spastic fashion sense is another thing she inherited from her father. She loves bright colors and shiny, sparkling bling.

"Okay, please bring at least one short sleeve shirt and shorts, just in case."

"No! If I'm hot, I'll wear my swimsuit and jump into Papa's pool."

"Kaydee, it's not even April yet. The pool will probably be too cold."

"Then it's not too hot for my Tutu shirt and sparkly pants."

I release a sigh of frustration. Learning to pick my battles with Brigg is coming in handy with Kaydee, as well.

"How's it going in here?" Mason asks.

"She's all packed up, finally."

"Mom didn't want me to wear my Tutu shirt because I might be too hot, but I'm so gorgeous, it will just match my face."

Mason laughs.

"She's more determined than I ever was," I whisper so that only Mason can hear and pull the suitcase behind me into the hallway.

He grabs my wrist and mouths, "thank you." He leans in toward my ear and whispers, "You are just as determined. Thank you for encouraging her to speak out. She will never know what it is like to be silenced the way you were. Thank you for letting her use her voice."

I fight back tears and snippets of memories that I've been trying to avoid. Between my flourishing counseling practice and Brigg's worsening symptoms, I'm afraid to cry. I encourage my clients to cry and "lean into" their emotional responses in order to complete the emotional cycle, and yet I can't seem to follow my own counsel.

I'm not the first, nor will I be the last person who ends up in the counseling profession, searching for answers to their own dysfunction. I've become pretty good at separating my own life from that of my clients, and my clients appear to be improving, which makes avoiding my own issues easier. I can't seem to heal myself, so I help others heal.

I'm also too busy to see a counselor. Besides, I already know what they would say to me. They'd remind me to practice self-care, eat well, exercise, and take up yoga. I'm too familiar with all the treatment modalities to let my guard down in session. The last two times I sought counseling, I ended up providing them with resources for continued education. So much for countertransference. Not that it was entirely their fault. I have a hard time being vulnerable when my goal is to be the smartest counselor in the room, which I often was. At least book smart, that is.

I drive Kaydee to Austin, trying to tune out the Disney songs that are blasting through the car. The girl thrives in chaos. Despite not being able to spell or read very well, she mastered the Pandora App on my iPhone and hijacked all my stations to play Disney music. Once at the airport, I get my escort gate pass, and we head to the terminal. I can't tell if she's more excited or more nervous.

"What's that?" She points at the large display of arrivals/departures. Before I can answer she points at something else and asks, "What's that?" And again, I only get a few words into an answer before she asks yet another question. This goes on until we reach her departure gate, at which point she asks for my phone and disappears into games. I zone out. The bone-deep exhaustion is really starting to wear on me.

The boarding announcement pulls me from my thoughts.

"The plane is ready for you. Phone time is over," I coax.

We approach the desk where a flight attendant is waiting for the unaccompanied minor travelers to gather around. Kaydee is so excited that the flight attendant is talking to *her* instead of to me that she forgets to say goodbye and skips down the sky bridge.

I sigh, resigned to the fact that it's too late to change my mind. "You're being silly," I continually scold myself. "Hundreds of kids spend a week away from home with their grandparents. She is going to love this." I can't get my mind to quiet. The dissonance is obvious, despite my inability to acknowledge that's what it is.

I didn't feel like I could justify stopping this visit. How am I supposed to tell my Dad that I don't trust him with his own granddaughter? He's never overtly said or done anything hurtful, and Kaydee has been waiting for her chance ever since Hayden went four years ago. I'm confident he won't sexually abuse her… his paranoia about being falsely accused ensures he'll never even be alone with her. Still, I feel like I've swallowed a hot coal. The anxiety aggravates my acid reflux.

I pull my phone out. Kaydee left me with 8% battery. "She's boarded," I text my Mom.

A few hours later Mom texts back, "I've got her."

"Have a fun week with my daughter," I respond, then to my surprise, tears begin to pour down my face. I hate crying, and it usually catches me off guard. I feel like a complete wreck; the words, "people cry when they are weak," play on repeat in my head even though I know better.

"Abi! We are going to be late for school. Let's go!" I inhale deeply, trying to keep my voice calm. Mason and I were thrilled when we got the phone call four years ago to come to a hospital in Katy, Texas, to meet our baby girl. Her chubby mocha cheeks and dark curly hair had melted my heart at first sight, and she instantly became a mama's girl.

The morning routine is plagued with lost shoes and tantrums. Even at four years old, she is textbook for Attention Deficit Hyperactivity Disorder (ADHD), which isn't surprising since she was born addicted to drugs and has mild microcephaly. Unfortunately, she's still too young for the medications that will help with ADHD, so we muscle through, just like we do every day. I exhale very slowly, counting to six and repeating my morning mantra, *her teacher will take over soon, her teacher will take over soon.*

I'm feeling more rushed than usual this morning, despite the fact that things have gone relatively well. I am attributing my anxiety to the fact that Kaydee will be arriving home late morning. So far, her visit seems to have gone smoothly, but I can't shake the feeling that shit is about to hit the fan.

"I like being late because then I get to go to the office and get a paper to give to my teacher, and she says, 'Thank you, Abi,' and I get to hug her in front of my class."

Abi's high-pitched voice distracts me from my nerves. She is struggling to get her backpack on because she has threaded her arm through the wrong strap. I remove the backpack, straighten the straps, then hold it back out to her.

"You should run for president when you grow up," I say as I pull her other arm through the other strap and adjust the bag to perch comfortably on her tiny frame. "Let's go," I demand, stepping behind her and firmly pushing against the outer pocket of her backpack. Heaven forbid I touch her body while nudging her forward. She could argue a point just for the sake of arguing, but touching her unexpectedly would send her into an overstimulation meltdown. She hasn't been formally diagnosed, but I suspect she has autism.

As usual, Abi resists the forward pressure between her shoulder blades, then gives in. "But I want a secret note to give to my teacher," she protests.

"I'll write one for you in the drop-off lane. Let's go."

I ignore the tension building as the kids push each other out the front door and scramble over one another into the van just to argue about which seat belt buckle goes to which seat.

I glance down at my chiming phone to see Mom's text: "She's boarded." I have a full day of clients, so Mason will pick Kaydee up from the airport after finishing his overnight call shift. "Hayden, please separate Landon and Abi before they kill each other back there."

"They aren't next to each other," Hayden calls back.

"Can you figure something out?"

"I'll try," he says, sounding less than confident.

Abi is like Brigg 2.0 except that few of the interventions that worked for Brigg were effective with her. Once again, I had been knocked off my self-proclaimed "expert parent" pedestal. Reduced to feeling like a complete failure as a mom was familiar territory for me. The expectation that the "alphabet soup" credentials at the end of my name somehow made me a better parent was being dashed to pieces just as my career in being paid for such expertise was beginning to really take off. I've come to embrace the fact that the more I learn, the more I realize how much I don't know.

On top of everything else, I had just been released from my "calling" as Young Women's president in our ward so that Mason could serve as the bishop, and almost immediately I was called to teach seminary again. Between the Army, church callings, college graduation, and stepping out of the stay-at-home mom gig and into my new career, I was definitely trying to function in too many roles to be truly successful in any of them. At Walden University, I'd learned that mental health professionals struggle with burnout earlier in their career than in other helping professions. I'm pretty sure I was burned out before I started my graduate program. Resting wasn't part of my skill set.

"Abi, stop touching me!" Landon's cries carry us into the drop-off loop at the side of Meadows Elementary School on Fort Hood.

"Abi, unbuckle and come up here so I can give you a secret note for Ms. Humphreys." I write "secret note from Abi" on lined paper and hand it to her. "Remember, go straight to your classroom and give that to Ms. Humphreys so that it doesn't get lost."

"Okay, Mama, I love you," she says, giving me a quick kiss on the cheek.

My first appointment isn't until 10 a.m., so I head home in order to catch up on some chores before starting my day at my practice.

Just as I turn right onto the main road, my Mom calls.

"Hey, Mom. How did Kaydee do?"

"I need to talk to you about something that happened. Is now a good time?" Mom's voice is shaky, and I brace myself.

"What's up?" I ask, trying to sound optimistic.

"Well…" She hesitates. I stay quiet. Usually, I'm not very good with silence, but I'm learning to recognize the value of therapeutic silence, especially when something difficult is about to be shared.

I hear Mom's sigh in my speaker. "Well, yesterday, Dad and I had planned to take Kaydee to the aquarium in Phoenix. Kaydee wore a long-sleeve dress with tulle sewn around the bottom seam. She paired that with her glittered sweatpants."

"Mmm-hmm," I respond.

"Well, I told her to change because she would be too hot, and she said she was comfortable. I explained that people might look at her funny because her outfit was silly…" her voice trails off.

I can feel the hot exhalation from my nose on my upper lip, one of my "tells" that I'm feeling defensive. I swallow hard to combat the flash of anger.

"It's one of her favorite outfits, she loves it," I reply. "She's definitely got Westbrook genes in her with all her crazy outfit combinations." I fake a chuckle, trying to ease the building tension.

"Yes, well, she told me she didn't care if people stare at her, and she promised not to complain that she was hot, so I conceded."

I'm pleasantly surprised and grateful.

"When Dad saw her," Mom continues, and the pace of her speech increases, "he told her she needed to change her clothing because her outfit was not appropriate for public. She told him she wears the outfit all the time in public. He told her that people would get the wrong idea, and that she was only wearing the outfit to get attention. She told him she didn't care what other people think."

My heart fills with pride at Kaydee's self-confidence and ability to stand up for herself. I'm also aggravated that Dad would pull his "people will get the wrong idea" bullshit.

"Well," Mom's words come faster, "Dad told Kaydee that he would not go to the aquarium if Kaydee decided she was going to wear that outfit. I stepped in then and told him the tickets had already been paid for and to just let it go, but he said he wasn't going to come with us unless Kaydee changed her clothes. Kaydee said that she was okay with that, so Dad stayed home."

I didn't realize I was holding my breath until I released it.

"I'm glad you and Kaydee still went. How was it?"

"We had fun. Most people who stared at her outfit were smiling, and lots of people told her she was very pretty in her Tutu shirt. She was very polite, not at all prideful with all the compliments, and she didn't complain about being hot. We enjoyed exploring, and then we went out for ice cream on the way home."

"Thanks, Mom. I appreciate your sticking up for her."

"Well, things were good until we got home. Dad was furious with her. He must have sat at home stewing about their conversation the entire time we were gone, because as soon as we walked in the door, he started to lecture her. He told her it was wrong to wear things that would get men to look at her or draw attention to herself. He told her she was a rude little girl. He told her it would be her fault if someone kidnapped her, made fun of her, or hurt her. Oh, Sarah, it went on for over an hour. He just wouldn't stop. When she didn't cow to him, he started yelling at her. It was awful."

A backdraft of fury hits me. My head is throbbing from my clenched jaw.

"He yelled at her for over an hour? What did you do?"

"Sarah, I'm so sorry. I just froze. Kaydee was so brave. She stood up for herself. She stayed so calm for most of the conversation. She has so much confidence… she reminds me of you in that way."

"What made him stop?" It's hard to swallow. I can feel my pulse in my fingertips. Gratefully I'm home. I shift the van into park and lean back.

"I did," Mom answers. "After ninety minutes or so, Kaydee broke down and started to cry. Once she started to cry, I told Dave he had said enough. He said he had a few more things to say, so I stood between him and her and said, 'No you don't, you are finished.' Then he stopped. Sarah, he's still furious. He refused to drive with us to the airport this morning. He said he didn't want to be around a brat like her. Kaydee told him that was okay with her because she didn't want to be around someone who was so mean over a shirt."

I can't focus. I recognize the signs of a flashback fighting to gain space in my brain. I have relived the May after my 16th birthday many times a day. The frequency had eased up in the past, with therapy, but not for very long. "Thank you for telling me."

"Are you mad at me, Sarah?"

I mumble, "I'll let you know when she lands," as I watch my trembling hand reach up to disconnect the call.

I never should have let her go.

Why did I let her talk me into it?

I blink several times, trying to clear my vision and get the images out of my head.

Dad's face inches from mine.

His spittle hitting my cheek.

He pushes me; I fall backward.

I hit the metal bed frame that jutted out past the box spring, pain exploding into my back.

Fire.

Throwing all of my journals into the fire.

The picture of Johnny kissing me melting into the flames that consume what is left of my dignity.

I lock my fingers into the old-fashion choir position and pull, creating opposing pressure meant to increase my blood pressure. It's no use. I have to escape the confinement of the van. I open the door to our duplex and step into the entry hall. I put my hand on the wall to help me feel balanced then ease my body to the floor. I lay flat on my back and begin to inhale and exhale deeply. It's not working.

I roll to my side and vomit onto my freshly washed hair.

AUTHOR'S NOTE

It's excruciating to recognize that I ignored my body's signaling and sent my daughter for a "fun" visit against my better judgment. The body shaming and emotionally abusive lecture was the first overtly offensive incident between my father and one of my daughters. My mother's lack of protection compounded the serious nature of this interaction.

Unfortunately, at that time in my life, I didn't have the capacity to go "Mama Bear" on my parents. I had spent the first decade of my marriage trying to be good enough for their approval, which I never received. Sometime around the birth of Kaydee, I had healed enough to no longer need it; however, I was not yet in a place to stand up to either of them, specifically to my father.

The Tutu shirt incident triggered my own trauma, and I melted into a flashback that negatively impacted my ability to function normally for several months. Once I got my bearings, I determined I would not allow any of my other children to get their "special week" with my parents. I didn't tell them that. I wasn't ready to make that boundary known. My plan was to make excuses to avoid future encounters. I reflect back on those earlier times and feel deep shame for placing my children in his occasionally unsupervised care, knowing what type of monster lived deep inside of him.

After this incident, I increased my protection of my children against my parents, in that I stopped allowing unsupervised interactions. Unfortunately, that wasn't enough to keep them safe, and approximately one year after the Tutu shirt fiasco, another event unleashed my inner Mama Bear, and I finally broke the cycle of abuse out loud.

BETTER HELP, HELPS

KILLEEN, TEXAS 2018

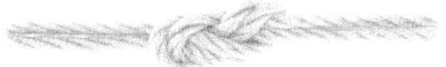

37 YEARS OLD

"You seem more anxious than normal." Mason's observation is accurate. Reaching across the dinner table for the salt, I pretend not to hear it.

It's been more than a decade since Michael and I lived down the street from each other. I hadn't heard from him in all that time; I figured he'd moved on. Three years ago, in a moment of loneliness, I had Facebook stalked him. He looked happy with his second wife, and Savannah was grown up. The pictures of his blended family showed they had seven children, one more than ours. I ended up sending him an apology, just to make myself feel better and regretted it as soon as I hit *send*. It had gone unanswered until today.

Thirteen years of silence, and then today's message, which could only be described as a small book. The desperation of his message concerned me so much that I contacted his younger brother, Luke, to check on him; I was worried Michael was suicidal again.

"Sarah..." Mason's firm voice is hard to ignore.

"I can't stop thinking about the message I received from Michael. It's got me rattled."

"It was cryptically weird, that's for sure," Mason admits.

"He was probably drunk," I reason. "He tends to write poetically like that, but this didn't make any sense. It's never been this difficult for me to extrapolate. It was poetic nonsense." I'm disappointed to find Michael still mired in unhappiness.

"Does he usually call you by your first and middle name?" Mason asks.

Sarah Elizabeth, it was never you, it could never be you. Don't ever think that.

Think what, exactly?

"That was a first," I answer Mason.

The fact that Mason can talk about this without any observable discomfort soothes my nerves.

"What did Luke say?"

"Not much. He thanked me, and we hung up. A few hours later, he texted me saying their mom had gone over to Michael's home, and he denied sending me any message at all. At least he's alive." I clear my throat, wanting to be upfront with my husband. "Luke texted me again, wanting proof that Michael had actually contacted me. I sent him screenshots. He wrote back and asked me why I felt the message was suicidal." It was kind of offensive. I reached out to try and help, and Luke all but accused me of lying.

"I told Luke I was a licensed professional counselor and sent him a ten-point analysis of Michael's message, explaining why I felt his message was a bid for help. Michael was showing classic red flags in the message with statements like 'I can't live without you in my life' and 'I have no place else to go in this darkness.'"

"Did you tell Luke you didn't want to be dragged into another situation with Michael?" Mason's voice is hesitant.

"I told him that I hadn't seen or heard from Michael since the affair in 2004 and that I don't have the energy to deal with the emotional fallout of being involved in Michael's life. I told him I wanted to step back. He got it. He said he's exhausted by Michael's needs, too. Apparently, Michael's second wife is a drug addict and abused his children. Sounds like he has addiction issues, too..." I control my tone, aware of how carefully Mason is observing me right now.

"You sound like you feel guilty for that," Mason says sharply. Neither one of us is touching our food anymore.

I huff, "I am responsible for *some* of his trauma. The research I've read indicates that lack of secure emotional attachments is the primary predictor of addiction."

"I thought addiction was about seeking out the next high to avoid withdrawal."

I clench my jaw, irritated that I have to slow down my thoughts in order to explain the addiction relationship to Mason. "I'd say seeking the high is more a symptom of addiction than the cause of it. Research demonstrates untreated trauma and abuse comes from a lack of, or damage to, primary attachments. The addictive behaviors also have a negative impact on current primary attachments, or any relationship for that matter."

"You are so hot when you talk clinical on date night."

I shoot Mason an exasperated scowl, and he chuckles.

"If Michael's addiction is because he doesn't have healthy attachments to his parents, what does that have to do with you?"

"'Primary attachment' doesn't just mean your parents. Maybe I should have said significant attachments, so it includes parents, close friends, intimate partners, siblings, etc... You and I are each other's significant attachments. And it doesn't have to be a person. The church is a significant attachment for you. Can you imagine what you'd go through if your church community shunned you or labeled you an apostate? It's common for people who go through that to struggle with addiction."

Mason looks uncomfortable. This dispute has become a common theme in our intellectual conversations about the church. Mason's default is to defend the church's position. "Don't you think some of those people struggle with addiction because the Holy Ghost has left them for sinning?"

"Are you serious, Mason? That's just ignorant. Give me one example, one, where Jesus abandoned someone in pain or struggle." My volume raises. I've been analyzing Michael's message all day.

"Wow, ignorant?" Mason's brow furrows, as he drums his thumb against the table. He's not getting it, and the more frustrated I get, the more I lose him.

"Look, sorry if I offended you," I soften. "Let me ask you a question. Do active members of the church struggle with addiction?"

"Well… of course, some do. What does that have to do with anything?"

"So, if an active member in good standing struggles with addiction and an 'apostate' struggles with addiction, which one has the Holy Ghost abandoned? How does walking away from the church *cause* addiction?"

"I dunno. The scriptures teach that God cannot look upon sin with the least degree of allowance. The Holy Ghost departs from us when we turn our backs on the church."

"That's a bunch of bullshit, a fear tactic the church uses to keep people *in*. How many of the people you've seen leave the church end up abusing alcohol? How many become addicts? Use and abuse look *very* different. To be completely honest, I see a much higher prevalence of addictive behaviors within orthodox members than I do in those who leave the church."

"We've kind of veered off topic here. What does this have to do with your feeling guilty about Michael's addiction?"

"I was a significant attachment in Michael's life, both in high school and in 2004. Both times that attachment was abruptly severed, increasing the risk for addictive behaviors. For him, substances; for me... overspending." I sit back in my booth and continue to pick at my food.

Mason sighs, "I think you need to go talk to someone, someone who can handle counseling a counselor."

I huff at Mason's observation. "You're probably right, and yes, it's much harder to counsel a counselor. Even for me. Especially with your deployment right around the corner. Why is it that both times Michael and I have made contact, you deploy?"

"It terrifies me, Sarah. I'd feel much better if you didn't engage with him while I'm gone."

"I'm too busy with work to engage with him, but I have a professional obligation to make sure he gets connected to services in his area for his suicidal ideation. I will keep you in the loop. I promise."

"I still don't like it."

Six months without Mason has flown by. In the time he was gone, I opened my private practice, adopted our youngest son, Tyler, who was almost three at the time, and did everything in my power to maintain my sanity while raising seven children. Mason was too busy serving as bishop from overseas to engage with the family consistently anyway. I hardly noticed how little Mason and I talked during his deployment… probably because I was too busy catching up with Michael.

Once life calmed down after Michael's initial crazy, mile-long message sent in a drunken haze, I heard from him again. I couldn't help but take pity on him. His first wife, Megan, had passed away in 2010 from breast cancer. He told me she passed just a year after they had finally worked through their marital struggles due to our affair in 2004. He became a single father of three with no real family support close by due to his military service.

He'd explained that the Army gave him a compassionate reassignment to Sierra Vista in Arizona, but that still wasn't close enough to his family to manage the day-to-day stuff and continue his career. Four months later, he remarried, and it had been a disaster.

A whiff of gasoline from the lawn mower stings the back of my throat as Mason opens the sliding glass door and passes me on his way to the living room where the toddlers' protests continue.

"You're stupid. Ouch! Mom-m-m-m," Landon wails.

"No, Abi," Mason raises his voice over Landon's screaming.

Landon and Abi are still adjusting to Tyler, who loves to play hard and hide under tables. The three of them epitomize *Love and War.* Either they are playing beautifully or torturing each other. The extremes in the dynamics of their free time are exhausting.

My conversations with Michael had been strictly platonic, and I had told Mason I was providing Michael with resources to help him get sober again. So it's not like I hid the communication, but I didn't exactly tell Mason about our renewed friendship. Mason was rarely available for meaningful conversation, unless it was church related, versus Michael who seemed to devour every moment I was able to give. It had felt good to be the priority in someone's life.

"I want Mom," Landon demands curtly.

"Mom is covered in salmonella," Mason counters.

I smile.

Mason distracts them with story time, which he reads them from the last word to the first word at breakneck speed. The kids find it hilarious.

I cut the bag of frozen broccoli open and notice my right hand is tremoring. I shake it out and stretch my neck by leaning my head side to side. After dinner, I have my second telehealth appointment with my new counselor, Luis, from Better Help.

I'm so busy in my own counseling practice that I never have time for me until after the kids go to bed. Besides, I feel uncomfortable sharing my past with a local counselor when I'm working so hard to build a strong network of clinicians for patient referrals and professional consultations. Better Help feels like a safe option for therapy for myself since my counselor doesn't practice anywhere near Killeen. The evening appointment availability and autonomy of the digital experience fits my hectic life and my budget.

The first session was pretty normal. Luis asked me all the usual questions. I explained the strained relationship dynamics with my parents and sent him the file of nasty emails my father and I had exchanged so that Luis could see for himself, without my bias of how toxic my family of origin is. While my relationship with Dad wasn't the focus of our sessions, I felt like the reference point was a good place to start, considering I was still struggling with symptoms of c-PTSD; however, I *was* incredibly nervous about his assessment of the rekindled friendship that Michael and I had developed while Mason was deployed.

I had kept my promise to Mason. While he was away, I communicated with Michael only through Facebook Messenger. I assumed the role of "educated friend" and advised Michael on how to seek mental health care in his community. I validated his struggles with his wife, Isabel, and provided accountability for his alcohol consumption. I was extremely careful not to cross into "counselor mode," but I also wasn't his Alcoholics Anonymous sponsor, as I had set and honored strong boundaries that limited his contact with me. I sent him a copy of *Unbroken Brain: A Revolutionary New Way of Understanding Addiction* by Maia Szalavitz, which he claimed had helped him understand himself in a new way.

I'm proud of myself for keeping Mason in the loop every step of the way this time like he had asked, and for making sure things were platonic with Michael. I know Mason was nervous, but like always, he respected my right to make my own choices; I was relieved when he said he felt like my help was appropriate and healing for both Michael and me.

Despite Mason's approval, I was concerned that Luis would see through my firm exterior to the hidden desire for more intimacy than I was allowing with Michael. I may have behaved well but couldn't shake how much love and desire for physical intimacy was still there.

Mason joins me in the kitchen. "Do you need any help, sweetheart?" He always kisses the back of my neck when I'm cooking.

"Nope."

"How are you feeling about your appointment tonight?"

I sigh. "The delay from Luis's poor internet connection is something I'm going to have to get used to."

"That's not a feeling. That's an analysis."

I laugh. "Are you shrinking me?" That's what the kids ask when they feel like I'm counseling them instead of parenting them.

"I've learned from the best." He waits for me to answer his question about my feelings.

"I feel nervous and afraid of being exposed."

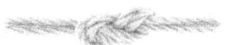

An hour later, I settle back and listen to Mason cleaning up after dinner and our children playing in the cul-de-sac with the neighbor kids while I wait for Luis to join our meeting on the Better Help App. I open the Facebook Messenger App and scroll through the recent conversation I had with Michael. As I do, I notice that the tremor in my hand is more pronounced, shaking my iPhone.

When Luis appears on my screen, my face moves up to a smaller box. It's interesting to be able to see both my and Luis's non-verbal expressions at the same time.

When the audio catches up, I hear Luis's deep bass voice ask, "Before we get started, do you have any questions from last week?"

"Were you able to get through all those emails?" I ask. I'm eager to hear Luis's professional assessment.

"I'm about two-thirds of the way through them." He shakes his head. "You weren't kidding when you said it was intense."

"What are your thoughts so far?"

"Well," he leans closer to the camera, his face growing larger on my small phone, "you were very honest and concise in expressing your feelings. I observed your Dad's responses and agree with you. He appears emotionally abusive."

"In what way?" I'm cataloging whatever Luis says to share with Mason, later.

"I will answer that, but also, you asked me to call you out on switching to counselor mode. I feel like 'in what way?' is a good question, but also borders on being a 'counselor question.' Which role do you feel you are in right now?"

"Mostly curious." I want to make sure that I didn't switch into a place of manipulation or abuse in my responses to him. "I'm asking as a client without putting up my counselor resistance."

"I agree." He backs away from the camera. I watch him for a few seconds, he appears to be searching for the right words. "September 26, 2018, was pretty to the point; I'm talking about the email you sent him. It was gentle, loving, but also clear. His reaction was arrogant, self-righteous, and accusatory. After that, your emails are longer, more emotional, like you're trying to force him to reconsider the past from your perspective, or at the very least, in a more honest light."

I try to consider what Luis has said without being defensive. "So, you think that my initial contact was fine, but later I became a little manipulative?"

"No, not necessarily manipulative. I understand why you try, Sarah, but you floodlighted him. There were too many things at once. I think it overwhelmed him and forced him into a fight or flight response, so he defended himself. He defended himself by being offensive, by justifying, reframing, accusing, finger-pointing, lying, romanticizing... he flits from one defense mechanism to another as desperate people tend to do."

I'm quiet for a minute, trying to digest what Luis has said and use it to self-evaluate. "Yeah, it was too much for him. The dam broke, and it all came out in a rush. I don't know if I could have done it differently in the moment, but I agree, the sheer amount of issues I addressed at once was traumatizing for him, and his survival brain intensified his toxic responses."

"This being an email exchange, with days between responses and time for him to process, it might have been reasonable for you to expect a more tempered response, but the reaction was fierce, nevertheless. You kept trying after that... same effort, same results. Yes, it's too much info. But before it was too much info, you made very reasonable and gentle efforts to bridge the gap in that September email. I'm really impressed by your ability to be accountable for your role in the toxic family dynamics with your parents."

"Thank you, I appreciate the compliment." I shift uncomfortably, trying not to let my pride seep in and take over my focus. "Being able to own my part is the result of a lot of hard work. It helps that I came prepared to be held accountable. I'm not certain I would do as well in the heat of the moment."

"True insight for all humankind. Preparing oneself to address the emotion first and be accountable is something we all struggle with."

I nod. "I'm tempted to get all geeky about the research supporting your statement, so we need to shift gears."

"Good recognition of counselor mode. No geeks allowed. Are you ready to talk more about your prolonged feelings of sorrow regarding your relationship with your high school sweetheart? What is his name again?"

I feel like I have a good enough handle on my anxiety to talk about this now. I take a deep breath, envisioning myself filling with focused energy and confidence. It helps. "His name is Michael, and sure, that's a good shift for me."

I pause and take a deep breath in then blow out slowly through my mouth to soothe my survival brain. I repeat this exercise two more times.

"I feel guilty for the pain I caused his first wife, Megan, and subsequently his three children. While I know their relationship was already strained, the affair didn't help. Michael told me that a year before her cancer diagnosis, they had finally gotten to a good place. I'm happy they were able to work through the mess we caused but can't shake the feeling that if I had never gone back to the hospital on that day, they would have had more happy years before she passed away."

Luis nods and says nothing, waiting for me to continue.

"All three of his children struggle, which makes sense. Their mother passed when they were so young, and Isabel, their stepmom, was horrifically abusive. I know that the added intensity of Megan and Michael's struggles because of me will have had an impact on their development and thus, their current day functioning. I hold some responsibility for that, and it's starting to consume me. My complex PTSD is flaring up again." I remember seeing Savanah for the first time, playing out front while her daddy watered the lawn. Would her life have been any different if I'd never contacted him?

"Do you feel the same guilt toward your own family?"

"Only a little. After I 'confessed my sins' to the bishop, Mason felt like nothing more needed to be said and we moved on, hardly talking about Michael again. After we adopted Brigg, I became so absorbed by his special needs that any residual trauma from the affair just slipped into the background. Mason and I came together stronger after his deployment to Iraq. He and I do 'hard' really well together." I shift into a more comfortable position; I can faintly hear the kids playing happily outside.

"What I'm hearing you say is that you don't feel like the strain of the affair lasted very long in 2004 due to being absorbed by Brigg's medical care. Is that accurate?" Luis leans closer to his phone, making his forehead look huge.

"Yes, but more than Brigg's care. I was a single mama, constantly afraid to get *that* knock on my door. I was stressed for many reasons. I feel like Mason's deployment affected Eric the way it affects most toddlers his age. He wondered when Daddy would be home from work, and I threw myself into being his mother and father. Six weeks into Mason's deployment, Eric got a new brother, whom he loved. Eric was so excited to give Brigg to his daddy so they could share…" My voice trails off, and I smile at the memory of Eric telling newborn Brigg how awesome Mason was.

"Eric would try to comfort Brigg's prolonged crying spells by telling him not to worry, he would have a daddy soon. I think, in a way, Eric worked out the trauma of Mason being gone by repeating to Brigg the things I said to Eric."

"You feel Eric had healthy supports and outlets to work through his responses to the challenges in your home."

I nod.

"That makes sense. Do you think Megan and Michael were able to provide those same types of supports for their children?"

"The way Michael describes it, they were volatile with lots of yelling and arguing. He said Megan needed to control everything in a way that bordered on abuse. To be honest, I have no idea. I'm not responsible for how they chose to treat each other. I just wish I could apologize to Megan, truly apologize. I want her to know that all these years later, I still feel so much pain for causing her such anguish. I want her to know my sorrow for my actions is genuine. But it's too late. Even if she was alive, I'm not sure it'd be helpful."

"You are Mormon, correct?" It's a question that I never have an easy time answering.

"Sort of, I mean I attend the Mormon Church with my family each Sunday. I teach the adult Sunday School class, but my heart isn't in it anymore. I'd say, I'm Mormon with a lot of caution tape wrapped around me. Or maybe I wrap that tape around the church. Either way, I believe in many of their teachings, but the culture is toxic, and I'm still working out how that all works for me. Why?"

"Do you believe in prayer?"

"I don't pray in the formal manner taught by the LDS Church—more a meditative style of prayer. I speak out loud to God while I'm driving a lot."

"Do you think Megan can hear you when you do that?"

I take a sharp breath in. I've never thought of it that way. "The church teaches that only God can hear our thoughts, but angels and demons alike can hear anything I speak out loud."

"Have you thought about voicing your apology out loud in a similar way to how you pray? Honoring our spirituality can be very effective at healing old wounds."

"I haven't." I'm intrigued by the suggestion.

"Do you think it would be healing for you? That Megan would hear and possibly accept your apology?" A flicker of hope lightens the heaviness of guilt.

I do believe that I can speak out loud to those who have passed before me, and that they will hear me. I've read about how people who have near-death experiences report feeling overwhelming love from a source I identify as God or Jesus. I wonder if Megan would be able to understand the depth of my emotions for what I have done if I speak my apology out loud. The warmth of hope deepens, and I feel as if God approves this method.

"I will try," I promise.

My session with Luis ends, and I walk to my room. I add thoughts of what I want to say in this prayer in the notebook that sits on my night-stand. A few days later, I cancel my appointments for the day and go for a long drive by myself. It only takes me a few minutes to tell Megan what I need to say. A spiritual high engulfs me as love descends upon me from heaven. I hear a whispered voice, "Give my children all the love you can from afar." I promise that I will, and for the first time since 2004, I forgive myself for sleeping with Megan's husband.

AUTHOR'S NOTE

I cannot even count how many times during my master's program we were taught that in order to preserve our ability to feel compassion for our patients and in order to prevent burnout, counselors should seek counseling for our own well-being. We were advised of the importance to talk to someone outside the situation in order to experience clarity of thought and gain perspective. When I found myself in need of counseling, I was afraid to let the other counseling professionals in my area know that I was struggling with a trauma bond that had the potential to destroy my relationship with my clients. I feared it would hurt my reputation as a practitioner. I utilized an online platform for therapy for a variety of reasons, not the least of which was to safeguard my privacy and protect my reputation.

FORT HOOD, TEXAS

NOVEMBER 2018

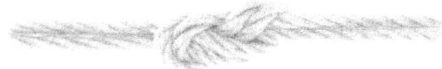

37 YEARS OLD

"What are you doing?" Mason asks as he saunters into the living room.

I drop the Kristen Hannah book that I'd just started reading into my lap. He's leaving me alone with the kids most of the weekend for his bishop duties, which makes me boil. Not only did he have to provide anesthesia to people with serious war injuries while in Afghanistan, the church thought it would be a great idea to keep him serving as the bishop of our ward. He had loved it, which irritated me because he was oblivious to the fact that he wasn't spending much quality time with our family.

"What do you think I am doing?"

"Reading the last chapter to find out what happens before you read the story. That's pathetic!" I know his teasing is good-natured, but it makes the simmer of anger grow.

"How is that any different from all the other good books I've read?" I turn the page and try to ignore him, content to pout that once again I haven't been consulted about or featured in his weekend plans.

"It's not. Don't you have any self-control?"

"Nope. If I read the first few chapters to know the plot then skip to the end, it makes it easier for me to put the book down when motherhood calls." I lift the book higher to avoid eye contact and ignore the sounds of children getting out of bed.

"Hey, Sarah. Can you please help me with breakfast this morning? I only have an hour before I have to go help the Batton family unload their U-Haul." I bristle when he says *have to*, as if he didn't volunteer for it.

"That's the same amount of time I have every weekday to get all seven kids up and out the door before I head to work. If I can do it, so can you." I don't even try to hide the apathy in my tone.

I feel like I've been hanging on for years, single parenting an ever-growing number of children while in graduate school and juggling part-time work as an intern, while the Army or the church got the best of Mason. Now that he actually has some free time for us, he's giving it to the Batton family or anyone else who asks for it, expecting me to hold down the fort alone and praising me for my righteousness in doing so, so he can fulfill his calling to the Lord. I'm done doing it alone.

I lift the book back up to my face and pretend to tune out the sounds of Kaydee trying to break up the noisy toddler wrestling match. Tyler's piercing scream and a loud thump ends our battle of the wills.

Mason sighs loudly and barks from the bottom of the stairwell, "Do I need to come up there, or can you two figure this one out on your own?" Like soldiers, the kids shut up and file down the stairs immediately.

"Do you want pancakes or waffles for breakfast?" Mason asks the kids. Like my mother, Mason doesn't believe in serving cold cereal for breakfast.

I roll my eyes. I survive the morning routine because of cold cereal.

"I want cereal," Abi demands.

"Too bad," Mason counters.

"I'm telling Mom you won't give me cold cereal for breakfast," Abi threatens.

"Go ahead, Abi. I don't have patience for your attitude this morning."

"Mom! Dad doesn't have my attitude!" Abi yells as she heads back upstairs looking for me.

"Mom is down here," Landon calls to her. "I want pancakes."

"You got it, buddy."

My stomach churns. I'm not a fan of pancakes, which Mason knows but never seems to consider when he's making breakfast.

Mom used to serve pancakes at least twice a week all the years I was growing up. Once I got married, I vowed to end the soggy, sticky bread breakfast. Unfortunately, Mason loves pancakes. For me, violent nausea induced by the smell of pancakes was a better pregnancy diagnostic tool than peeing on a stick. Through all three pregnancies, Mason would stand over me, asking through a mouth full of pancake, if I was okay while I retched bitter green bile into the kitchen sink. The pancake-stomach-turnover had become a permanent part of my existence since birthing Landon, the youngest of our biological children. Mason wasn't trying to be an asshole. It just didn't occur to him that banning pancakes for nine months was an option to manage my morning sickness. Obliviousness to anyone else's emotional needs is Mason's "character flaw."

491

"Mom," Abi's voice carries through our military base housing unit.

"I'm downstairs in the living room," I call back up to her, feeling slightly guilty about all the noise this early on a Saturday. The *Comanche II* Army housing development is one step up from a ghetto as far as I'm concerned. The duplexes are boxy, and the walls are paper thin.

"Daddy is making me eat pancakes, and I want cold cereal," Abi whines as she climbs into my lap.

"How about I snuggle you for a few minutes and then you go eat your pancakes. After breakfast we can go play at the park while Daddy helps the Batton family move in."

Distraction has become my go-to parenting intervention lately. I'm too overwhelmed for anything else, including the black mold issue growing in our bathroom that Fort Hood housing maintenance just keeps painting over.

Mason was "called" to be the bishop of our Killeen congregation six months before he got his orders to deploy to Afghanistan for Operation Enduring Freedom. He accepted the volunteer position (equivalent to a Catholic priest or Christian pastor) because declining isn't the "right" thing to do. Not that he would want to decline. Being called to be the bishop was a status symbol indicating an extra level of worthiness. Mason had hoped to be a bishop for several years. At least his hope came from a place of loving to serve others and not from a "holier than thou" attitude.

"Your family will be blessed by your sacrifice," the stake president had promised us both when Mason accepted the calling as bishop of the ward.

The stake president wasn't interested in "releasing" Mason when he went to war, claiming that the Lord had provided modern-day technology for situations such as these. Mason left for Afghanistan, and in true Mormon military ward fashion, he continued to lead the congregation through WhatsApp.

Mason loved being bishop, and he was a good bishop. I hated it. He was too busy helping other people's families to notice how much his own family needed him. He missed out when the kids celebrated successes and when they had struggles, even major struggles. Their support came mostly from me. I opened my counseling practice while he was gone, and business was thriving. Still, we were having financial problems due to the house we were renting out. When I expressed my concerns to him now that he was home from Afghanistan, he decided more service to others was the way to ensure security of resources. After all, the prophets had taught us that safety and security were to be found in obedience to the Lord's principles and that the more we gave to the church, the more our lives would be blessed. Frankly, I was burned out, and Mason was so emotionally disengaged that he was missing out on our lives.

"Sarah," Mason calls from the kitchen. "Tag, you're it. Can you wash Abi's hands? She keeps dipping her fingers in the syrup and then typing on the computer's keyboard."

Our game of "tag" had become code for your turn or I'm going to lose it on the child. We tagged out on Abi more often every day. She has ADHD, and at five years old, she's still too young for medication. At least, that's what the psychiatrist says.

He might change his opinion if he was the one responsible for making sure she stayed alive. I fold over the corner of the page to mark my place in my book and set it on the end table.

Miss Sticky Fingers is busy rapping the keyboard and screaming, "Buttons! I have to touch all the buttons!"

"How about we wash your hands and go to the park? I'll push you on the swings." Hopefully, she won't notice the resignation in my voice.

Making sure our parenting style is shame-free and nonviolent is getting harder the longer Mason is absent, physically and mentally. Numbness from burnout had pushed me into autopilot since right before the deployment. Even though Mason is home now, his mind and heart seem to be with the church. Is it too much to ask that our family come first for a change? He's more like my roommate than my partner. We're contributing to a shared household as two individuals rather than as one unit; we're supposed to be in this together.

I push the statistics of abuse and neglect created by single-parent homes out of my mind as I pin Abi between my body and the counter and let her play with the soap suds and running water. I haven't crossed into adding to those statistics, but I've been closer to it than I like to admit.

After breakfast, Mason takes the three oldest boys with him to help with the move so that they can practice their "priesthood duties," and I take the youngest four across the street to the community park behind the duplexes. I watch the kids run and play, wondering how my life would be different if I'd married a nonmember.

SO THAT'S WHY

JANUARY 2019

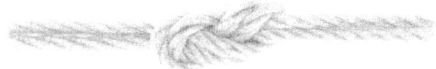

37 YEARS OLD

"Stop picking your brother's nose." I clench the muscles in my jaw.

"But his boogers are de-wish-us."

"Abi-*i-i-i*-i, that's so gross," Hayden gags in the backseat of my giant van.

Hayden reaches over the seat, grabbing her five-year-old hands and holds them gently above her head.

"Gotcha!" he says playfully. "Now you can't pick anybody's nose."

I make eye contact with him in the rearview mirror and mouth *thank you* as I pull into the half-moon drop-off area of the kid's school, ignoring the thick tuft of dark hair sticking up at the back of his head.

The teacher's aide slides our giant van door open. "Good morning, Westbrooks!"

Her bright voice is a welcomed sound indicating only one more school to go before I'll be kid-free. I never thought I'd still be dropping preschoolers off at 38. We adopted Tyler, our youngest, only six months ago. "Seven is the number of perfection, no more kids," has become my morning mantra.

Hayden climbs over the center console before we head to the middle school. As soon as I am kid-free, I dial Mom's number. It's been our routine for years. I talk, she half listens, and then we start our day. If I don't call her, I get anxious, feeling like I've done something dreadfully wrong. Lately, our conversations leave me frustrated and angry.

The time difference gives us about an hour every weekday morning to chat uninterrupted.

"Morning, Sarah. Did you survive?"

"Barely. Hayden has been really helpful at making sure the car ride is tolerable. I wish they could put Abi on medication for her ADHD. It'd make all our lives better."

"She is the busiest child I have ever experienced," Mom agrees with me.

"So, how did your counseling session go?"

Mom started seeing a counselor again after Dad bloodied Abi's lip and after the email drama between Dad and me. We agreed not to talk about anything having to do with Dad, but Mom asks for my input since I am in the field as well, even though she never takes my advice.

"Good… hard." She hesitates. "Well, I don't want to dishonor your father by telling you this, but I think it's important for *you* to have context."

"Hmmmmmmm," I say, trying to disguise the deep breath and prolonged exhalation preparing for whatever it is she is going to say.

"Well, during our couple's session on Monday, Dad said he thought the reason he pushed you away when you were going through puberty had to do with your being too big and his feeling claustrophobic."

I laugh. "I don't buy that."

"Neither do I, and I don't think the counselor did either, but then we shifted to reasons we thought may have contributed to your hypersexuality as a child."

"We don't have to talk about it, Mom, if it makes you uncomfortable."

"It'll be fine, you have a right to know. I told her how you said it was normal for kids to self-stimulate, but yours was more similar to a child who had experienced some type of sexual abuse. I told her what you said, that you have no recollection of that type of abuse at all."

She falls silent again.

I wait, anxious to hear the rest of this story, and Mom's awkward slow rolling leads me to believe it's a big revelation.

"Well, she asked if you had ever watched pornography or if anyone had ever had sex in front of you, and well… please don't judge me, Sarah. When your Dad wanted sex, nothing stopped him. Even when I said no, he forced me to anyway."

I grind my teeth, increasing the building pressure in my head.

"Well, Dad and I lived in a one-bedroom apartment, and you shared the bedroom with us. I was too afraid to leave you in the living room."

"Mom, what happened?"

"Dad refused to wait until you were asleep for us to have sex. I didn't like it because you would watch us. Even when we turned your swing to face the wall, you would twist around and watch."

"How old was I when you moved me out of the bedroom?"

"Not until Joey was born, so you had to be around two."

I pull into my office parking lot, bile rising in my throat.

"So, I watched you and Dad have sex regularly?"

"Yes. I'm so ashamed. I'm sorry, Sarah. I didn't know it would matter so much or that it might impact you in that way."

I bite hard on the forefinger on my clenched fist. "I'm at work. I need to go." I swallow the acid rising from my stomach, fighting the nausea.

"I love you," she sniffs. "Are you mad at me?"

"Gotta go." I hit the red phone button on my steering wheel and lean forward.

I'm flooded with memories of Mom telling me how Dad demanded sex of her, how she would have sex to soothe his anger, how she gave him sex to get what she wanted.

"Until I was two," I whisper in disbelief. "Oh my God."

"When do you get a lunch break?" I text to Mason. "I need to talk for a few minutes."

I wait for the three rotating dots to indicate that he's texting back and startle when the phone rings instead.

"My case is delayed this morning. I have about thirty minutes. What's up?"

"My Mom just told me she and Dad had sex in front of me regularly, while I was awake, until Joey was born."

"That's… weird, and well, wrong."

"Mason, it explains why I was so hypersexual as a young child. I masturbated to deal with anxiety, depression, to get my way… it's what my parents modeled for me."

"Are you sure about that, Sarah? That seems like a stretch. You were only two."

"My brain would have been developing rapidly. Something like a million neural connections a second. Prior to two, I would have been learning most from observing and experiencing the interactions between sensations and responses. Mom used sex to help regulate and soothe Dad's uncomfortable moods. When he was mad, they bumped uglies, and when he was anxious, depressed, overwhelmed. Sex in front of Sarah. Hey, Sarah, look at how to make Daddy like you again. Hump, hump, hump." I lean my head back so I don't slap myself, my flying hands matching the sarcasm.

"Why didn't they just wait 'til you fell asleep?"

"My Dad? Wait?"

"Okay, dumb comment."

I let the truth of Mom's disclosure settle in. "God, it makes so much sense now."

When Dad came home from work grumpy, I would rub my pubic bone against him trying to ease the tension. He would push me away and tell me I was disgusting.

God, they really fucked up my sexual development.

AUTHOR'S NOTE

Expression of sexuality, such as engaging in masturbation, is not an indicator that a child has been exposed to inappropriate sexual stimuli; self-stimulation is a normal part of healthy child development. On the contrary, *hyper*sexual behavior suggests a degree of abnormality and is cause for concern. Often, social factors are associated with excessive, compulsive sexual behavior, like physical sexual abuse, or as was the case with me, exposure to explicit images and viewing material.[24]

In families that share sleeping space, children may be present while the parents are intimate. Even in families with separate sleeping spaces, children may walk in on adults engaged in sexual activity. These scenarios differ from what my mother disclosed. In the former, the children usually are asleep for the sexual interaction, and in the latter, the interaction terminates until the child is no longer present. What my mother described to me was a situation in which, from birth to age two, I was repeatedly present and actively watching, with both parents' full knowledge, for the entirety of their sexual interaction.

During the first few years of life, a child learns through observing, mimicking, and exploring their environment.[25] Repetition is an effective way to help children learn and develop. This can be used to model healthy and unhealthy behavioral patterns. I assume my mother was a victim of sexual assault at times in her marriage, and because she would use sex to sooth my father's unpredictable moods (often in front of me) I learned early how to utilize sexual stimulation to soothe myself and others.

---

24   Levine., P. A., & Kline., M. (2007). *Trauma through a child's eyes: Awakening the ordinary miracle of healing: Infancy through adolescence.* North Atlantic Books. Pages 69-70

25   Cozolino, L. J. (2017). Part 4. In *The Neuroscience of Psychotherapy: Healing the Social Brain* (3rd ed., pp. 201-279). W.W. Norton & Company. Pages 201-279

FORGIVENESS IS A SYMPTOM

MARCH 2021

40 YEARS OLD

I can tell Mom is trying to hide her disapproval of Dad's action, but the edginess of her tone on the other end of our phone call gives her away. "It's been over two years, Sarah." She clears her throat. "Dad wasn't feeling well that day. You put too much on him by coming here with all your kids."

I roll my eyes. They had insisted I come to their house since I was in Arizona with Mason's family, and I honored their wishes. Now she's using that against me to blame me for Dad's poor behavior. My body shakes with frustration. All I want is for Dad to take accountability for his actions. Some things never change no matter how much I wish, dream, or long for it.

"You need to forgive him," Mom's comments break into my thoughts.

My body stiffens. I hate that my parents demand forgiveness. I've been a counselor for almost a decade. Forgiveness is a by-product of healing. Without accountability on their part for how badly things had gone, and without observable change in how Dad interacts with my kids, forgiveness doesn't feel possible.

"Forgive and forget. It will help you feel better." Mom speaks with a tone of authority, like there was no other option.

"I'm uncomfortable with the demand that I forgive Dad in order for our relationship to heal." I turn my blinker on, glance over my right shoulder and switch lanes so I can pull over. I can tell this conversation is going to take more focus than I can give while driving. I hear the vocal changes in my voice, indicating I've switched into the therapist mode anyway. I pull the car off to the side of the road.

"Dad has forgiven you. You need to forgive him so that things can go back to normal," her voice pleading.

"I don't want things *back to normal*. It was toxic for me." I put the car in park and rub my eyes struggling to keep my breathing even. I hate it when I shift into the little girl mode, begging for them to accept me and make things safe.

"Don't you think you're overreacting?"

I bite the inside of my cheek to stop myself from snapping at her. This isn't the first time she's minimized the severity of Dad's behaviors. Next, she'll be telling me what a "good man" he is. I need to go to the heart of this issue like I do with my clients, hoping she can finally admit that Dad's behaviors are manipulative at best, and abusive at worst.

"No, Mom, I think I'm honoring a boundary that makes you and Dad uncomfortable."

"Sarah, enough therapist speak," she snaps back without absorbing my words. "Dad apologized. You need to forgive him."

I think back to the day it all came to a head. It was August 2018. I had just assumed custody of Tyler. The kids and I were staying in Grandma and Grandpa T's vacant home directly behind my parent's home. Mom forbade us from eating in her parent's house because there was carpet under the dining room table. I promised I'd have the carpets professionally cleaned if there were any spills. She demanded that "if we *had* to come" then we had to eat all of our meals at her house.

It was stupid. I hadn't had to visit them at all… we were comfortable staying with Mason's younger brother and his wife. Grandma T had said she didn't care if we ate in her house, but I gave in to Mom and Dad because telling them no felt overwhelming. I was sure that if we didn't come, pouting would follow. With Mason in Afghanistan, I just didn't have the energy to put up with it.

I couldn't return home to Killeen, Texas, with the kids until the legal pathway for Tyler's adoption gave me permission to take Tyler out of the state of Arizona. Once again, I'd felt trapped by my parents' demands of me. Even as an adult, I was stuck in the never-ending circle of trying to please them through compliance, and never doing anything right.

To make matters worse, we all got lice. I was pretty sure we had picked it up at the family reunion just two weeks before. It didn't really matter. I had shown up to my parents' house and shaved all the boys' hair completely off. Chemical treatments and a nit comb helped us get rid of the infestation in Kaydee and me. Abi was the only one of us that escaped bug free.

Three days into our stay, Abi pranced into the living room after a morning of swimming, swiped a tortilla chip off of Eric's lunch plate, and popped it in her mouth.

Dad leapt from his recliner, screaming, "You are not allowed to eat in my living room!"

We'd been eating in front of the TV for days, and he had had no issues with Eric, who was sitting next to him, munching away.

Dad grabbed Abi by the back of her head, his large fingers digging into the soft tissue around her neck, and used his other hand to cram his finger into her mouth to forcibly remove the tortilla chip.

"Stop manhandling my daughter!" I screamed. I'd spent decades avoiding conflict with my father by submitting to his will over matters large and small. It was witnessing this grown man, over a chip, use violence against my daughter's tiny four-year-old body that finally broke his hold on me.

He let go, stunned, then stormed into his bedroom, slamming the door behind him, saying nothing.

I was livid and trembling as I wrapped Abi in a hug and cleaned up her bloody lip. It was then I realized seven-year-old Landon was hiding in the corner behind the couch, shaking uncontrollably and hyperventilating. We left and went back to Grandma and Grandpa T's house.

As soon as we walked in the door, Eric exclaimed, "Whoa, that was weird. I thought it was okay to eat in the living room."

We returned to Mom and Dad's for dinner because I'd given my word that we would have our meals at their house. Dad came out of his bedroom to go "check on things" at Grandma and Grandpa's house before joining us at the table. It was a quiet meal, heavy with tension and over as quickly as the kids could eat. Back at Grandma and Grandpa T's, I found a note from him waiting for me on my pillow.

While I'd hoped for an apology, I didn't expect one, not from him. I was shocked to find that he was accusing me of being the one who man-handled my children. The examples he gave were of times when I had had to physically restrain Brigg for his or the other children's safety due to fits of psychosis.

Amazingly, our Interstate Compact on the Placement of Children was approved late the following day, giving us permission to leave Arizona. As soon as I got the email from the attorney with clearance, I packed and left within the hour.

For several days, when I should have been consumed solely with help-ing two-year-old Tyler adapt and feel safe in his new home, I was consumed by thoughts of my father's behavior. I also obsessed over other incidents, starring Dad, that had left me feeling like my daughters were not physically or emotionally safe in his presence.

Images of him clawing food out of Abi's mouth played on repeat in my dreams. During the day, I processed the anger I had stifled when he had subjected Kaydee to comments at the family reunion about her changing body being "chubby" and suggestions that she needed to diet at only 11 years of age. I found myself trapped in the same emotions that gripped me in my teen years as a result of his emotional, and eventually, physical abuse.

Once I had collected myself enough to focus and respond in a calm and intentional manner, I sent him an email. In what I thought was a lov-ing but firm manner, I shared my concerns about his behavior and con-cluded that he was no longer allowed to be with my children, specifically my girls, without supervision.

That one email kicked off a rapid exchange that went on for almost a year, with my father masterfully deflecting any responsibility and my flood-lighting him by offering too much evidence in an attempt to be under-stood. Finally, I gave up trying to get him to comprehend how his physical and emotional abuse and need to always be "right" negatively impacted me as a child and teen, and how it continued to impact my children.

"Sarah? Are you still there?" Mom's voice cuts into my memories.

"Yes, Mom, I'm still here. You are right. Dad said 'I'm sorry if you ever felt unloved.' That is not apologizing for what he did to Kaydee or Abi. He also said if he had to do the entire Michael thing from high school again, he'd do it the exact same way, and he blamed me for the relationship problems you and he have had since I was born."

"He was angry. Forgiveness is an action word, Sarah. Once you forgive him, he'll feel safe around you again."

Seriously. She is worried about that man feeling safe around *me* after everything he had done to me and my children. My Mom's need to protect the abuser instead of my children grates my Mama Bear protective instincts.

"With all due respect, Mom, I disagree. Working on healing is an active process, and forgiveness is the natural by-product of healing. I'm still working on healing." Her inability to see my Dad in an honest light or to stop defending him to everyone else's detriment is the exact reason I need space from her so that I can heal.

"But I miss our morning conversations," she laments. "We almost never talk anymore."

I had missed talking to Mom in the mornings… for years, talking to Mom was how I started my day. No matter what chaos life brought, that connection was constant. Not having that constant is, at times, disorienting, but it's also freeing. I didn't realize until we stopped calling that those conversations were like sand in my shoe. I always walked away from them feeling aggravated and edgy.

"I miss us, too, Mom, but for now, the distance needs to stay in place." I know I sound like I'm talking to a patient in clinic in my attempts to protect myself from being sucked back into their dysfunction.

"How does it help us heal from this, if we don't talk about it?"

"Mom, I don't talk to you every day because I'm tired of your being punished for having a relationship with me. You read what Dad wrote. He blames me for *all* of your marriage struggles." I'm frustrated that Mom doesn't understand that I'm not willing to be the reason she takes crap from Dad. "Every time we have a conversation, he's in the background demanding your attention, and when we talk the next day, you vent about how angry he was that we talked. He claims I'm putting you in the middle of this. That is not my intent, so I need to step back."

"But you do try to come between Dad and me. You want me to take your side." I just want her see the situation for what it is, instead of what Dad tells her to think it is.

"That's not true," I answer. "All I want is to be understood. You told me a few months ago that you had decided you were going to stay married to Dad. If that is what works for you, then I am truly happy for you. Unfortunately, he gets grumpy and unbearable every time you and I talk on the phone, and if you are married to Dad, you have to deal with it. That gets in the way of your having a healthy relationship with either one of us. When you don't talk to me, he's happier, which makes you feel like things are going well."

"But it's not okay for him to do that."

"I agree, and yet after a year, it hasn't gotten any better. In fact, it's gotten much worse. So, I made a choice. If I step away from you, you and Dad are happier. I choose your happiness. It hurts, but it hurts me more that you get punished when I'm in your life, so I said goodbye."

"I feel like I am losing you."

She is losing me and I am losing her, but knowing our relationship hurts her is not acceptable.

"I can no longer participate in a relationship where you get hurt by my presence." I wish she could see how painful this is for me as well.

"What about counseling? I'm willing to do counseling with you."

"You and I don't need counseling. You, Dad, and I do. I'm willing to participate and pay for it, but Dad needs to be there, and we all need to be in a place where we can hear each other and work to understand, rather than blame and seek validation for who is right and who is wrong."

"Your Dad is afraid to do counseling with you." Her comment doesn't shock me. Dad has said many times I'm a master manipulator, and since I am a counselor, he seems convinced that I have some secret superpower another professional won't be able to identify.

"Well, I agree that nothing gets solved without us talking about it."

"I miss you, Sarah." I hear her voice crack.

"I miss you, too, Mom, but we aren't able to work through this on our own without making this much worse. I guess we'll have to wait."

THERE, NOT HERE

JUNE 2021

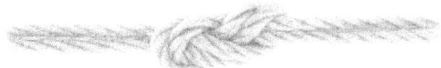

40 YEARS OLD

Leaving Michael's tiny Phoenix apartment, I berate myself for stepping into this again. He'd baited me, claiming he needed help only I could provide. I can't even say that I was caught off guard or didn't see it coming; this was completely predictable. I slide into the front seat of my silver 4Runner. How am I supposed to tell Mason the worst has happened *again*? He's dealing with enough trying to figure out how to have a mixed-faith marriage since I officially left the church six months ago. Why am I so fucking weak?

"This is not the way you handle feeling isolated in your relationship, Sarah. You know better. Use your skills." I scold the steering wheel.

Sticky shame slides up my throat. I need a new therapist. I'm obviously not equipped to navigate another affair on my own.

I back out of my parking spot and drive mindlessly to the corner gas station. Tears run down my face, my limbs are still shaking. I pull close to the pump, put the Runner in park, and cut the engine.

"Fuck, Sarah.

"Fuck.

"Fuck.

"Fuck!

"You need to end this! No excuses." I punch the steering wheel, tearing the skin on my knuckles.

"What the fuck is the matter with you?"

You and Michael share a bond because of the trauma you share. Jerry's words replay in my mind. *That's powerful stuff.*

Aside from Jim, Jerry was the best counselor I'd ever had, but he died unexpectedly from a heart attack just as I was starting to let my defenses down and do the "work."

Jerry had nudged in his direct manner when we first started. I remember him saying to me, *If you want to be the counselor in this relationship, I have some stuff I'd like to get off my chest.* He helped me wade through my past so that I could understand why I kept turning to Michael. I figured out that while my teenage mind fantasized that Michael would save me, the truth was even he had deserted me when things became tough. Mason is the only man who stayed by my side during the tumultuous storm of my journey toward healing.

"Jerry," I looked out my car window up toward the fluffy white clouds "if you can hear me, I need help." Tears run down my face. "I am destroying the people I love most. Please help me."

Write, Sarah. Write. Those were the words that I heard in my heart in response.

Jerry reinforced that writing slows the mind so that the frontal cortex can manage the strength of the amygdala's response.

Write to teach, write to create, write to heal.

I fill my gas tank and punch the "home" button on my GPS. The whole time I'm driving away from my self-made hell in Phoenix, I berate myself out loud. Just outside the city, when I'm finally numb, I pull the car off the road to a scenic overlook.

I climb out and sneeze. I'm only allergic to the sun in Arizona. One more reason to stay away from this God-forsaken Mormon desert. I dig around the trunk of my SUV, looking for my notebook and pen, my pale skin cooking. I break into a sweat.

Finally, my fingers brush against the spiral metal binding. I pull the notebook out then shove my suitcase deeper into the trunk. I pull myself into the back of the SUV and sit cross-legged, leaving the hatch open and praying for a breeze. It's hotter inside the car than out, but I'm protected from the sun's searing rays.

There, Not Here

I scrawl at the top of the page. I take a slow deep breath, ensuring that my exhalation takes longer than my inhalation. I wait for the words to come.

Inhale.

Long slow exhale.

Inhale.

Long slow exhale.

I open my eyes, place my pen on the lined paper and focus on the sound of pen scratching words onto the page.

Young love and laughter
Stolen moments in secret
Firsts, awkward
Then vulnerable, safe
There, not Here

Agency stolen
Abuse, isolation
Love taken
"Gifts" given, unwanted
There, not Here

Pretend smiles, an act to please
Unrighteousness dominion, grief
Escape the prison
Longing to be free
There, not Here

New chapter in life
Captor's approval
Learning again how to love
It's broken, no trust
There, not Here

Vows made in a temple
But not understood
Trauma still lingers
Liberated, not free
There, not Here

Hiding in darkness
Your presence still lingers
Trying to be perfect
The stage disappears
There, not Here

You come out of nowhere
A shock to my system
Confusion, agony
Old feelings ignited
There, not Here

Once given, then taken
Shame in disclosure
Hurting the innocent
Cultural demands, forced reparations
There, not Here

You enter my dreams
Like a thief in the night
Holding, caressing remembered
So real but not right
There, not Here

Nightmares ensue
Running, screaming
No longer secure
I'm fragmenting, you're haunting
There, not Here

Out walking
Kids smiling
Your voice in the wind
Startled, can't see you
There, not Here

Shopping for groceries
Mundane and routine
Your scent, shared with others
My mind tricking me
There, not Here

Flashbacks, jumpy
Heart pounding in chest
Dizzy, world spinning
Is this my last breath?
There, not Here

Friendship a failure
Emotions too strong
Tightening of boundaries
Always
There, not Here

Again, hearts are broken
The innocent wronged
Trauma consumes me
Please stay
There, not Here

How to escape this
Will I ever find peace?
No closure, no ending
I'm unraveling
There, not Here

God be with me
My desperate plea
Silence, no answer
I travel alone
There, not Here

I reread the words. My mind is clear. I am walking away from the trauma that is there and into my safe haven with Mason and my children. Things may not be perfect, but I finally understand what Mason means when he says, "I choose you, every day."

I crawl out of the hatch and wipe the sweat from my face, neck, and arms with the bottom of my shirt. I look at the desolate empty land then remove my shirt, grateful for the hot air on my exposed skin. I dig through my suitcase again, searching for a clean shirt and shorts. The desert sucks the sweat from my sticky skin, leaving behind a film of itchy salt crystals.

I glance around quickly once more before changing my shorts, close the hatch, and climb back into the driver's seat. I turn the ignition on and let it idle while I step back out, taking in the cloudless sky, feeling lighter. The poem had freed me from the ensuing darkness.

Once the SUV's interior has had enough time to cool down, I climb back in, readying myself for the journey ahead.

"I'm coming home, Mason, to Missouri. For better or worse. I will own my mistakes. I can't promise I won't stumble again, but I choose you." I hear the conviction in my voice and send my gratitude for Jerry's words up to the heavens.

It's time to conquer this demon.

I CHOOSE YOU

JUNE 2021

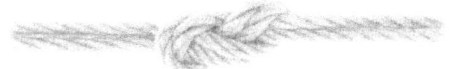

40 YEARS OLD

I stumble into the house, tugging my bright parrot-covered suitcase behind me.

"Welcome home, beautiful. How was Arizona?" Mason greets me, arms open wide.

I walk into his embrace and crumble. A 20-hour drive right after cheating on Mason was too much time to wallow in my thoughts. I'm ragged.

"Whoa, Sarah. What's going on? Did your Dad say something?" The fact that Mason's mind jumps to my parents deepens my shame.

I shake my head.

"What do you need? I made breakfast for dinner. I can make you an omelet."

"Not hungry, but thanks for offering." I step away from him.

He reaches for my hand, then stops.

"Why are your knuckles so swollen? It looks like you got into a fight."

"In a way I did."

"What did you hit?"

"Mostly the steering wheel… I… Michael…" I can't find the words. I glance over my shoulder at the kids, who are staring at us. "Later."

Mason checks the clock on the stove.

"Hayden, I need you to make sure the kids finish their dinner. Have them take showers and give them their meds at eight before bed."

"Sure thing, Dad," Hayden says, squinting at me.

I abandon the suitcase to hug each of my children.

"Are you sad?" Tyler asks.

"I need sleep. I drove the whole time the moon was up last night until right now. Can we play Connect Four after breakfast tomorrow?"

"We are eating breakfast right now," Abi protests, using her spoon to draw shapes in the syrup lake on her plate. "Can you play with us right now?"

"No, baby girl. Mama needs to sleep, otherwise my grumpy parts will come out." I pull a piece of white fuzz from her braids.

Mason shifts from foot to foot. "I'm going to take Mama for a walk. I'll read you bedtime stories when I get back, or Hayden will read to you at eight." He shifts his gaze to Hayden, who nods.

Mason follows me up the driveway. Fireflies sparkle like flying sequins all around us. We walk in silence for several blocks. I take in the beauty of the wildflowers and the buzz of the cicadas' song.

"I went to Michael's house." I hang my head as the quiet words leave my lips.

Mason stops walking, waiting, his jaw tightening in a hard line. "And?"

"Things went too far."

"Did you have sex?"

I turn my head away. "Yes."

Color drains from his face. "And your hands?"

"I was mad at myself. I pulled over and took my anger out on a tree somewhere in New Mexico."

"Why?" he chokes out. "Why do you keep going back?"

Jerry asked me the same question before he passed away. "What keeps you turning toward Michael when your trauma is triggered?"

You'd think after a decade of being a professional counselor, I'd know the answer to that. Academically, I understand that I feel emotionally connected and safe with Michael even though he really isn't safe for me. But it feels that way. I have never felt judged by him, but I also feel like shit for hurting Mason.

"I honestly don't know. I wish I did."

"I'm so tired of this Michael shit. I choose you Sarah, but you can't seem to choose me back."

"What is that even supposed to mean?" I snap at him.

I hear the control in his voice, but I'm watching his body zing with electricity. He's fidgeting so much he looks like he's about to come out of his skin.

Each time I've told Mason about indiscretions with Michael, he's said "I choose you, Sarah. Every day, I choose you, and I will continue to choose you." It's annoying. I want him to get mad and yell so that I don't feel so guilty and so I can yell back.

"It means I recognize that you come with heavy baggage, and I love you enough to work with you on that."

He stops walking and falls silent. I glare at him; he enabled this. He's honored my friendship with Michael over the years, despite continued betrayals. When I tried to be completely transparent, he refused to read any of the messages between us, choosing to trust me.

I know I'm being irrational. Jerry had helped me realize that Mason was managing the issue the best way he knew how, and that his choice to trust me was healthy, even if I wasn't honoring that trust. He told me to stop blaming Mason for my choices. I remember Jerry's words: It's not Mason's job to babysit you.

"It means I'm not going to add to your trauma by abandoning you like every other man in your life has," his voice gets louder, "including Michael. But even I have limits, Sarah, and you are pushing them."

My shoulders lower with his words. "I won't fight you if you need to leave."

His lips press firmly together.

"Mason, I get it, and so will everyone else. No one will blame *you* if we get divorced."

"Oh, hell no!" He kicks a rock that ricochets off a tree. "Don't you think I'm about to take the easy way out."

"Divorce is not easy," I snap back. I hate feeling like he is stuck with me out of some stupid religious obligation. "You choose to stay because you hate change. You stay because you're afraid of being alone," I accuse.

He leans toward me. "You know what?" His eyes lock onto mine. "That's true, I do hate change and I don't want to be alone, but *it... is... not...* the reason I stay."

I force myself to stare into his hurt, wounded eyes, fighting the urge to run.

"I stay, Sarah, because I know you don't want to hurt me, but you are hurting me."

Don't move, I order myself. This is important for him to say and me to hear.

"I feel inadequate at meeting your needs," his voice cracks, and it grows louder as he says, "and I'm pissed that you won't even give me the chance to meet your needs."

"Can't or won't?" I bite back. "You don't have the tools. I've asked you more times than I can count to go see a counselor and learn how to deal with emotions so that you can connect with me, *really* connect with me." Heat rises in my face. If he could connect with me, I wouldn't feel so empty and I wouldn't be running off to Michael. "I love you. I want to be married to *you,* but you shut down anytime I try to talk to you about my past. You can't handle my trauma."

Mason steps back, his face wounded.

"Sorry, that wasn't entirely fair," I mumble. "I need to move or my anxiety will hijack my brain."

Mason reaches for my hand, and I pull it away. He deflates and slides his hand into his front pocket.

"I can't stand that Michael provides something for you that I'm not." His voice is quiet again. "I know you're not doing this because you don't love me, or that you're trying to hurt me."

I swat at a bug in front of my face, refusing to make eye contact.

"I need you to end all contact with him."

"I'm not going to a bishop this time. I left the church. I need you to know I won't do that."

"I know, Sarah," he says softly. "I won't ask you to. I get the church's discipline system didn't help you heal, not the way it was supposed to. Just know that Jesus can heal your trauma and fix both of our pain. I will place my faith in that, but I need you to work through whatever is driving you to do what you do and stop this."

"I don't know how to forgive myself. I'm disgusted, I can't get past this shame." Bitterness rises into my mouth.

He stands there quiet for a while then finally says, "What do you think Jerry would say to you?"

"I pulled over for a bit on my way home. I sorta prayed and heard Jerry's voice in my mind, telling me to write."

He swats at a fly. "So, write." He takes a breath, "If that's what you need to heal, then do it."

I laugh at the irony. "Soooo, I don't have to tell the bishop, but I get to tell the world?"

"You don't *have* to tell anyone. You're *choosing* to share it with the world. It's your story to share when and if you want to. I need you to do things differently, Sarah. I told you that I need you to end contact with Michael."

We walk in silence to the end of our street and gaze at the Osage River flowing peacefully behind the canopy of green.

"It's me I don't trust with my trauma, Mason. The first time I connected with Michael was because I felt abandoned by my parents. I'm not sixteen anymore. Just because he met a need for me then doesn't mean I need him to meet that need now. I feel trapped."

"I feel trapped, too. Not trapped in our marriage, but in this never-ending cycle of pain. It's an infected wound that won't heal. Just when you think you're ahead of it, something bursts open and leaks into everything. It's like we are in a constant state of emergency intervention. I'm exhausted."

"That's kinda morbid," I say.

"*This IS* morbid."

"I will cut ties with Michael. You're right. It's way past time for that."

"I need you to honor that commitment."

"I get it. I will."

We start walking home, slowly, hand in hand.

"Mason, just because I've left Mormonism doesn't mean Mormonism has left me. I'm so used to obeying and 'checking off the boxes' that I tend to turn off my brain when it comes to Michael. I need to figure out how to reclaim my authenticity. I need to start thriving, not just surviving. I need to heal."

Mason pulls me to a stop and turns to face me. His hazel eyes seem to see me differently. He leans forward and kisses my forehead.

COURAGE

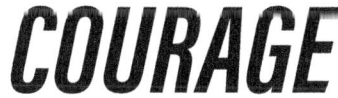

JUNE 2022

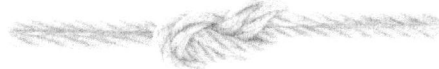

41 YEARS OLD

I reach for my phone and read the text from Mason, which says, "I just need time to cry."

I inhale deeply through my nose and purse my lips for the drawn-out, steady exhale, focusing on the low whistle coming from my lips. *One-two-three-four-five-six, deep inhalation.* I slow my thoughts in preparation to be present for Mason without becoming defensive.

It's been almost a year since I last saw Michael. We've had a few brief conversations, with Mason's permission, but only for fact-checking purposes while I write this book. Jerry's heavenly counsel to write had released the burden of pain for me. I knew it would hurt Mason to read it. I tried to prepare him before emailing him the manuscript.

"This is the most honest thing I've ever done" is my opening message in the email.

Years ago, when I told him what happened, I painted broad strokes, letting his imagination fill in the rest. Now that he's read the manuscript, he knows what happened, along with my thoughts and feelings. I can no longer hide behind vagaries, and he can't let his imagination pull the punch.

"Landon," I call down the basement stairs to my 11-year-old. "Can you help Tyler start a movie?"

"Sure, can we play on something, too?"

I smile. Landon is persistent. "Sure, just this time."

With the kids distracted, Mason and I can be alone. I return to kitchen clean-up. I need to keep my body moving so that my panic won't consume me.

Mason's text scares me. I wonder if the grief could be too much for him? Will he decide divorce is what is best for him now that he knows the full truth? I'll honor his choice, just as he has honored mine over and over again, despite the pain it's caused him. What if being completely honest is what breaks us? It feels like we have so much more to lose now than ever before.

Remus's welcoming bark lets me know Mason is home. I rinse out the rag and wash my shaking hands.

"Feel with him. Be steady," I remind myself in a whisper.

He walks through the door. His eyes are bloodshot; he looks haggard.

"I love you," I say, my voice cracking.

He gives a quick nod and walks past me to our bedroom. I'm jumping out of my skin. I wait a moment and then force myself to follow him.

"Do you want to be alone, or can I hold you?" I ask from the doorway.

He shrugs, climbing into our bed. He draws his knees into his chest then releases a sob.

I lock the door behind me and curl into him on the bed. I feel his body shudder against mine.

He stays in the fetal position, gasping through tears.

I hold him and stroke his hair for half an hour, fighting the urge to say something.

Finally, he reaches for my hand. "Thanks for being here. I needed to cry."

"Do you want to talk?" I ask, tentatively.

He shakes his head, then speaks, anyway.

"You told Michael he could have a key to our home."

I cringe in shame.

"You told him he could come and go as he pleased after I deployed." His voice falters.

"I know."

"Or that sexual contact with Michael only stopped because Megan found out."

There's nothing I can say without it sounding like an excuse.

"You let me think he raped you."

As much as I feel shame over this, it's outweighed by the relief of just being honest.

"I know, I'm…"

"Don't apologize." He rolls over and faces me.

"Sorry, I didn't mean to apologize. Shit, sorry."

He raises his eyebrows at me. "You're pathetic."

We chuckle, and he pulls me in for a hug.

"I really am sorry, Mason." I hope he can feel my sincerity.

"P-A-T-H-etic," He teases gently. "Sarah, I didn't know." His voice falters, and I feel the guilt rising again. "This is so different from what I thought." He stretches. "But I still don't understand why you kept going back. He's like heroin for you."

"In a way, I *am* addicted to him."

He shakes his head. "I can't handle much more of Michael in our life. I want to beat the shit out of him, but then you'd feel like you needed to rescue him again."

I give him a weak smile. "That's probably true, and I'd hate myself for it."

He pulls away from me. I stare into his face; his whiskers accentuate his solemnity. He stares at the ceiling.

I hesitate. "I'm glad you hate him. It helps me recognize the depth of your love for me. I've never had that before, so thanks," I say weakly.

"Michael is… untrustworthy," he breathes deeply while he considers his words. "You're the only one who sets boundaries in your relationship, and he consistently crosses them. He has nothing to lose and everything to gain. He doesn't think of anyone but himself. Not me, not our children, not even you."

"I've crossed the boundaries I've set more times than I can count, Mason. You are right. Michael has everything to gain, but I need to adhere to the commitments I've made to you and to myself." The truth feels prickly in my throat.

Mason rolls on his side and props himself up on his elbow. He leans forward and kisses my cheek.

"I still choose you, my love. Every day, I *choose* you."

His words fill me with gratitude. I blink rapidly, clearing my vision.

"I choose you, too. Every day." I melt into his embrace.

"I think the 'courage' tattoo you want on your forearm is fitting."

"But you hate tattoos."

"Yes, I do. But *you* find power in them, and I can honor that. This book, your story, sharing it with me is one thing. Being vulnerable like that with the world, *that's* courage."

"Courage is not simply one of the virtues, but the form of every virtue at the testing point."
~C.S. Lewis[26]

---

26   C.S. Lewis, *The Screwtape Letters* (London: Geoffrey Bles, 1942), no.29.

EPILOGUE

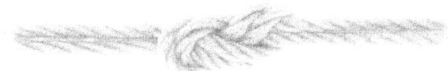

Being honest with myself is something that still takes daily effort. I can't promise Michael won't infiltrate my life again, which is both terrifying and exhilarating. Speaking my vulnerability out loud can be excruciating. I will forever be grateful for the work that Brené Brown has done on shame and belonging, as it continues to shape my life. No one heals without pain; and yet, the connective beauty of healing is worth the effort. Brené's *Power of Vulnerability* presentation was the catalyst for helping me identify my "shame gremlins" and work through my own trauma. I recommend and use her work in my own practice regularly.

Regarding the toxic culture of the Mormon Church: Bill Reel, from *Mormonism Live*, once said to me, "Belonging is not allowed, so fitting in is all we can do." He went on to explain to me that the Mormon Church does not allow space for individual authenticity, so the best we can do is try to fit in with the rest of the crowd.

For me, the feeling of belonging in my family of origin was fractured in 1997 when my parents discovered my sexual relationship with Michael. I am still working through the trauma from those years of abuse. The unconditional love demonstrated by my Army family helped me develop the empathy that was not modeled for me in childhood.

It's easy to feel disgusted by my parents' actions. It's a response that I've had to work through many times. I do not condone abuse in any form, but I realize that they did the best they knew how to do with the skills they had. What hurts me the most is my father's repeated statements that if he had to do it all over again, he'd do it the same way. He refuses to acknowledge the harm he caused me. His actions separated me from my peer group, my religious group, my siblings, my mother, and until recently, from my authentic self.

My mother has apologized many times for her inability to stand up for me and protect me from the abuse. It was not a skill she had when I needed it the most. Forgiveness for her lack of action came naturally after her genuine apology and years of therapy. I recommend reading *Why Won't You Apologize?* by Harriet Learner for more information on the healing power of an effective apology. It has changed the way I apologize and has helped me recognize more fully how impactful an apology can be to someone in pain.

In 2018, I stood up to my father for the first time. Since then, our relationship has deteriorated, and the closeness my mother and I once shared is collateral damage. I miss our daily conversations and our friendship. The depth of our grief mirrors the depth of our love. It is hard to recognize that someone you care for deeply will be happier without you in their life. The physical pain of losing my mother in this way is indescribable. Unlike with death, there is no closure for losing a mother who is still alive.

When I am with my father, I turn into a person I dislike very much. I revert to a younger, more reactive, and less rational Sarah. Bessel van der Kolk outlines that phenomenon in his book, *The Body Keeps the Score: Brain, Mind, and Body in the Healing of Trauma*, another book I highly recommend. It is painful and often necessary to distance yourself from people who are toxic to you. Most people identify my father as a "good man." Through his example, I learned how to work hard, how to love serving others, and how to use creativity to engage small children. I have learned to honor his goodness from afar, as both he and I become toxic when we are together.

I saw a meme on Facebook recently that said:

> *Never underestimate a cycle breaker. Not only did they experience years of generational trauma, but they stood in the face of the trauma and fought to say, "This ends with me." This is brave. This is powerful. This comes at a significant cost. Never underestimate a cycle breaker.*
>
> *~Unknown*

I feel that truth in my soul. I'm not a perfect parent, obviously. I know that my children will have their own struggles to work through as a result of my mistakes, but I find peace in knowing and accepting that I did the best I knew how to do. I hope my children will feel comfortable coming to me so that we can heal together as they do better with their families than I did with them.

Affairs can cause irreparable damage to a marriage. I have seen the tragedy unfold before my eyes many times with my clients and with my own experience. I have also seen people grow closer to their partners during the post-affair healing process. I thank Drs. John and Julie Gottman as well as Dr. Sue Johnson for teaching me the skills needed to heal my relationship with Mason. Without their research and insight, I don't think Mason and I would have survived. I advise seeking a qualified licensed counselor/therapist with specialty training in trauma, attachment, and relationships as you strive to heal from your own betrayal.

Clearly, life is a journey, and I'm still traveling. I know that sharing my story will alter my relationships. I will lose some, gain some, and rediscover my personal tribe. There is beauty in the context of sharing and embracing those who travel differently than you do. I am still learning. I invite you to love without condition, withhold judgment, and develop empathy, so that we can extend grace and understanding for those in struggle.

Last, trying to fit into the Mormon culture became an exhausting chore that eventually led to a nervous breakdown. I left Mormonism for good in early 2021. I share my journey and experiences exiting the Mormon Church in my podcast *Unpacking Mormonism: And Other Religious Trauma* and plan to write a book with the same title. I hope both will help you find understanding and healing for yourself and your loved ones. I can't wait to see y'all there for our live events. For updated information or to be included in my monthly newsletter, please visit www.daisygirlcommunications.com or www.sarahwestbrookbooks.com.

With much love,

Sarah

Printed in Dunstable, United Kingdom

66671974R10312